Aesthetic Head and Neck Surgery

McGraw-Hill Plastic Surgery Atlas

Aesthetic Head and Neck Surgery

McGraw-Hill Plastic Surgery Atlas

Samuel J. Lin, MD, FACS
Assistant Professor of Surgery
Site Director, Combined Harvard Plastic Surgery Residency
Divisions of Plastic Surgery and Otolaryngology
Beth Israel Deaconess Medical Center
Harvard Medical School
Boston, Massachusetts

Thomas A. Mustoe, MD
Lucille and Orion Stuteville Professor of Plastic Surgery
Feinberg School of Medicine
Northwestern University
Chicago, Illinois

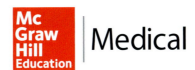

New York   Chicago   San Francisco   Lisbon   London   Madrid   Mexico City
Milan   New Delhi   San Juan   Seoul   Singapore   Sydney   Toronto

Aesthetic Head and Neck Surgery: McGraw-Hill Plastic Surgery Atlas

Copyright © 2013 by The McGraw-Hill Companies, Inc. All rights reserved. Printed in China. Except as permitted under the United States Copyright Act of 1976, no part of this publication may be reproduced or distributed in any form or by any means, or stored in a data base or retrieval system, without the prior written permission of the publisher.

1 2 3 4 5 6 7 8 9 0   CTP/CTP   18 17 16 15 14 13

ISBN 978-0-07-159771-5
MHID 0-07-159771-9

This book was set in Sabon by Thomson Digital.
The editors were Brian Belval and Cindy Yoo.
The production supervisor was Sherri Souffrance.
The illustration manager was Armen Ovsepyan.
Project management was provided by Charu Bansal, Thomson Digital.
The designer was Eve Siegel; the cover designer was Anthony Landi.
China Translation & Printing Services, Ltd., was printer and binder.

This book is printed on acid-free paper.

Library of Congress Cataloging-in-Publication Data

Aesthetic head and neck surgery / [edited by] Samuel J. Lin, Thomas A. Mustoe.
       p. ; cm. – (McGraw-Hill plastic surgery atlas)
    Aesthetic head and neck surgery
    Includes bibliographical references and index.
    ISBN 978-0-07-159771-5 (alk. paper)
    ISBN 0-07-159771-9 (alk. paper)
    ISBN 978-0-07-163265-2 (ebook)
    ISBN 0-07-163265-4 (ebook)
    I. Lin, Samuel J. II. Mustoe, Thomas A. III. Title: Aesthetic head and neck surgery. IV. Series: McGraw-Hill plastic surgery atlas.
    [DNLM: 1. Face–surgery–Atlases.   2. Reconstructive Surgical Procedures–methods–Atlases.
3. Cosmetic Techniques–Atlases. 4. Neck–surgery–Atlases. WE 17]
    617.5'2059–dc23
                                                            2012048538

McGraw-Hill books are available at special quantity discounts to use as premiums and sales promotions, or for use in corporate training programs. To contact a representative please e-mail us at bulksales@mcgraw-hill.com.

Managing Editor

Ahmed M. S. Ibrahim, MD
Research Fellow
Division of Plastic and Reconstructive Surgery
Beth Israel Deaconess Medical Center
Harvard Medical School
Boston, Massachusetts

Contents

Contributors

Omid Adibnazari, BS
Medical Student
University of Central Florida College of Medicine
Orlando, Florida

Olubimpe A. Ayeni, MD, MPH, FRCSC
Attending Plastic Surgeon
Southlake Regional Health Centre
Newmarket, Ontario

Alfonso Barrera, MD, FACS
Clinical Assistant Professor
Department of Surgery, Division of Plastic Surgery
Baylor College of Medicine
Houston, Texas

Richard A. Bartlett, MD, FACS
Clinical Assistant Professor of Surgery
Harvard Medical School
Boston, Massacusetts

Branko Bojovic, MD
Assistant Professor of Surgery
Department of Surgery, Division of Plastic Surgery
University of Maryland Medical Center
Baltimore, Maryland

Rodger H. Brown, MD
Assistant Professor of Surgery
Department of Surgery, Division of Plastic Surgery
Baylor College of Medicine
Houston, Texas

Jamal M. Bullocks, MD
Clinical Assistant Professor
Department of Surgery, Division of Plastic Surgery
Baylor College of Medicine
Houston, Texas

Jerry W. Chang, MD
Private Practice
New York, New York

Christopher T. Chia, MD
Attending Physician
Department of Plastic Surgery
Manhattan Eye, Ear and Throat Hospital
New York, New York

C. Spencer Cochran, MD
Clinical Assistant Professor
Department of Otolaryngology-Head
   and Neck Surgery
University of Texas Southwestern
   Medical Center at Dallas
Dallas, Texas

Bruce F. Connell, MD, FACS
Private Practice
Santa Ana, California

Jason S. Cooper, MD
Attending Staff, Division of Plastic and
   Reconstructive Surgery
Department of Surgery
Massachusetts General Hospital
Boston, Massachusetts

Sean T. Doherty, MD
Attending Plastic Surgeon
Boston Plastic Surgery Associates
Concord, Massachusetts

Lee E. Edstrom, MD
Professor of Surgery
Surgery (Plastic)
Organization/Rhode Island Hospital/Lifespan,
   Brown University
Providence, Rhode Island

Kenton Fong, MD
Private Practice
Campbell, California

Ryan Michael Garcia, MD
Resident Physician of Plastic Surgery
Division of Plastic, Maxillofacial and Oral Surgery
Duke University School of Medicine
Durham, North Carolina

Ronald P. Gruber, MD
Clinical Assistant Professor
University of California
San Francisco, California
Adjunct Clinical Assistant Professor
Stanford University Medical Center
Palo Alto, California

Jack P. Gunter, MD
Clinical Professor, Department of Plastic Surgery
Clinical Professor, Department of Otolaryngology-Head
   and Neck Surgery
University of Texas Southwestern Medical Center
   at Dallas
Dallas, Texas

Bahman Guyuron, MD, FACS
Chairman, Plastic and Reconstructive Surgery
University Hospitals Case Medical Center
University Hospitals Rainbow Babies and
   Children's Hospital
Cleveland, Ohio

Daniel A. Hatef, MD
Resident Physician of Plastic Surgery
Department of Surgery, Division of Plastic Surgery
Baylor College of Medicine
Houston, Texas

John B. Hijjawi, MD, FACS
Associate Professor
Department of Plastic Surgery
Medical College of Wisconsin
Milwaukee, Wisconsin

Nathaniel L. Holzman, MD
Chief Resident
Department of Plastic and Reconstructive Surgery
Lahey Clinic Medical Center
Burlington, Massachusetts

Kenneth B. Hughes, MD
Private Practice
Los Angeles, California

David M. Knize, MD
Associate Clinical Professor of Surgery
University of Colorado School of Medicine
Denver, Colorado

Bernard T. Lee, MD, MBA
Acting Chief, Division of Plastic and
   Reconstructive Surgery
Department of Surgery
Beth Israel Deaconess Medical Center
Harvard Medical School
Boston, Massachusetts

Samuel J. Lin, MD, FACS
Assistant Professor of Surgery
Site Director, Combined Harvard
   Plastic Surgery Residency
Divisions of Plastic Surgery and Otolaryngology
Beth Israel Deaconess Medical Center
Harvard Medical School
Boston, Massachusetts

Alyssa Lolofie, BS
Research Student
Department of Ophthalmology
John A. Moran Eye Center
University of Utah
Salt Lake City, Utah

Hamid Massiha, MD
Professor of Plastic Surgery
Department of Surgery
Medical School, Louisiana State University/
   Medical Science Center
New Orleans, Louisiana

Alan Matarasso, MD
Clinical Professor of Surgery
Albert Einstein College of Medicine
Bronx, New York
Attending Surgeon
Manhattan Eye, Ear & Throat Hospital
Lenox Hill Hospital
New York, New York

Scott R. Miller, MD, FACS
Private Practice
La Jolla, California

Thomas A. Mustoe, MD
Lucille and Orion Stuteville
   Professor of Plastic Surgery
Feinberg School of Medicine
Northwestern University
Chicago, Illinois

Martin I. Newman, MD, FACS
Department of Plastic Surgery
Head of Clinical Research
Associate Program Director,
   Plastic Surgery Residency Program
Educational Director
Cleveland Clinic Florida
Associate Clinical Professor
Florida International University
Diplomate, American Board of Surgery
Diplomate, American Board of Plastic Surgery
Weston, Florida

Brian M. Parrett, MD
Attending Plastic Surgeon
The Buncke Clinic, California Pacific Medical Center
San Francisco, California

Malcolm D. Paul, MD
Clinical Professor
Aesthetic and Plastic Surgery Institute
University of California, Irvine
Newport Beach, California

Byron Poindexter, MD
Private Practice
Reston, Virginia

Diana C. Ponsky, MD
Assistant Professor of Plastic and
   Reconstructive Surgery
Assistant Professor of Otolaryngology-Head
   and Neck Surgery
Case Western Reserve University-University Hospitals
Cleveland, Ohio

Amr N. Rabie, MD
Associate Professor of Otolaryngology-Head
   and Neck Surgery
Department of Otolaryngology
Ain Shams University, Faculty of Medicine
Cairo, Egypt

Stephen L. Ratcliff, MD
Attending Anesthesiologist
North Houston Anesthesiologists
Houston, Texas

Emily B. Ridgway, MD
Division of Plastic Surgery
Dartmouth Hitchcock Medical Center
Lebanon, New Hampshire

Renato Saltz, MD, FACS
Medical Director Saltz Plastic Surgery
First Vice-President ISAPS
Past President ASAPS
Salt Lake City and Park City, Utah

Brooke R. Seckel, MD, FACS
Chairman Emeritus, Assistant Professor
Plastic Surgery
Lahey Clinic, Harvard Medical School/
   Lahey Clinic Medical Center
Boston, Massachusetts

David Shafer, MD, FACS
Plastic Surgeon
Department of Plastic Surgery
Shafer Plastic Surgery
Manhattan Eye, Ear and Throat Hospital of North
   Shore-Long Island Jewish Health System
New York, New York

Fred E. Shapiro, DO
Assistant Professor of Anaesthesia
   Harvard Medical School
Department of Anesthesiology,
   Critical Care and Pain Medicine
Beth Israel Deaconess Medical Center
Boston, Massachusetts

Douglas M. Sidle, MD, FACS
Assistant Professor
Feinberg School of Medicine
Department of Otolaryngology-Head and Neck Surgery
Division of Facial Plastics and Reconstructive Surgery
Northwestern University
Chicago, Illinois

Robert Sigal, MD
Private Practice
Reston, Virginia

Robert C. Silich, MD, FACS
Assistant Clinical Professor of Surgery (Plastic)
Department of Surgery, Division of Plastic Surgery,
   New York Presbyterian Hospital
Weill Cornell Medical Center
New York, New York

Meryl Singer, MD
University of Colorado Denver
Denver, Colorado

Sumner A. Slavin, MD
Clinical Associate Professor of Surgery
Department of Surgery, Division of Plastic Surgery
Beth Israel Deaconess Medical Center
Harvard Medical School
Boston, Massachusetts

Henry M. Spinelli, MD, FACS
Clinical Professor of Surgery (Plastic) and
   Neurological Surgery
Department of Surgery and Neurological Surgery
Joan and Stanford I. Weill Medical College
   of Cornell University
Attending Surgeon
New York Presbyterian Hospital
New York, New York

Samuel Stal, MD
Former Chief, Division of Plastic Surgery
Professor of Surgery
Baylor College of Medicine
Texas Children's Hospital
Houston, Texas

Ithamar Nogueira Stocchero, MD
Clinical Director
Centro Médico Viver Melhor
São Paulo, São Paulo

Kimberly A. Swartz, BA
Medical Student
University of Florida
Gainesville, Florida

Edward O. Terino, MD, FACS
Medical Director
Plastic Surgery Institute of Southern California
Agoura Hills, California

Charles H. Thorne, MD
Associate Professor of Surgery (Plastic Surgery)
NYU School of Medicine
Manhattan, New York

George Weston, MD
Private Practice
Reston, Virginia

Michael J. Yaremchuk, MD, FACS
Clinical Professor of Surgery
Program Director, Harvard Plastic
   Surgery Residency Program
Director, Craniofacial Surgery
Division of Plastic and Reconstructive Surgery
Massachusetts General Hospital
Boston, Massachusetts

Preface

Plastic surgery is a relatively young surgical specialty that has always been characterized by innovation, underwritten by basic surgical principles that have resulted in a variety of approaches to yield a successful surgical outcome. In the last two decades there has been an enormous evolution in techniques to gain predictable natural results in facial aesthetic surgery. Among the many textbooks available, there is a lack of ready-to-use information on the essentials of surgical technique.

Aesthetic Head and Neck Surgery is geared toward providing high-yield information on surgical techniques covering the broad spectrum of aesthetic facial surgery to the surgical trainee and plastic surgeons early in their career. This book focuses upon aesthetic procedures about the head and neck in an atlas format and has world experts who have graciously detailed their surgical pearls and favorite reliable techniques in an easy-to-read format, clearly illustrated with well-selected before and after examples.

The book is intended to allow quick review of a variety of surgical techniques to achieve an aesthetic outcome encompassing the entire spectrum of approaches.

We hope you enjoy the book and find it useful as at reference. We look forward to seeing you at the meetings!

S.J.L. and T.A.M.

Chapter 1. Forehead Anatomy

Samuel J. Lin, MD, FACS; Amr N. Rabie, MD

LAYERS AND ATTACHMENTS

The forehead occupies the upper third of the face. It is bordered superiorly by the hairline and inferiorly by the glabella (medially) and the eyebrows overlying the supraorbital ridge (laterally). When making an incision, careful consideration should be made in terms of choosing to place the incision either within the hairline or in a pretrichial location. A hairline approach is indicated when the patient's hairline is low, if the patient is satisfied with their eyebrows, and if the patient's main concern is aesthetic result. To avoid injuring hair follicles, this incision should be beveled. The pretrichial approach can be used when the patient's hairline is high, if the patient wants to alter the appearance of his or her eyebrows, or if the patient wants to avoid even minimal hair loss. To escape altering the natural hairline, the incision should be made in very close proximity to the hairline in a "stair-stepped" manner. Finally, incisions should be closed in layers with fine sutures to evade unsightly depressions.

The 5 layers of the scalp (skin, subcutaneous tissue, galea aponeurotica, loose areolar connective tissue, and periosteum) continue into the forehead; however, the skin of the forehead is very thick in comparison to the rest of the face and is rich in sweat glands and sebaceous glands. The galea aponeurotica splits into superficial and deep planes at the origin of the frontalis muscle to enclose the muscle. In the midforehead region, the deep plane itself splits to encapsulate the galeal fat pad, and caudal to this level, splits again to form the glide plane space of the brow. The deep galeal plane, the subgaleal space, and the periosteum are separate layers, except in the lower part of the forehead where they become fused and fix to the frontal bone. During reconstructive surgery, excellent exposure can be achieved via the coronal approach where the flap is lifted in a subgaleal plane above the temporalis fascia laterally and the periosteum medially (Fig. 1-1). Care should be taken to avoid injury to the frontal branch of the facial nerve and the supratrochlear and supraorbital nerves and vessels.

NERVE SUPPLY AND BLOOD SUPPLY

The supratrochlear and supraorbital nerves pierce the frontalis muscle to reach the anterior scalp and provide sensory innervations to the forehead and the anterior scalp. During upper facial surgical rejuvenation, it is vital to respect the course of these nerves. The supraorbital nerve passes through the supraorbital foramen and divides into a deep lateral branch and a medial superficial branch. The medial superficial division lies in the galeal fat pad superficial to the corrugator muscle, whereas the deep lateral division exists deep to the galeal fat pad and runs along the floor of the glide plane space deep to the corrugator muscle. The terminal branch of this deep division pierces the galea close to the coronal suture to provide sensation to the frontoparietal scalp. The supraorbital

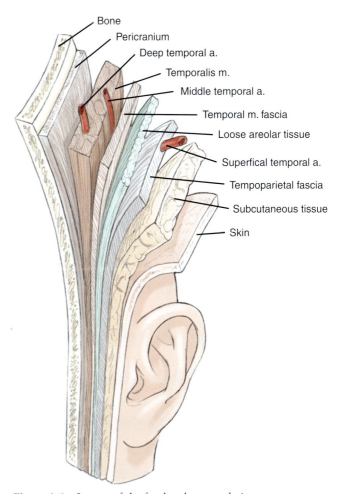

- Bone
- Pericranium
- Deep temporal a.
- Temporalis m.
- Middle temporal a.
- Temporal m. fascia
- Loose areolar tissue
- Superfical temporal a.
- Tempoparietal fascia
- Subcutaneous tissue
- Skin

Figure 1-1 Layers of the forehead, coronal view.

nerve also provides small eyelid branches, which supply the upper eyelid. The supratrochlear nerve exits the orbit medial to the supraorbital notch and above the trochlea. The nerve then passes through the corrugator and frontalis muscles at the supraorbital rim toward the skin. It is important to note that care should be taken during corrugator resection to avoid damage to the nerve. This nerve provides sensation to a vertical strip of forehead and the medial upper eyelid. It is also imperative to be wary for the frontal branch of the facial nerve, which runs within the temporoparietal fascia in the temporal region, where it crosses the sentinel vein and then enters the frontalis muscle and the deep part of the orbicularis muscle just above the level of the supraorbital rim. It provides motor fibers to the muscles of facial expression of the forehead and eyebrows. To avoid injury to the frontal branch during elevation of facial flaps, elevation should be done either deep to the superficial musculoaponeurotic system (SMAS) or in a subcutaneous plane. Also, it is important that this branch be identified during rhytidectomy. For the surgeon, in addition to being cautious regarding the frontal branch of the facial nerve in the region of the temple, it is important to notice the superficial temporal artery and the sentinel veins. The superficial temporal artery (STA) is a terminal branch of the external carotid artery; it arises within the substance of the parotid gland then ascends to cross the zygomatic arch anterior to the tragus. The STA then becomes invested in the superficial temporal fascia above the arch (Fig. 1-2). It gives multiple branches, the most important of which in this scenario is the frontal branch, which remains above and parallel to the nerve along its course. Both the frontal branch of the STA and the sentinel vein are key surface landmarks, which indicate fairly accurately the subcutaneous position of the frontal branch of facial nerve. Additional blood supply to the forehead region includes the supratrochlear and supraorbital arteries, along with the temporal and occipital arteries. The supratrochlear vessels pass through the orbit superior-medially and run in a cephalad direction; the supraorbital arteries pass through the supraorbital foramina and provide the primary arterial supply to the forehead. The occipital arteries arise from the posterior scalp and the temporal arteries from the lateral scalp, and provide a negligible blood supply to the scalp.

MUSCLES OF THE FOREHEAD

The mimetic muscles of the forehead play a role in the aging process. Rhytides are dynamic in origin with vertical wrinkles appearing across the glabella, horizontal wrinkles across the forehead, and oblique wrinkles in between the eyebrows. The main mimetic muscles of the forehead are the frontalis, the corrugators, the procerus, and the orbicularis oculi muscles (Fig. 1-3). The frontalis muscle forms the frontal belly of the occipitofrontalis; it is a large, flat, bilateral muscle that spans the entire fore-

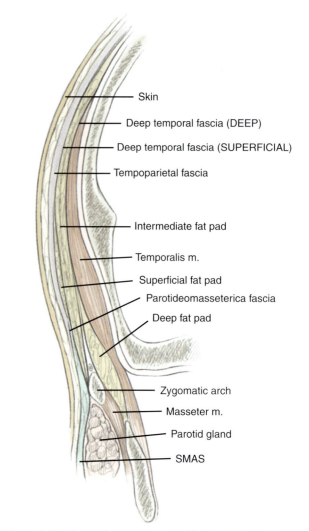

Figure 1-2   Coronal cross section of forehead (lateral).

- Skin
- Deep temporal fascia (DEEP)
- Deep temporal fascia (SUPERFICIAL)
- Tempoparietal fascia
- Intermediate fat pad
- Temporalis m.
- Superficial fat pad
- Parotideomasseterica fascia
- Deep fat pad
- Zygomatic arch
- Masseter m.
- Parotid gland
- SMAS

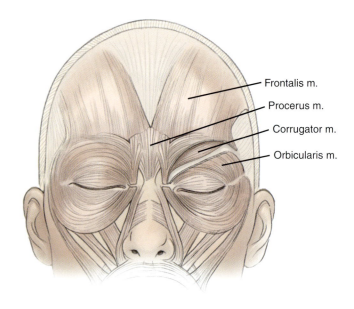

Figure 1-3   Origins and insertion of the main forehead muscles.

- Frontalis m.
- Procerus m.
- Corrugator m.
- Orbicularis m.

head. It takes origin at the superior aspect of the scalp, its fibers are directed vertically and insert into the galea aponeurotica. Thickening and lengthening of the frontalis muscle results in horizontal forehead lines called "worry lines," which can be as simple as minor mimetic lines or as apparent as skin folds. These "worry lines" can be treated either by peeling, which includes a variety of options—laser resurfacing, chemical resurfacing, dermabrasion, radiofrequency treatment—or through the use of Botox and skin fillers (both permanent and nonpermanent). Autologous fat transfer is another approach; this technique, however, may yield better results when applied to the lower two-thirds of the face as opposed to the forehead, perhaps because of the strong tension of the skin in this region. If 2 or more deep forehead wrinkles exist, the rhytides can be excised, adapted, and sutured in layers; in time, the scar will appear as a single wrinkle. A more conventional approach is an endoscopic forehead lift, which enables the surgeon to lift the forehead through 3 to 5 incisions, each measuring 1 to 2 cm in length. The monitor magnifies the anatomical structures by 10 times and the light source and endoscope has very small diameters, sometimes as small as 2.7 mm. It is vital to avoid injury to the supratrochlear and supraorbital nerves during an endoscopic forehead lift. It is important to note that the frontalis muscle causes elevation of the eyebrows. Injury to the temporal branch of the facial nerve will result in loss of forehead motion and unilateral brow ptosis. The corrugator muscle originates just above the nose from the medial orbital rim and is inserted into the frontalis muscle and skin of the eyebrows. Together the procerus and orbicularis oculi muscles act to close the eyelids and form oblique and transverse glabellar or frown lines across the forehead, which become more prominent with corrugator and procerus hypertrophy. When depressor muscle tone (corrugator and procerus muscles) surpasses the elevator muscle tone (frontalis muscle), the lower forehead skin starts to descend; this occurrence is especially common if the patient is a "frowner." The procerus muscles exhibit vertical fibers that extend from the radix of the nose to the lower forehead. The orbicularis oculi surround each orbit acting as a sphincter for each eye.

LIGAMENTS

The orbital ligaments represent the true dermal-to-periosteal retaining system of the upper face, whereas the periosteal zone of adhesion, which is an adherence of the deep galea to periosteum, represents the false retaining system of the upper face. The orbital ligaments are taut, white fibers measuring 6 to 8 mm that lay adjacent to the temporal crest and fusion line. It is important for the surgeon to avoid trauma to the sensory nerve, small artery, and large veins that are present in this area. The periosteal zone of adhesion is a wing-shaped band

measuring 1.5 to 2.5 cm in width. This area extends from the nasofrontal junction to the orbital ligaments at the zygomaticofrontal junction. Subperiosteal release of the periosteal zone of adhesion and the orbital ligaments will cause the glide plane space and the galea fusion band to elevate, as well as resulting in mobility of the forehead and brow soft tissue; hence, for elevation to be pertinent, cephalic fixation must be done within the deep galea.

PITFALLS

During the creation of the optical cavity in endoscopic forehead lift, discontinue blind dissection 2 cm above the eyebrows; further dissection should be done under endoscopic visualization to avoid injury to the supraorbital nerves.

In 15% of patients, the supraorbital nerves reach the forehead through a bony canal above the orbital rim.

Close the incisions with staples if they lie in a hair-bearing area, or with intradermal sutures if they are in front of the hairline.

PEARLS

Be wary for the frontal branch of the facial nerve that runs within the temporoparietal fascia in the temporal region where it crosses the sentinel vein and then enters the frontalis muscle and deep part of the orbicularis muscle just above the level of the supraorbital rim; to avoid injury of the nerve during elevation of facial flaps, elevation should be done either deep to the SMAS or in a subcutaneous plane.

SUGGESTED READING

De la Torres JI, Gardner PM, Vasconez LO. Forehead endoscopy. In: Peled IJ, Manders EK, eds. *Esthetic Surgery of the Face*. London, UK: Taylor & Francis; 2004:29-31.

Janis JE, Potter JK, Rohrich RJ. Brow lift techniques. In: Fagien S, ed. *Putterman's Cosmetic Oculoplastic Surgery*. 4th ed. Philadelphia, PA: Saunders Elsevier; 2008:67-77.

Larrabee WF Jr, Makielski KH. Facial musculature. In: Larrabee WF Jr, Makielski KH, eds. *Surgical Anatomy of the Face*. New York, NY: Raven; 1993:49-59.

Larrabee WF Jr, Makielski KH. Forehead and brow. In: Larrabee WF Jr, Makielski KH, eds. *Surgical Anatomy of the Face*. New York, NY: Raven; 1993:123-128.

LaTrenta GS. Surgical approaches to the forehead and brow. In: LaTrenta GS, ed. *Atlas of Aesthetic Face & Neck Surgery*. Philadelphia, PA: Saunders Elsevier; 2004:78-81.

LaTrenta GS. The aging face. In: LaTrenta GS, ed. *Atlas of Aesthetic Face & Neck Surgery*. Philadelphia, PA: Saunders Elsevier; 2004:62-63.

Panfilov DE. Forehead. In: Panfilov DE, ed. *Aesthetic Surgery of the Facial Mosaic*. Berlin, Germany: Springer; 2007: 133-138.

THE UPPER EYELID

The eyelid functions to protect the globe, regulate the light reaching the eye, and aids in maintaining the tear film and tear flow. Operating on the eyelid requires comprehensive understanding of its anatomy (Figs. 2-1 and 2-2).

Surface Anatomy of the Eyelid

The upper eyelid extends from the lid margin to the eyebrow. The superior palpebral sulcus (skin crease) is approximately 8 to 11 mm superior to the eyelid margin and is formed by the attachment of the superficial insertion of levator aponeurotic fibers (7 to 8 mm in men and 9 to 11 mm in women). In Asians, the superior palpebral sulcus is absent or displaced inferiorly. The highest point of the normal adult upper eyelid margin is just nasal to the center of the pupil. The normal curvature of the upper eyelid is made by the shape of the tarsus combined with the curvature of the globe. During adolescence, the upper eyelid margin is placed at the limbus, whereas in adults it is 1.5 mm below the limbus. A useful method to describe the eyelid position is the margin reflex distance (MRD), which is the distance in millimeters from the corneal light reflex to the lid margin; for the upper eyelid, it measures 4 to 5 mm. It can be measured using a ruler or it can be estimated, keeping in mind that the midway point between the corneal light reflex and the limbus is approximately 2.5 mm. The MRD is a vital part of the eyelid examination. A drooping upper eyelid, known as ptosis, and an upper eyelid positioned above the limbus is termed *lid retraction*. The posterior lid margin is sharp and is applied to the globe, while the anterior lid margin is curved and holds the eyelashes.

The palpebral fissure is a fusiform space extending between the upper and lower lid margins and measuring approximately 28 to 30 mm in length and reaching up to 9 mm in height. Ideally, the 2 palpebral fissures are separated by 1 palpebral fissure width. The level of the lateral canthal angle differs with ethnicity; in whites it is 2 mm higher than the medial angle, whereas in Asians it is 3 mm higher.

The eyelids are divided into 2 anatomical lamellae. The anterior lamella is made up of the skin and the orbicularis muscle, and the posterior lamella contains the tarsus and the conjunctiva. There is a gray line on the lid margin that marks the junction of the lid lamellae.

Skin and Subcutaneous Tissue

The skin of the eyelid is among the thinnest in the body, and it contains relatively little adipose tissue. It is attached loosely to the orbicularis oculi muscle, but firmly to the region of the canthal ligaments, particularly the medial canthus. The meibomian gland openings are located at the mucocutaneous junction at the free lid margin, apart from the eyelashes, and the skin hairs are very fine. There are 3 to 4 eyelash rows in the upper eyelid.

Orbicularis Oculi Muscle

The muscles of the eyelid may be divided into protractors (orbicularis muscle) and retractors (levator and Müller's muscles). The orbicularis oculi muscle is one of the facial expression muscles; it is formed of thin sheets of concentrically arranged muscle fibers. It is innervated by the temporal and zygomatic branches of the facial nerve from its undersurface. It is divided into 2 parts— the orbital and the palpebral parts; the latter is further divided into the preseptal and pretarsal. The orbital part originates from the medial orbital margin and curves around the orbital margin, extending superiorly above the eyebrow and interdigitating with the frontalis

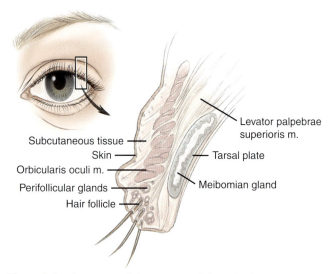

Figure 2-1   Anatomy of the upper eyelid: sagittal view.

Subcutaneous tissue
Skin
Orbicularis oculi m.
Perifollicular glands
Hair follicle

Levator palpebrae superioris m.
Tarsal plate
Meibomian gland

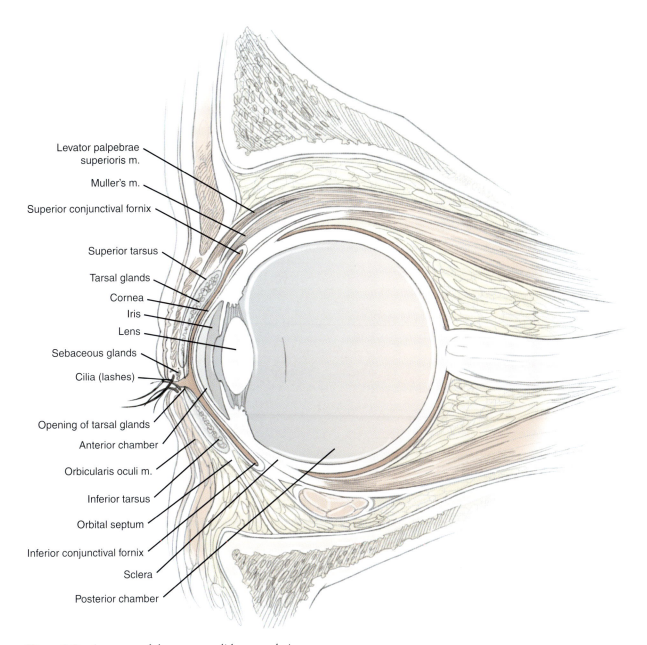

Levator palpebrae
superioris m.

Muller's m.

Superior conjunctival fornix

Superior tarsus

Tarsal glands

Cornea

Iris

Lens

Sebaceous glands

Cilia (lashes)

Opening of tarsal glands

Anterior chamber

Orbicularis oculi m.

Inferior tarsus

Orbital septum

Inferior conjunctival fornix

Sclera

Posterior chamber

Figure 2-2 Anatomy of the upper eyelid: coronal view.

and the corrugator supercilii muscle. It extends laterally to cover the temporalis fascia and inferiorly to cover the origins of the upper lip elevators. Clinically, it plays a role in voluntary lid closure (winking) and forceful lid closure.

The preseptal portion overlying the orbital septum with intervening fat pad, if sizeable, may be misinterpreted as being the preaponeurotic fat. Laterally, it is inserted in the Whitnall's lateral orbital tubercle (3 to 4 mm deep to the lateral palpebral raphe). Medially, it has 2 heads: the superficial head arises from the anterior rim of the medial canthal ligament and the deep head that is adherent to the lacrimal sac and fascia. Clinically, it contributes to voluntary and involuntary lid closure (blinking).

The pretarsal orbicularis lies anterior to the tarsus, and it is firmly adherent to the underlying tarsus and to the superficial insertion of the levator aponeurosis at the superior border of the tarsus. Its origin is formed of a superficial and deep head closely associated with the medial palpebral ligament. Its fibers run horizontally deep to the lateral palpebral raphe to be inserted in the lateral orbital tubercle through the lateral canthal tendon.

Levator Palpebrae Superioris

The levator palpebrae superioris is a thin triangular muscle, arising by narrow tendinous origin from the undersurface of the lesser wing of the sphenoid. Its insertion is formed of a wide aponeurosis that splits into 3 lamellae.

The superficial lamella blends with the upper part of the orbital septum and extends above the superior tarsus deep to the skin of the eyelid. The middle lamella is inserted in the upper border of the superior tarsus. The deep lamella blends with the sheath of the rectus superior muscle and is attached to the superior conjunctival fornix. The levator palpebrae raises the upper eyelid and is innervated by the abducens nerve.

Müller's Muscle

The Müller's muscle arises from the undersurface of the levator palebrae superioris muscle, approximately 15 mm above the upper tarsus border (its insertion). It is made up of smooth muscle fibers and innervated by the sympathetic nervous system. It functions to provide the upper lid an extra 2 mm of elevation (Fig. 2-2).

Submuscular Areolar Tissue

The submuscular areolar tissue consists of loose connective tissue. The eyelid may be divided into anterior and posterior portions through this plane, which is represented at the lid margin by the gray line. The levator aponeurosis traverses the submuscular areolar tissue plane; fibers from the levator aponeurosis pass through the orbicularis muscle to be inserted into the skin forming the lid crease.

The Tarsal Plate

The tarsal plates are made of dense fibrous tissue and are responsible for the integrity of the eyelid. The superior tarsus is crescentic in shape and is approximately 29 mm long, 1 mm thick, and 10 mm in vertical height centrally. Its lower border forms the posterior lid margin and its posterior surface is adherent to conjunctiva. The tarsal plate encloses approximately 30 meibomian glands that span the whole vertical height of the tarsus and open on the lid margin posterior to the gray line. The tarsus is attached to the orbital rim by the lateral and medial palpebral ligaments.

Orbital Septum (Palpebral Ligament)

The orbital septum is a membranous sheet attached to the edge of the orbit. Its circumference blends with the tendon of the levator Palpebrae superioris and the superior tarsus.

Medial Palpebral Ligament

The medial palpebral ligament measures approximately 4 mm in length and 2 mm in breadth. It is attached to the frontal process of the maxilla anterior to the lacrimal groove and is divided into upper and lower parts, each being attached to the medial end of the corresponding tarsus.

Lateral Palpebral Raphe

This structure is attached to the margin of the frontosphenoidal process of the zygomatic bone at the lateral orbital tubercle, passes medially, and divides into 2 slips, which are attached to the margins of the respective tarsi.

During lateral canthotomy to decompress the orbit to lower the intraorbital pressure, the inferior and superior crus of the lateral canthal ligament must be released from the tarsal plate.

Fat Pads

The fat in the upper eyelid is divided into two distinctive fat pads: the medial and the central. The medial fat pad is whitish and more fibrous, whereas the central pad is yellowish, less fibrous, and termed the *preaponeurotic fat pad*. The 2 pads are separated by the trochlea. The preaponeurotic fat pad is surrounded by thin translucent connective tissue capsule and lies directly superficial to the levator aponeurosis for which it serves as an important landmark.

Clinically, the medial fat pad may herniate through the orbital septum, forming a bulge underneath the trochlea. The medial fat pad is associated with the medial palpebral artery and the infratrochlear nerve, which is why it requires deeper anesthetic injection for its removal. Because of the fat pads' close proximity to the trochlea, superior oblique palsy has been reported during their dissection in blepharoplasty.

The retroorbicularis layer may contain significant amount of fat, which may be misinterpreted as being the preaponeurotic fat.

Palpebral Conjunctiva

The conjunctiva is made up of 2 components: the bulbar conjunctiva, which covers the globe extending to the corneal limbus, and the palpebral conjunctive, which lines the eyelid. The 2 conjunctival components meet at the conjunctival fornices. The superior fornix is stabilized by a suspensory ligament that arises from the conjoining of the superior rectus and the levator muscles. The conjunctiva is loosely adherent except at the limbus, the tarsus, and the superior tarsal muscle where it is firmly adherent to these structures.

Blood Supply

The eyelid is supplied by both the internal and the external carotid systems. The internal carotid contributes to the arterial supply of the eyelid through terminal branches of the ophthalmic artery medially and the lacrimal artery laterally, while the external carotid contribution comes from branches of the facial artery, the superficial temporal artery, and the infraorbital artery.

The lateral and medial palpebral arteries have superior and inferior branches that form arcades that lie on the anterior surface of the tarsus approximately 2 to 4 mm from the lid margin and supply the upper and lower eyelids. The lateral palpebral arteries are branches of the lacrimal artery (a branch of the ophthalmic artery).

The medial palpebral arteries are direct branches from the ophthalmic artery. Their branches run laterally to form superior and inferior arcades that anastomose with the lateral palpebral artery and with branches from the supraorbital and zygomaticoorbital arteries (superior arch). The inferior arch anastomoses with the facial artery. Additionally, branches from the superficial temporal, infraorbital, and transverse facial arteries supply the eyelids.

The veins of the eyelids are numerous and larger than the arteries. They drain either superficially into the veins on the face and forehead, or deep into the ophthalmic veins.

Nerve Supply

The supraorbital and supratrochlear nerves of the ophthalmic division of the trigeminal nerve supplies sensory innervation for the upper eyelid. The supraorbital nerve exits the orbit at the supraorbital foramen or notch, and supplies the upper eyelid and the forehead skin, except for a midline strip that is supplied by the supratrochlear nerve, which exits the orbit between the pulley of the superior oblique and the supraorbital foramen and passes close to the bone, ascends beneath the corrugator supercilii and frontalis muscles, and divides into its terminal branches that pierce these muscles.

Tips

- In Asians, the superior palpebral sulcus is absent or displaced inferiorly.
- The highest point of the normal adult upper eyelid margin is just nasal to the center of the pupil.
- The orbicularis oculi muscle is innervated by the temporal and zygomatic branches of the facial nerve from its undersurface.
- The lid crease is formed by the insertion of the levator aponeurosis into the skin of the upper eyelid.
- During lateral canthotomy to decompress the orbit, the inferior and superior crus of the lateral canthal ligament must be released from the tarsal plate.
- The retroorbicularis layer may contain significant amounts of fat, which may be misinterpreted as being the preaponeurotic fat.
- Just above the superior tarsal border, a peripheral arterial arcade arises from the marginal arcade and lies directly over the Müller's muscle and is susceptible to injury during surgery for blepharoptosis.

THE LOWER EYELID

The eyelid functions to protect the globe, to regulate the light reaching the eye, and to aid in maintaining the tear film and tear flow. Operating on the eyelid requires a comprehensive understanding of the anatomy (Figs. 2-3 and 2-4).

Surface Anatomy of the Lower Eyelid

The lower eyelid extends from the lid margin to below the orbital margin to join the cheek, forming 3 folds. The inferior palpebral crease corresponds to the lower edge of the tarsus; it is less prominent than the superior palpebral crease. This crease runs from 5 mm below the lid margin medially to approximately 7 mm laterally. The nasojugal crease runs inferolaterally at 45 degrees below the medial aspect of the inferior palpebral crease, overlying the interface between the orbicularis oculi and the levator labii superioris. The malar crease originates below and lateral to the lateral canthus and runs inferomedially to meet the lateral aspect of the nasojugal crease 15 mm below the midpoint of the lower eyelid margin.

The lower eyelid margin is found at the level of the limbus. The upper and lower eyelids meet at the medial and lateral commissures. The medial and lateral canthi are the angles formed at the medial and lateral commissures, respectively. The lateral canthus is more acute and positioned slightly higher than the medial canthus.

The caruncle and the plica semilunaris displace the medial commissure anteriorly, while the lateral commissure rests directly on the globe. The posterior lid margin is sharp and is applied to the globe, while the anterior lid margin is curved and holds the eyelashes.

The palpebral fissure is a fusiform space extending between the upper and lower lid margins, measuring approximately 28 to 30 mm in length and reaching up to 9 mm in height. Ideally, the 2 palpebral fissures are separated by 1 palpebral fissure width. The level of the lateral canthal angle differs with ethnicity; in whites it is 2 mm higher than the medial angle, whereas in Asians it is 3 mm higher.

The eyelids are divided into 2 anatomical lamellae: the anterior lamella comprises the skin and the orbicularis muscle, and the posterior lamella contains the tarsus and the conjunctiva. There is a gray line on the lid margin that marks the junction of the lid lamellae.

Skin and Subcutaneous Tissue

The skin of the eyelid is among the thinnest in the body; it contains relatively little adipose tissue. It is attached loosely to the orbicularis oculi muscle, but firmly to the region of the canthal ligaments, particularly the medial canthus. The meibomian gland openings are located at the mucocutaneous junction at the free lid margin, apart from the eyelashes, and the skin hairs are very fine.

Orbicularis Oculi Muscle

The orbicularis oculi muscle is one of the facial expression muscles; it is formed of thin sheets of concentrically arranged muscle fibers. It is innervated by the temporal and zygomatic branches of the facial nerve

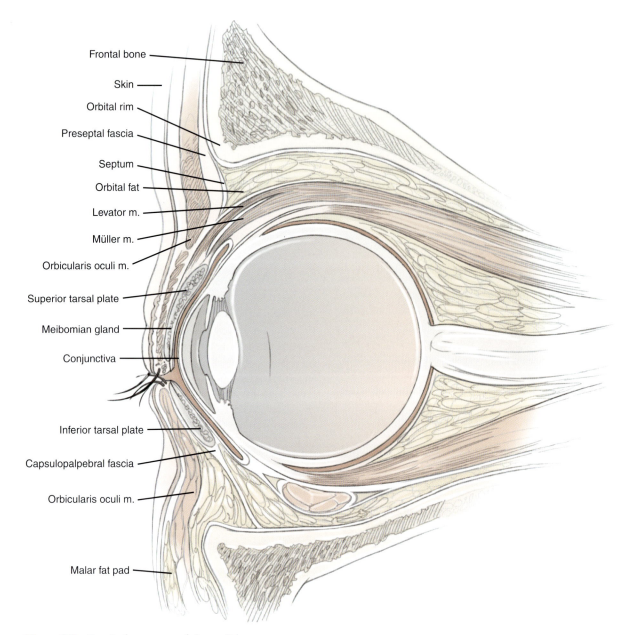

Figure 2-3   Surgical anatomy of the eyelids.

from its undersurface. It is divided into 2 parts: the orbital and the palpebral. The latter structure is further divided into preseptal and pretarsal. The orbital portion originates from the medial orbital margin and curves around the orbital margin, extending superiorly above the eyebrow and interdigitating with the frontalis and the corrugator supercilii muscle. It extends laterally to cover the temporalis fascia and inferiorly to cover the origins of the upper lip elevators. Clinically, this structure plays a role in voluntary lid closure (winking) and forceful lid closure.

The preseptal portion of the palpebral orbicularis oculi overlies the orbital septum with intervening fat pad; if sizeable, this structure may be misinterpreted as

being the preaponeurotic fat. Laterally, it inserts in the Whitnall's lateral orbital tubercle (3 to 4 mm deep to the lateral palpebral raphe). Medially, it has 2 heads: the superficial head, which arises from the anterior rim of the medial canthal ligament, and the deep head, which is adherent to the lacrimal sac and fascia. Clinically, it contributes to voluntary and involuntary lid closure (blinking).

The pretarsal orbicularis lies anterior to the tarsus, and is firmly adherent to the underlying tarsus and to the superficial insertion of the levator aponeurosis at the superior border of the tarsus. Its origin is formed of a superficial and deep head closely associated with the medial palpebral ligament. Its fibers run horizontally deep

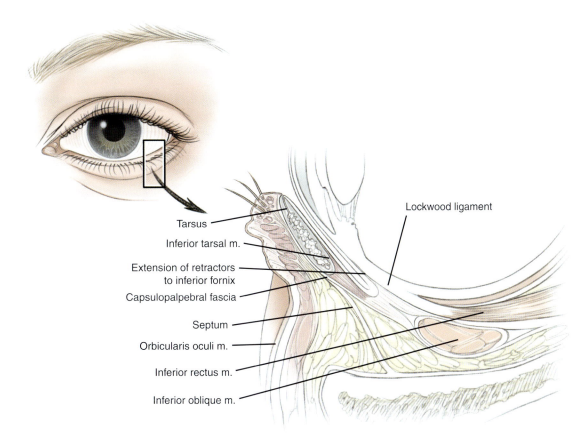

Tarsus
Inferior tarsal m.
Extension of retractors to inferior fornix
Capsulopalpebral fascia
Septum
Orbicularis oculi m.
Inferior rectus m.
Inferior oblique m.
Lockwood ligament

Figure 2-4   Anatomy of the lower eyelid: sagittal view.

to the lateral palpebral raphe, to be inserted in the lateral orbital tubercle through the lateral canthal tendon.

The lower eyelid retractors are the capsulopalpebral ligament, a fibrous extension from the inferior rectus muscle, and the inferior tarsal muscle (sympathetically innervated).

Submuscular Areolar Tissue

The submuscular areolar tissue consists of loose connective tissue. The eyelid may be divided into anterior and posterior portions through this plane, which is represented at the lid margin by the gray line.

Tarsal Plate

The tarsal plates are made of dense fibrous tissue and are responsible for the integrity of the eyelid. The inferior tarsus is approximately 25 to 30 mm long, 1 mm thick, and 3 to 5 mm in vertical height centrally. Its lower border forms the posterior lid margin, and its posterior surface is adherent to conjunctiva. The tarsal plate encloses 20 to 30 meibomian glands, spanning the whole vertical height of the tarsus and opening on the lid margin posterior to the gray line. The tarsus is attached to the orbital rim by the lateral and medial palpebral ligaments.

Orbital Septum

The orbital septum is a membranous sheet that connects the periosteum of the orbital margin with the lid. The attachment of the orbital septum to the orbital rim is known as the *arcus marginalis*. At the arcus marginalis 3 structures meet: the orbital septum, the periorbita, and the periosteum.

Medial Palpebral Ligament

The medial palpebral ligament measures approximately 4 mm in length and 2 mm in breadth. It is attached to the frontal process of the maxilla anterior to the lacrimal groove and is divided into upper and lower parts, each being attached to the medial end of the corresponding tarsus.

Lateral Palpebral Raphe

The lateral palpebral raphe is attached to the margin of the frontosphenoidal process of the zygomatic bone at the lateral orbital tubercle and passes medially, dividing into two slips, which are attached to the margins of the respective tarsi.

During lateral canthotomy to decompress the orbit to lower the intraorbital pressure, the inferior and superior crus of the lateral canthal ligament must be released from the tarsal plate.

Fat Pads

The fat pads of the lower eyelid are made up of a larger medial fat pad and a smaller temporal one, which are separated by fascial bands. The medial fat pad extends to the medial canthal area and is a single fat pad anteriorly, while posteriorly it is divided by the origin of the inferior oblique muscle. The lateral fat pad is more fibrotic and tends to prolapse less frequently. The lower eyelid fat pads are in direct contact with the extraconal orbital fat, which is why excessive traction may be transmitted to the deeper fat into the orbit, resulting in an intraorbital hemorrhage.

Palpebral Conjunctiva

The conjunctiva is made up of 2 components: the bulbar conjunctiva, which covers the globe extending to the corneal limbus, and the palpebral conjunctiva, which lines the eyelid. The 2 conjunctival components meet at the conjunctival fornices. The superior fornix is stabilized by a suspensory ligament that arises from the conjoining of the superior rectus and the levator muscles.

Blood Supply

The eyelid is supplied by both the internal and the external carotid systems. The internal carotid contributes to the arterial supply of the eyelid through terminal branches of the ophthalmic artery medially and the lacrimal artery laterally, while the external carotid contribution come from branches of the facial artery, the superficial temporal artery, and the infraorbital artery.

The lateral and medial palpebral arteries have superior and inferior branches, which form arcades that lie on the anterior surface of the tarsus, approximately 2 to 4 mm from the lid margin, and supply the upper and lower eyelids. The lateral palpebral arteries are branches of the lacrimal artery (a branch of the ophthalmic artery). The medial palpebral arteries are direct branches from the ophthalmic artery. Their branches run laterally to form superior and inferior arcades that anastomose with the lateral palpebral artery and with branches from the supraorbital and zygomaticoorbital arteries (superior arch). The inferior arch anastomoses with the facial artery. Additionally, branches from the superficial temporal, infraorbital, and transverse facial arteries supply the eyelids.

The veins of the eyelids are numerous and larger than the arteries. They drain either superficially into the veins on the face and forehead, or deep into the ophthalmic veins.

Nerve Supply

The maxillary division of the trigeminal nerve, through the infraorbital and the zygomaticofacial nerves, supplies most of the lower eyelid, except the for the most medial portion, which is supplied by the ophthalmic division, through the infratrochlear nerve, a terminal branch of the nasociliary nerve.

Tips

- The orbicularis oculi muscle is innervated by the temporal and zygomatic branches of the facial nerve from its undersurface.
- The lower eyelid fat pads are in direct contact with the extraconal orbital fat; this is the reason that excessive traction may be transmitted to the deeper fat into the orbit, resulting in an intraorbital hemorrhage.
- The lateral fat pad is more fibrotic and tends to prolapse less frequently.

SUGGESTED READING

Chen WP-D. *Oculoplastic Surgery: The Essentials.* New York, NY: Thieme; 2001.

Della Rocca RC, Bedrossian EH, Arthurs BP. *Ophthalmic Plastic Surgery: Decision Making and Techniques.* New York, NY: McGraw-Hill; 2002.

Gray H, Clemente CD. *Anatomy of the Human Body.* 30th American ed. Philadelphia, PA: Lea & Febiger; 1985.

Kakizaki H, Malhotra R, Selva D. Upper eyelid anatomy: an update. *Ann Plast Surg.* 2009;63(3):336-343.

Nerad JA. *Techniques in Ophthalmic Plastic Surgery: A Personal Tutorial.* Philadelphia, PA: Saunders Elsevier; 2010.

Chapter 3. Nasal Anatomy

Jason S. Cooper, MD

ANATOMIC CONSIDERATIONS

Rhinoplasty is indicated for patients with functional or aesthetic nasal deformities. Appropriate rhinoplasty candidates have specific concerns that can be visually appreciated and reasonable expectations that are achievable by a surgeon performing rhinoplasty. The degree of concern for one's deformity ought to be compatible with the nasal deformity. Rhinoplasty is avoided in patients whose expectations are beyond the surgical limitations of aesthetic improvement. If the deformity exceeds the surgeon's capabilities, the patient should be referred to a more experienced surgeon.

Understanding the interrelationship between skin, soft tissue, and structural support of nasal anatomy is critical to evaluating and devising an appropriate operative plan. A systemic approach to nasal analysis is equally important to preoperative planning. Standardized photography and computer imaging enable the surgeon to visualize the preoperative deformity, gauge the patient's level of understanding, and review possible anticipated outcomes. The operative plan is individualized to the patient's specific concerns, while operative maneuvers are adjusted to account for size and shape of the patient's face. Clinical analysis of nasal symmetry, shape, projection, tip rotation, and definition (skin thickness) clarify surgical techniques critical to attaining a mutually desirable result.

Soft-Tissue Envelope

The thickness of the nasal skin overlying the bony and cartilaginous framework of the nose is assessed prior to incision. Palpation helps determine the relative skin thickness in different locations of the nose. Nasal skin is usually thick over the bony dorsum, thinnest overlying the upper lateral cartilages (ULCs), and thickest over the nasal tip (Fig. 3-1). The sebaceous, oily quality of nasal tip skin can conceal the lower lateral cartilages (LLCs), obscuring subtle tip grafts and suturing techniques during the procedure. Bony and cartilaginous resection is modified to account for overlying skin thickness. Thin skin leaves small amounts of bony and cartilaginous resection visible. Thick nasal skin may mask changes to the dorsum or tip even after considerable osseocartilaginous resection. Resection of the nasal skin and thinning of the soft-tissue envelope should be done judiciously. The skin and soft-tissue enveloping the LLCs provide tip support. Dissections of the skin envelope from the LLCs lead to loss of tip support. Anticipatory maneuvers are used to strength tip support.

Blood Supply

Branches from the ophthalmic and facial arteries provide blood to the nose (Fig. 3-2). Columellar branches are transected in open rhinoplasty, leaving lateral and dorsal nasal arteries to supply blood to the nasal tip. To prevent injury to the lateral nasal arteries, extended alar resections are avoided during open rhinoplasty. Venous and lymphatic drainage is in the subcutaneous layer superficial to the arteries.

Nasal Bones and Cartilaginous Vault

The nose may be separated into vertical thirds based upon its underlying bony and cartilaginous framework. The upper third of the nose consists of the nasal bones, the middle third is composed of the ULCs, which constitute the midvault, and the lower third is composed of the

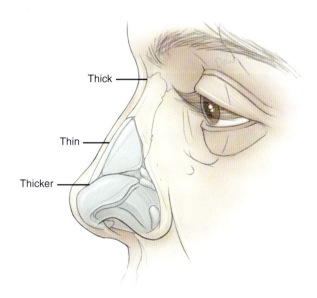

Thick

Thin

Thicker

Figure 3-1 Skin characterizations of the nose.

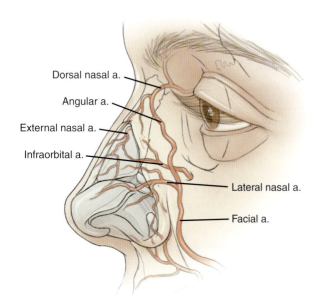

Figure 3-2   Blood supply of the nose.

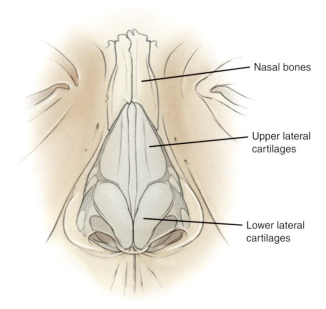

Figure 3-3   Nasal bones and cartilages.

LLCs. The nasal bones are fixed immobile structures, whereas the ULCs are partially mobile and the LLCs are freely mobile (Fig. 3-3). The mobility and function of the cartilages are considered when grafting, suturing, bending, or shaping of these areas.

The paired nasal bones articulate with the frontal bones superiorly, and the frontal process of the maxilla laterally. The nasal bones are thickest at the nasofrontal suture line, and taper as they join with the ULCs. Medially, the ULCs fuse with the septum. Inferiorly, the ULCs interdigitate with the LLCs; this junction is known as the *scroll area*, which is a tip-supporting structure. Caution is observed when making intercartilaginous incisions or performing a cephalic trim. Cephalic trim of the alar cartilages can damage the caudal portion of the ULCs, weakening the tip and midvault support. At least 6 to 8 mm of alar cartilage, depending on the patient, is left to prevent external nasal valve collapse.

The keystone area is created by the union between the nasal bone, ULC, and septum. This area should be the widest part of the dorsum. Here, the nasal bones overlie the ULC. The relationship between the ULC and septum is critical to maintaining proper dorsal contour. Internal nasal valve competence (formed by caudal portion of upper lateral cartilage with anterior septal edge) is contingent upon the width and stability of the ULCs, along with the width, stability, and height of the middle vault.

Nasal Tip

The lower third of the nose is composed of the LLCs known as the *alar cartilage*. The LLCs begin anterior to the nasal spine as widened medial crural footplates and narrow anteriorly medial to the anterior nostril margin. In profile, the intermediate crus is seen to ascend slightly from the medial crus. The intermediate crura span the infratip lobule, which is the soft-tissue region of the nose extending from anterior nostril margin to the nasal tip. The angle of divergence is the junction of the intermediate and lateral crura. The dome lies lateral to the angle and is composed of the lateral crus. The lateral crura extend laterally to meet the pyriform aperture at the hinge, which is composed of small accessory cartilages.

The integrity of tip support can be assessed by digitally depressing the nasal tip and observing the give of the tissue under the pressure of one's fingertip, along with the recoil of the tip back to its resting position. The majority of tip support is derived from the strength of LLCs, the LLC–septum attachment, and the scroll attachment. Minor contributing structures to tip support include the interdomal ligament, sesamoid complex, membranous septum, cartilaginous dorsum, nasal spine, and the alar attachment to skin and soft tissue. Tip projection is also dependent upon dorsal height. Therefore, when the dorsum is resected or trimmed, the nasal tip will lose projection. Nasal facial analysis is critical to anticipating tip projection in conjunction with other goals.

Airway Obstruction

When evaluating a patient for rhinoplasty, the most common correctable causes of nasal obstruction include septal deviation, mucosal/bony turbinate hypertrophy, and an incompetent nasal valve. The internal nasal valve is the main regulator of nasal airflow in the nose and is composed of the septum, ULC, and anterior aspect of the turbinate. The angle between the septum and the ULC should be, at minimum, 10 to 15 degrees to maintain internal valve patency. In ethnic populations the interval valve typically has an obtuse angle, thus it is less frequently a cause of airway obstruction, although in certain individuals it may manifest as nasal obstruction. A Cottle test can be performed by digitally distracting the middle vault laterally; improved airflow suggests internal nasal valve incompetence. A cotton-tip applicator can be inserted into the nostril to push the ULC laterally to assess internal nasal valve patency. The turbinates describe 3 or 4 bilateral extensions from the lateral nasal wall. During inspiration, up to two-thirds of upper airway resistance is produced by the anterior tip of the inferior turbinate in the area of the internal nasal valve.

PITFALLS

The relationship between the ULC and septum is critical to maintaining proper dorsal contour and avoiding internal nasal valve collapse. Altered dorsal contour as seen by an inverted V deformity has become a telltale sign of rhinoplasty, whereas internal nasal valve collapse leads to functional airway obstruction. The junction between ULC and septum is fused, they are not separate entities. The ULC should be cut sharply and carefully dissected from the septum. Inadvertent tears in the septal mucosa or ULC can set the stage for cicatricial contracture of the internal nasal valve. Resection of the ULCs equal to or less than dorsal septal cartilaginous resection is recommended. Overresection of the ULCs creates an inverted V deformity. The patient with short nasal bones and thin skin overlying the ULCs is particularly prone, as thin skin lacks the ability to hide this technical error.

SUGGESTED READING

Cochrane S. Clinical analysis. Paper presented at: 26th Annual Dallas Rhinoplasty Symposium; March 6-8, 2009; Dallas, TX.

Gorney M. Patient selection in rhinoplasty: patient selection. In: Daniel RK, ed. *Aesthetic Plastic Surgery: Rhinoplasty*. Boston, MA: Little, Brown; 1993.

Jackson LE, Koch RJ. Controversies in the management of inferior turbinate hypertrophy: a comprehensive review. *Plast Reconstr Surg*. 1999;103:300.

Lam SM, Williams EF. Anatomic considerations in aesthetic rhinoplasty. *Facial Plastic Surg*. 2002;18(4):209.

McKinney P, Johnson P, Walloch J. Anatomy of the nasal hump. *Plast Reconstr Surg*. 1986;77:404.

Rees TD. In: *Aesthetic Plastic Surgery*. Philadelphia, PA: Saunders; 1980.

Rohrich RJ, Gunter JP, Freidman RM. Nasal tip blood supply: an anatomic study validating the safety of transcolumellar incision in rhinoplasty. *Plast Reconstr Surg*. 1995;95(5): 795-799; discussion 800-801.

Rohrich RJ, Krueger JK, Adams WP Jr, Marple BF. Rational for submucous resection of hypertrophied inferior turbinates in rhinoplasty: an evolution. *Plast Reconst Surg*. 2001; 108(2):536-544; discussion 545-546.

Chapter 4. Midface Anatomy

Jason S. Cooper, MD

PERTINENT ANATOMY

The midface refers to the central third of the face. This area is defined superiorly by a horizontal line above the zygomatic arch to the lateral canthus. Inferiorly, the midface extends from the inferior border of the tragal cartilage to the oral commissure (Fig. 4-1). The midcheek is bordered laterally from the frontal process of the zygoma to the oral commissure and medially from the lower lid above to the nasolabial fold. There are 5 basic layers of the midface: the skin and the subcutaneous layer, the musculoaponeurotic layer, loose areolar tissue (ie, spaces and retaining ligaments), the fixed periosteum, and the deep fascia (Fig. 4-2). The superficial musculoaponeurotic system (SMAS) layer contains the intrinsic muscles of the midcheek, while the loose areolar layer features the retaining ligaments that fix the overlying tissues to the facial skeleton. The retaining ligaments of the midcheek

are the orbicularis, zygomatic, and lateral orbital thickening ligaments. Spaces exist between these fibrous attachment points, enabling soft-tissue movement for mimetic animation and facial expression. The retaining ligaments course through the SMAS and attach within the dermis. Much debate exists regarding how much of a role attenuation or laxity of these fibrous connections leads to midface aging (ie, soft repositioning, wrinkles, creases, and grooves).

Midface Aging

Facial aging is a very complex nonlinear process involving the facial skeletal, soft tissues, muscles, and skin. Correction of the midcheek, tear trough, and lid-cheek junction are believed (by some surgeons) to be fundamental to midface rejuvenation. The tear trough, or nasojugal groove, is a natural depression within the midface extending inferolaterally from the medial canthus. The tear trough is short (no more than 3 cm in length) and terminates approximately in the midpupillary line. The palpebromalar groove or lid-cheek junction is located inferior and parallel to the infraorbital rim. It stretches laterally from the tear trough as an indentation becoming more apparent with facial aging. The youthful lid-cheek junction has a high convex contour that extends up to the lower lid at the infratarsal crease and overlies the lower lid septum orbitale, the orbital rim, and part of the upper cheek. The nasolabial fold is a cutaneous skin crease. This fold varies considerably from person to person. Three types of fold may be distinguished: convex, concave, and straight. Lip elevator muscles (within SMAS layer) have been reported to be directly responsible for the shape and depth of the fold. In the absence of functioning lip elevators, as in facial palsy, the nasolabial fold disappears. Midfacial muscle variability exists at the cellular and anatomic level. An anatomic study by Pessa found that the risorius and zygomaticus minor muscles are present in a small minority of individuals. However, the levator alae nasi, levator labii superioris, and zygomaticus major were uniformly present.

Skeleton of Midcheek

The craniofacial skeleton continues to grow with age. Continued remodeling of the facial skeleton may be summarized by clockwise rotation of the maxilla relative to

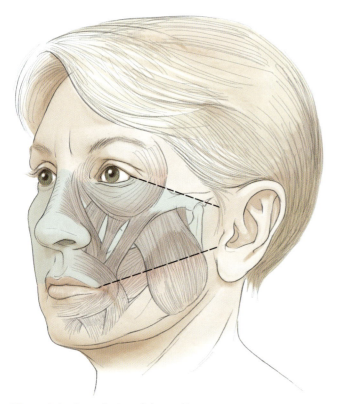

Figure 4-1   Boundaries of the midface.

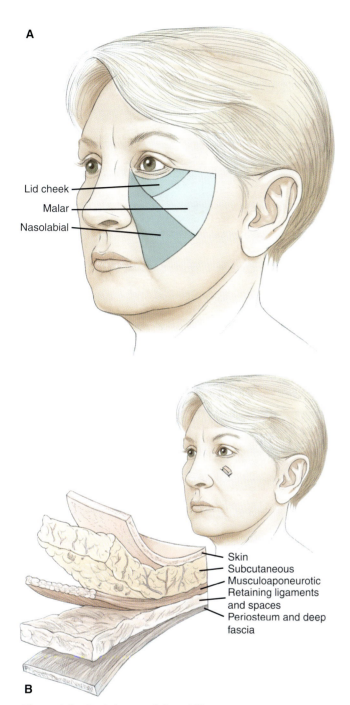

A

Lid cheek

Malar

Nasolabial

Skin
Subcutaneous
Musculoaponeurotic
Retaining ligaments
and spaces
Periosteum and deep
fascia

B

Figure 4-2   Basic layers of the midface.

portion of the zygoma projects forward as a platform over the upper and outer recess of the oral cavity. This platform serves as an attachment for the zygomatic muscles and ligaments. The orbital rim is the supporting structure for the soft tissues of the midface. Age-related skeletal remodeling directs the vector of change of the soft tissues inferior and posterior, mimicking the changes of the inferior orbital rim. The lower eyelid may become loose as a result of normal skeletal aging whereby the surface area available to support the lower lid diminishes.

Ligaments of the Midface

Preservation of taut retaining ligaments is essential to preventing inferior repositioning of soft tissues, a key feature of midface aging. The zygomatic ligament, orbital retaining ligament (ORL), and lateral orbital thickening (LOT) are known collectively as the retaining ligaments of the midface. The zygomatic ligament consists of a fibrous septa found at the medial border of the zygomaticus minor muscle. This ligament extends laterally to a junction between the arch and body of the zygoma. The zygomatic ligaments fix the malar fat pad and the skin of the cheek to the underlying zygomatic eminence (body). The ORL varies in length from 1 to 1.6 cm, and, ultimately, it merges laterally with LOT. The LOT is a triangular condensation of the SMAS in continuity with the temporoparietal fascia and orbicularis muscle fascia. The role of the ORL in the development of a tear trough and descent of the lid-cheek junction remains controversial. In the past, the retaining ligaments were thought to be

the cranial base. (Fig. 4-3) The anterior surface of the midcheek skeleton provides the base for the attachment of the muscles of the lower lid and the upper lip, as well as the related ligaments that support the midcheek soft tissue. The midcheek skeleton is formed by the zygoma, anterior surface of the maxilla, and the lacrimal bone. The body of the zygoma contributes to the orbit laterally, while its maxillary process forms part of the medial orbital rim along with the lacrimal bone. The maxillary

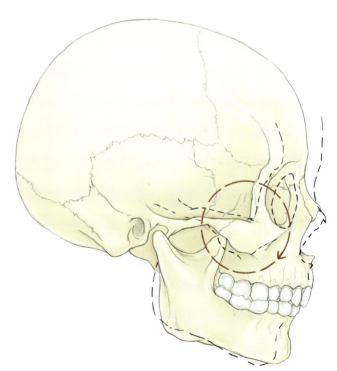

Figure 4-3   Remodelling of the facial skeleton.

solely responsible for midface aging. However, Lambros and Pessa have highlighted the roles of subdermal fat loss and skeletal remolding as other causative factors. Lambros used photographs of the same patient over time to demonstrate that the lid-cheek junction does not actually descend with age. Clinical studies by Pessa suggest a more versatile model of midface aging by incorporating skeletal remolding.

PEARLS

A combination of nonlinear changes of midface occur involving ligamentous laxity, gravity, muscle weakness, and ptosis in conjunction with age-related rotation of the maxilla.

SUGGESTED READING

Accioli de Vasconcellos JJ, Britto JA, Henin D, et al. The fascial planes of the temple and face. In: Eisenmann-Klein M, Neuhan-Lorenz C, eds. *Innovations in Plastic and Aesthetic Surgery*. New York, NY: Springer-Verlag; 2008:146-148.

Flowers RS. Tear trough implants for correction of tear trough deformity. *Clin Plast Surg*. 1993;20(2):403-415.

Gamboa GM, de la Torre JI, Vasconez LO. Surgical anatomy of the midface as applied to facial rejuvenation. *Ann Plast Surg*. 2004;52(3):240-245.

Hamra ST. Arcus marginalis release and orbital fat preservation in midface rejuvenation. *Plast Reconstr Surg*. 1995;96(2):354-362.

Lambros V. Observations on periorbital and midface aging. *Plast Reconst Surg*. 2007;120:1367-1376.

Mendelson BC, Jacobson SR. Surgical anatomy of the midcheek: facial layers, spaces and the midcheek segments. *Clin Plast Surg*. 2008;35(3):395-404, discussion 393.

Mendelson BC, Muzaffar AR, Adams WP Jr. Surgical anatomy of the midcheek and malar mounds. *Plast Reconstr Surg*. 2002;110(3):885-896.

Pessa JE. An algorithm of facial aging: verification of Lambros's theory by three-dimensional stereolithography, with reference to the pathogenesis of midfacial aging, scleral show, and the lateral suborbital trough deformity. *Plast Reconstr Surg*. 2000;106(2):479-488.

Pessa JE, Zadoo VP, Adrian EK, Yuan CH, Aydelotte J, Garza JR. Variability of the midfacial muscles: analysis of 50 hemifacial cadaver dissections. *Plast Reconst Surg*. 1998;102(6):1888-1893.

Rubin LR, Mishriki Y, Lee G. Anatomy of the nasolabial fold: the keystone of the smiling mechanism. *Plast Reconstr Surg*. 1989;83(1):1-10.

Chapter 5. Eyebrow Anatomy

Amr N. Rabie, MD; Samuel J. Lin, MD, FACS

GENERAL CONSIDERATIONS

The proper position and design of the eyebrow is relative and depends on a number of factors, including racial, cultural, and other factors. Measurements, marks, and parameters should only be used as a guide when planning for surgery, as they are not absolutely correct for every individual's facial features. Nevertheless, it is widely regarded that the female brow is located above the superior orbital rim, is arched with its peak above the lateral limbus, and thins laterally, whereas the male brow is heavier in hair density, more inferiorly placed, and is more horizontal. With age, the brow will start to move below the rim, which will result in redundancy and folding of the skin of the upper eyelid, as well as narrowing of the space between the eyebrow hairs and the lashes, which leads to a frowning appearance. The skin of the eyebrow is hair-bearing, thick, and rich in sweat and sebaceous glands. The eyebrow fat pad lies between the periosteum and deep fascia, and enhances motility of the eyebrow. The fat pad extends inferiorly to the periorbital septal plane; through this fat pad, dense attachments secure the brow to the supraorbital ridge. It is very important during blepharoplasty procedures that the eyebrow fat pad be distinguished from the postseptal fat and the preaponeurotic fat. During rejuvenation procedures where the brow fat pad is manipulated, the surgeon must be careful not to give the female patient a masculine appearance, or, more commonly, give the male patient a feminine appearance. The eyebrow functions as an essential protective component for the eye; it keeps dust and sweat away from the eye and also acts as a stationary defense against eye injury through its overhang. The eyebrow also serves to portray facial mood and expression; a flat eyebrow indicates fatigue, elevation suggests surprise or sadness, a downward slant expresses anger, and a proper arch denotes happiness and attractiveness.

MUSCLES OF EYEBROW ANIMATION

The frontalis muscle is responsible for elevation of the eyebrow, it is the primary elevator of the eyebrow; hence, care should be taken to avoid injury during a brow lift procedure. It is a paired muscle that is a continuation of the occipitalis muscle and the galea aponeurotica. Its vertical fibers are inserted into the supraorbital dermis and its insertion does not go beyond the fusion line. The corrugator supercilii muscle is a paired muscle that arises from the periosteum of the superior orbital rim and is inserted via oblique fibers into the dermis of the medial eyebrow skin, and by way of lateral interdigitations into the medial portion of the orbicularis oculi muscle. Contraction of the corrugators will result in medial and inferior displacement of the eyebrow, as well as vertical oblique lines of the glabella.

The procerus muscle is the primary eyebrow depressor; contraction of the procerus causes medial and inferior displacement of the medial eyebrow along with a transverse line at the nasal radix. Its origin is the nasal bones and upper lateral cartilages and is inserted through vertical fibers into the dermis of the glabella along the medial border of the frontalis. In cases of brow ptosis, the frontalis muscle activates and attempts to compensate in an attempt to elevate the descended eyebrows, which may result in muscle hypertrophy, causing forehead furrows. As the patient ages, brow ptosis occurs as a consequence of absence of a fibrous connective tissue bond that exists between the subgaleal periosteum and the deep galea in the upper two-thirds of the forehead, which prevents soft-tissue descent. Lateral eyebrow ptosis can also be attributed to descent of the unsupported temporal tissue mass over the temporalis fascia as a result of gravity. It is often characterized by migration of the brow skin into the superior lid region creating skin excess, malposition of the brow, lateral hooding, and loss of the normal supratarsal definition. It is vital that ptosis or laxity of the eyebrows be detected before an upper-lid blepharoplasty is performed, as failure to correct laxity will inevitably impair the outcome of the blepharoplasty. Eyebrow elevation is typically different on each side of the face and at each point along the brow. During brow elevation, it is important that the frontalis muscle not be weakened so as to maintain an elevated brow position. Weakening of the medial portion of the corrugators causes medial brow elevation and correction of the glabellar frown lines, while the lateral portion produces some lateral brow elevation and hence should be preserved. When the procerus is weakened, medial brow elevation is achieved because it is the primary depressor. In a majority of cases, to restore good-looking eyebrow configuration, elevation is required more laterally than medially. In the end, the surgeon must be able to distinguish between eyebrow and eyelid abnormalities; patients may have subbrow fat pad thickening and/or lateral brow ptosis, which may be associated with upper-lid dermatochalasis and herniated fat, which blepharoplasty alone cannot repair. To improve aesthetic results, patients who have brow ptosis may undergo browpexy or suspension at the time of blepharoplasty.

NERVES (MOTOR AND SENSORY) AND VESSELS

Before performing any procedures that involve debulking or positioning of the eyebrow, it is vital that the surgeon be oriented with the course of the frontal branch of the facial nerve, as well as of the supratrochlear and supraorbital neurovascular bundles. Muscles of the eyebrow are supplied by the facial nerve; the frontal branch of the facial nerve provides motor innervations to the frontalis and corrugator muscles, while the buccal branch of the facial nerve innervates the procerus. The frontal branch of the facial nerve arises from the main facial nerve trunk; it lies within the superficial temporal fascia as it crosses the zygomatic arch where it is most likely to be injured. It then perforates the temporoparietal fascia to travel below that level. Finally, it runs along a line that extends from 1 cm below the tragus to a point 1.5 cm above the eyebrow to enter the undersurface of the frontalis muscle. Injury to the facial nerve will result in paralysis of the frontalis muscle. The supratrochlear and supraorbital nerves provide sensory innervations to the forehead region including the eyebrows. They arise midway between the apex and base of the orbit from the frontal nerve, which is the largest branch of the ophthalmic nerve. The smaller of the two, the supratrochlear nerve, passes beneath the frontalis and corrugator muscles while providing branches that pierce these muscles. It sends filaments to the conjunctiva and skin of the upper eyelid, and supplies the skin of the lower part of the forehead close to the midline. The supraorbital nerve is found one finger breadth from the lateral side of the nose or at the midpupillary line; it passes to the forehead, where it divides into medial and lateral terminal branches. The medial branch perforates the frontalis muscle, while the lateral branch perforates the galea aponeurotica. The supraorbital nerve supplies the integument of the scalp up to the lambdoid suture. The supraorbital artery and vein pass through the supraorbital foramen or notch to emerge from the orbit; they penetrate the frontalis muscle and appear superficial to the muscle in the subcutaneous fat. The supraorbital vessels supply the forehead. The supratrochlear vessels perforate the corrugator muscles to reach the subcutaneous fat; they branch widely to supply the forehead and anterior scalp. The location of the supraorbital and supratrochlear neurovascular bundles are found 22 and 11 mm, respectively, from the midline of the nasofrontal junction. It is possible to palpate their boney notches or foramen to determine their course, which is especially important for avoiding injury to these neurovascular bundles in any of the procedures used for brow suspension. The development of rhytids has a profound effect on periorbital aesthetics; they result from prolonged hyperactivity of the periorbital and forehead musculature. During brow lift procedures, resection or transection of the offending muscles can prevent dynamic accentuation of rhytids from muscle activity and improve the general appearance. An alternative is the use of chemodenervation (botulinum toxin); however, chemodenervation does not provide a permanent solution, and the patient will require several sittings to maintain results.

FASCIA AND ATTACHMENTS

The superficial temporal fascia which contains the facial nerve is an extension of the superficial musculoaponeurotic system (SMAS), which consists of loose areolar tissue that separates it from the deep temporal fascia. The superficial temporal fascia is continuous with the galea. The deep temporal fascia is made up of a superficial layer and deep layer; it is marked by division of its periosteal reflection along the superior temporal line, which is connected to the temporal region of the subperiosteal and subaponeurotic spaces, this zone of transition lies along the anterior crest of the temporal bone. The deep temporal fascia is continuous with the periosteum of the skull. The attachment of these fascial planes to the brow tissue and their union to the skull form the fusion line and orbital ligament. The orbital ligament can limit movement of the superficial temporal fascia and binds the lateral eyebrow to the orbital rim.

AESTHETIC CONSIDERATIONS

There is a mathematical basis for eyebrow beauty where certain measurements can be made and used to help achieve the surgical goals. A useful system to use, which defines proportions considered to be beautiful, is the Divine Proportion. This is also known as the Golden Proportion, Golden Ratio, or the Golden Cut. The Golden Proportion states that when the relationship between 2 objects is 1:1.618, the appearance will be attractive and pleasing. For an attractive feminine eyebrow (Fig. 5-1), the vertical distance between the lower and upper eyelids (the eye aperture) in forward gaze is related to the distance between the arch of the eyebrows and the upper eyelid by the Golden Ratio (1:1.618). However, for an attractive masculine eye brow (Fig. 5-2), the relation is inversed (1.618:1). As these parameters vary from patient to patient, so will the height of the attractively positioned eyebrow. Moreover, the Golden Proportion defines the position of the peak of the attractive eyebrow (Fig. 5-3); the peak divides the eyebrow by the Golden Proportions

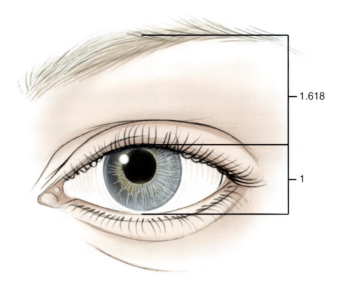

Figure 5-1   The Golden Proportions for an attractive female's eyebrow. The aperture of the eye in forward gaze to the distance between the arch of the eyebrows and the upper eyelid is 1:1.618.

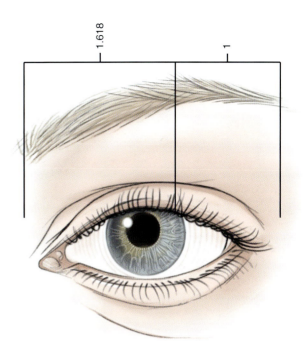

Figure 5-3   The Golden Proportions define the position of the peak of the attractive eyebrow.

(the ratio of the lateral portion to the medial portion is 1:1.618). Despite the fact that these measurements assist in establishing realistic surgical results, experience, perception, and the natural artistic intuitiveness of the plastic surgeon becomes more important in achieving a better outcome. For these surgeons, measuring comes second to "seeing."

SUGGESTED READING

Camirand A. Periorbital rejuvenation. In: Peled IJ, Manders EK, eds. *Esthetic Surgery of the Face*. London, UK: Taylor & Francis; 2004:43-50.

Janis JE, Potter JK, Rohrich RJ. Brow lift techniques. In: Fagien S, ed. *Putterman's Cosmetic Oculoplastic Surgery*. 4th ed. Philadelphia, PA: Saunders Elsevier; 2008:67-77.

Larrabee WF Jr, Makielski KH. Forehead and brow. In: Larrabee WF Jr, Makielski KH, eds. *Surgical Anatomy of the Face*. New York, NY: Raven; 1993:123-128.

LaTrenta GS. The aging face. In: LaTrenta GS, ed. *Atlas of Aesthetic Face & Neck Surgery*. Philadelphia, PA: Saunders Elsevier; 2004:62-63.

Marten TJ. Hairline lowering during foreheadplasty. *Plast Reconstr Surg*. 1999;103(1):224-236.

McCord CD Jr. Endoscopic-assisted eyebrow surgery. In: Chen WPD, Khan JA, McCord CD Jr, eds. *Color Atlas of Cosmetic Oculofacial Surgery*. Philadelphia, PA: Butterworth-Heinemann; 2004:25-31.

Ricketts RM. Divine proportion in facial esthetics. *Clin Plast Surg*. 1982;9(4):401-422.

Spinelli HM. The eyebrow and lacrimal gland. In: Spinelli HM, ed. *Atlas of Aesthetic Eyelid & Periocular Surgery*. Philadelphia, PA: Saunder Elsevier; 2004:136-145.

Tolleth H. Concepts for the plastic surgeon from art and sculpture. *Clin Plast Surg*. 1987;14(4):585-598.

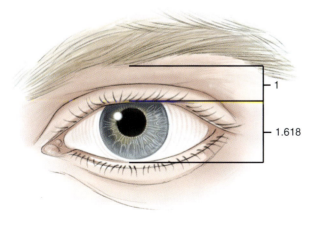

Figure 5-2   For an attractive male eyebrow, the Golden Proportions are inversed. The aperture of the eye in forward gaze to the distance between the arch of the eyebrows and the upper eyelid is 1.1618:1.

Chapter 6. SMAS/Facial Retaining Ligaments

Brian M. Parrett, MD; Samuel J. Lin, MD, FACS

A complete knowledge of facial anatomy and its changes with aging is essential to successfully perform rhytidectomy. The face can be divided into 5 anatomical concentric layers; these layers are, starting with the outermost layer: skin, subcutaneous fat, the superficial musculoaponeurotic system (SMAS)/muscle layer, a thin and transparent layer of fascia, and the facial nerve branches (Fig. 6-1). The third layer, or SMAS layer, is the most critical layer in regards to facelift anatomy.

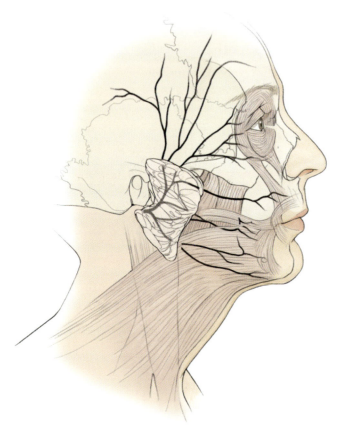

Figure 6-1 The facial nerve begins deep beneath the parotid gland and then, medial to the parotid gland, becomes more superficial, just deep to the SMAS, parotidomasseteric fascia, and the platysma muscle.

SUPERFICIAL MUSCULOAPONEUROTIC SYSTEM (SMAS)

The SMAS is a discrete fascial layer that separates the overlying subcutaneous fat from the underlying parotidomasseteric fascia and the facial nerve. Its thickness varies from one region of the face to another. It is thicker over the parotid and thins over the masseter muscle, buccal fat pad, and malar region. It becomes thin and attenuated medially in the cheek. The SMAS can be fibrous, muscular, or fatty, depending on the location within the face. It is continuous with the platysma muscle in the neck, the frontalis muscle in the forehead, and the superficial temporal fascia in the temporal region. The muscles of facial expression are essentially part of the SMAS layer (frontalis, orbicularis oculi, zygomaticus major and minor, and platysma muscle) and function as a single unit in producing movement of the facial skin.

The parotidomasseteric fascia lies under the SMAS layer and over the facial nerve branches. This is analogous to the superficial cervical fascia in the neck and the subgaleal fascia in the temporal region. These layers are very thin and the facial nerve branches lie directly beneath them.

The facial nerve branches innervate the facial muscles on their deep surfaces with 3 exceptions: the buccinator, mentalis, and levator anguli oris muscles are innervated via their superficial surfaces. Consequently, dissection in the subcutaneous plane, superficial to the SMAS/muscle layer, is safely performed. Dissection deep to the SMAS requires special care and experience.

For a facelift to be effective, manipulation of the SMAS layer is often required. In general, the SMAS layer can either be excised and reapproximated, or it can be plicated. The SMAS over the parotid gland is relatively immobile compared to the SMAS beyond the gland. In a SMASectomy procedure, a strip of SMAS is excised and the mobile SMAS is sutured to the immobile SMAS. SMAS plication can be performed, especially in thinner patients, without excising any SMAS. SMAS dissections vary in extent and are discussed in later chapters.

FACIAL RETAINING LIGAMENTS

The facial retaining ligaments are areas where the anatomic layers become condensed, less mobile, and anchored from deep, fixed facial structures to the overlying dermis (Fig. 6-2). The retaining ligaments of the face were first described by McGregor with the zygomatic cutaneous ligament (McGregor's patch), and Furnas and Stuzin have since reported their clinical experience and anatomic studies. Stuzin et al described 2 types of retaining ligaments. First, there are osteocutaneous ligaments, which are fibrous bands that run from periosteum to dermis; this is exemplified by the zygomatic and mandibular ligaments. A second system of supporting ligaments is formed by coalescence between the superficial and deep facial fascia in specific regions (parotidocutaneous and masseteric cutaneous ligaments) that also have fibrous septa extending to the dermis.

The retaining ligaments support facial soft tissue in normal anatomic position, resisting gravitational change. As people age, the support from the ligament system becomes attenuated, leading to descent of facial tissue adjacent to these regions. This results in the stigmata of the aging face, such as jowling and prominent nasolabial folds. The retaining ligaments are important in facelift surgery as they can cause anatomic disorientation with dissection of false planes into the dermis; they are useful anatomic landmarks during facial dissections, and their tethering effects must be released for maximal upward movement and redraping of facial skin.

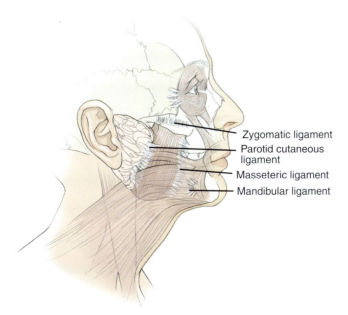

Figure 6-2 The locations of the facial retaining ligaments are shown. Attenuation and the tethering forces of these ligaments lead to the stigmata of facial aging and thus should be corrected during rhytidectomy procedures.

ZYGOMATIC CUTANEOUS LIGAMENT

The zygomatic ligament is located in the cheek, anterior and superior to the parotid gland. The zygomatic ligaments originate from the periosteum of the malar region as a series of fibrous septa that begin laterally, where the zygomatic arch joins the body of the zygoma, with similar fibers overlying the malar eminence. These fibers insert into malar skin and fix the malar pad to the underlying zygomatic eminence. A typical grouping is a bundle of white, firm fibers located 4.5 cm in front of the tragus and 5 to 9 cm posterior to the zygomaticus minor muscle. A second bundle may be found anterior to the first bundle. The length of the zygomatic ligament is 1.6 to 3.4 cm with a width of 2.7 to 3.4 mm (Fig. 6-2). A branch of the zygomatic branch of the facial nerve and a branch of the transverse facial artery travel in the midportion of the ligament.

The zygomatic ligaments suspend malar soft tissue over the zygomatic eminence and loss of zygomatic ligament support allows for inferior descent of the malar pad, causing nasolabial fold prominence. To diminish prominent nasolabial folds, attention should be directed at repositioning the malar soft tissue to its previous position.

MANDIBULAR LIGAMENT

Furnas reported that the mandibular ligaments originate from bone along a line approximately 1 cm above the mandibular border that extended along the anterior third of the mandibular body, appearing as a linear series of parallel fibers. A second tier of fibers is often aligned 2 to 3 mm above and parallel to the first tier, and interdigitates among the platysma muscle fibers. The ligament has a length of 2.2 to 3.2 cm and a width of 2.5 to 3.4 mm. During a facelift, the mandibular ligament is identified in the parasymphyseal region and extends from the bone to the overlying skin, fixing the parasymphysial dermis to the underlying mandible. The posterior limit of the mandibular ligament is palpable as a firm, sharp border that forms the anterior border of the jowl (Fig. 6-2).

The mandibular ligament has a tethering effect on the anterior jowl area. This is surgically important, because without release of the mandibular ligament, there is an inability to adequately lift the skin in a vertical direction.

PREAURICULAR PAROTID CUTANEOUS LIGAMENT

The posterior border of the platysma recedes into a fascial condensation that attaches to the overlying skin, resulting in a firm adherence between the platysma/inferior parotid fascia and dermis of the inferior auricular regions. Recent anatomical studies localize the preauricular cutaneous ligament in the anteroinferior auricular region, vertical preauricularly, with a length of approximately 2.6 to 3 cm and a width of 2.2 to 2.5 mm (Fig. 6-2). These attachments must be completely divided during a facelift to obtain adequate flap mobility. Cutaneous branches of the great auricular nerve are often found within this ligament.

MASSETERIC CUTANEOUS LIGAMENT

The masseteric cutaneous ligament is a fibrous structure extending between the parotidomasseteric fascia and skin of the middle and anterior cheek, extending along the entire anterior border of the masseter. This is essentially analogous to the platysma cutaneous ligament described by Furnas. The direction of the ligament is vertical and oblique. The zygomatic branch of the facial nerve is in close proximity to the ligament. The length of the ligament is 1.8 to 2.7 cm and the width is 1.2 to 1.8 mm in men; in women, the length is 1.6 to 2.4 cm and the width is 1.1 to 1.5 mm.

The masseteric cutaneous fibers are important as they support the soft tissue of the cheek superiorly above the mandibular border. A loss of masseteric ligament support allows for the inferior descent of facial fat below the mandibular border, leading to the formation of jowling. Repositioning of the descended fat pads above the mandibular border culminates in a young face and restores cheek support.

SUGGESTED READING

Furnas DW. The retaining ligaments of the cheek. *Plast Reconstr Surg*. 1989;83(1):11-16.

Ozdemir R, Kilinç H, Unlü RE, et al. Anatomicohistologic study of the retaining ligaments of the face and use in face lift: retaining ligament correction and SMAS plication. *Plast Reconstr Surg*. 2002;110(4):1134-1147.

Stuzin JM, Baker TJ, Gordon HL. The relationship of the superficial and deep facial fascias: relevance to rhytidectomy and aging. *Plast Reconstr Surg*. 1992;89(3):441-449.

Chapter 7. Facial Nerve Danger Zones

Nathaniel L. Holzman, MD; Sean T. Doherty, MD; Brooke R. Seckel, MD, FACS

The most feared complication of facelift surgery is catastrophic injury to one of the major facial nerve branches. Injury can result in permanent facial deformity, numbness, dysethesia, and pain. Even a limited neurologic recovery can leave the patient with an undesirable aesthetic outcome, as well as discomfort. A thorough understanding of the nerve anatomy is paramount to avoiding injury. This chapter discusses the facial anatomic zones in which the major facial nerve branches are most susceptible to injury as described by Seckel (Fig. 7-1). Each of the seven sections highlights nerve origins, anatomic course, consequence of injury, and techniques for safe surgical dissection.

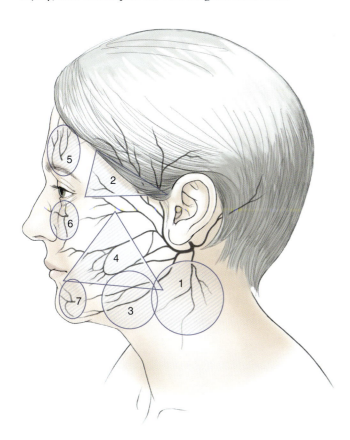

Figure 7-1 Side view highlighting the seven Facial Danger Zones.

ZONE 1

Facial danger zone 1 describes the region where the great auricular nerve is most susceptible to injury. With the patient's head turned to the opposite side, a vertical line can be drawn, 6.5 cm in length, from the caudal edge of the external auditory canal. Centered around this point, a 3-cm radius circle is drawn. In this defined region, approximately 9 cm below the caudal edge of the external auditory canal, the great auricular nerve emerges at the posterior border of the sternocleidomastoid muscle, and becomes highly susceptible to injury, as it then runs superficial to the muscle belly. Injury to this nerve results in numbness or painful dysesthesia to the lower two-thirds of the ear, as well as the adjacent neck and cheek.

For safe dissection, after completing the postauricular incision, maintain a thin dissection plane just deep to the subcutaneuous fat, but superficial to the deep cervical fascia and sternocleidomastoid muscle. To identify the proper plane, retract the ear lobule forward and locate the two postauricular branches of the great auricular nerve that lie at the superior border of the dissection. Another tool for identifying the great auricular nerve is to visualize the external jugular vein throughout the dissection. Note the great auricular nerve will lie 0.5 to 1 cm posterior to this vessel. When plicating the platysma-superficial musculoaponeurotic system (SMAS) layer, careful attention must be paid to avoid compression of the nerve. One way of avoiding a painful compressive neuropathy is to utilize the Hamra technique of tightening the platysma-SMAS layer via excision and repair of platysma bands anterior to the nerve.

ZONE 2

Danger zone 2 encompasses a triangular area through which the temporal branch of the facial nerve courses from its emergence beneath the parotid gland to the frontalis muscle. Laterally, a line is drawn from a point 0.5 cm inferior to the tragus to a point 2 cm superior to the lateral eyebrow. Inferiorly, a line is drawn along the zygoma to the lateral orbital rim, and medially, a third line connects the point 2 cm above the lateral eyebrow to the lateral orbital rim. It is here that the temporal branch of the facial nerve is most susceptible to injury when lying just below the temporoparietal fascia-SMAS layer. Nerve injury results in ipsilateral frontalis paralysis causing unilateral brow ptosis and asymmetric forehead animation.

To avoid injuring the temporal branch of the facial nerve, one must maintain the dissection within Marino's mesotemporalis plane. The superior plane is developed by dissecting in the subtemporoparietal fascia-SMAS layer from the scalp to the zygoma. Inferiorly, the plane is maintained subcutaneously in the supra-SMAS layer from the mandibular ramus to the zygoma. Oftentimes, the nerve can be seen coursing inferiorly to the frontal branch of the superficial temporal artery.

ZONE 3

The marginal mandibular branch of the facial nerve is most susceptible to injury in zone 3. In a region where the SMAS layer thins, the nerve courses anteriorly to the depressor anguli oris muscle and is vulnerable to injury. This zone, with a 2-cm radius, is centered around a point on the mandibular body that lies 2 cm posterior to the oral commisure. At this site of a thin SMAS layer, the nerve also courses anterior to the facial artery and vein. The astute surgeon must be cognizant of injury to these vessels, as well. Injury to the marginal mandibular branch of the facial nerve results in denervation of the depressor anguli oris muscle. At rest, this appears as a unilateral pout, and asymmetry is further exacerbated when the patient smiles or grimaces.

Visualization is key to avoiding nerve injury in this region. This is optimized with adequate lighting, appropriate retraction, and meticulous hemostasis. If bleeding develops from facial artery or vein branches, attempts to avoid cautery should be exhausted. If electrocautery is deemed necessary, one should only utilize bipolar cautery.

ZONE 4

Coursing through facial danger zone 4 are the zygomatic and buccal branches of the facial nerve. This zone lies in a plane deep to the platysma-SMAS layer and parotid fascia, and superficial to the masseter muscle and Bichat's fat pad (Fig. 7-2). It is bordered posteriorly by the parotid gland, anteriorly by the zygomaticus major muscle, and inferiorly by the mandibular body. Injury to these nerves results in the paralysis of the lip levator muscle groups, including the zygomaticus major and minor muscles. Clinically, there is a considerable facial asymmetry that is demonstrated by unilateral sag of the upper lip and oral commisure on the affected side. There are multiple interconnections between these 2 nerves that mask their injuries. For example, the buccal branch is the most common

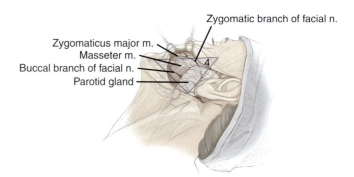

Figure 7-2 Deep view of Facial Danger Zone 4 showing location of the Buccal branches of the Facial Nerve.

injured nerve during facelift procedures, but often goes undiagnosed. Although these overlapping innervations protect against permanent nerve damage, persistent involuntary twitching and paralysis does happen.

Injuries generally occur during sub-SMAS or composite rhytidectomy. If performing a more invasive facelift procedure, the vertical spreading technique can be employed to minimize the risk of nerve injury. This involves rotating the scissors in a gentle vertical spreading motion when at the anterior border of the parotid gland. This enables the dissection of the SMAS off the zygomatic and buccal branches of the facial nerve. Surgical experience is a notable factor in avoiding injury during this dissection.

ZONE 5

After emerging from the bony foramina, the supraorbital and supratrochlear nerves are most susceptible to injury in facial danger zone 5. This zone incorporates a circle, with a 1.5-cm radius, centered on the supraorbital foramen. The supratrochlear nerve is rather susceptible to injury as it does not course deep to the corrugator muscle, like the supraorbital nerve, but rather courses through it. Injury to these nerves can result in numbness or painful dysesthesia of the ipsilateral upper eyelid, nasal dorsum, medial forehead, and scalp.

Typically, injuries to these nerves occur during a coronal brow lift. When approaching the supraorbital rim during the dissection, the surgeon must be acutely aware of the neurovascular pedicle that lies at the junction between the lateral third and middle third of the flap. Also, if excision of a portion of the frontalis muscle is planned, an island of tissue surrounding the neurovascular pedicle should be left intact.

ZONE 6

The infraorbital nerve, a branch of the second division of the trigeminal nerve, lies within facial danger zone 6. A vertical line, drawn from the supraorbital foramen through the medial limbus and the infraorbital and mental

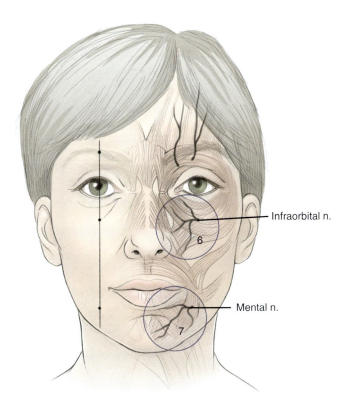

Infraorbital n.

6

Mental n.

7

Figure 7-3   Frontal view Sensory Facial Danger Zones 6 and 7 showing course of Infraorbital (Zone 6) and Mental (Zone 7) Nerves.

foramina to the second mandibular premolar allows for easy identification of facial danger zones 6 and 7 (Fig. 7-3). Zone 6 is a circle, with a 1.5-cm radius, centered on the infraorbital foramen. Numbness to the ipsilateral eyelid, cheek, lateral nose, and upper lip can result from nerve injury. Injury is unlikely during the typical subcutaneous or sub-SMAS facelift, but can occur during an extended subperiosteal facelift or midface advancement surgery.

ZONE 7

The mental nerve lies in facial danger zone 7. The emergence of this sensory branch of the third division of the trigeminal nerve can be located in a circle, with 1.5-cm radius, centered at a point on the midmandibular body. This point is located on the vertical line, described in the previous section, below the second mandibular premolar. Injury results in numbness of both the mucosal and cutaneous surfaces of the lower lip and chin. This can lead to

difficulty with speech and handling of food boluses, as well as the inability to avoid trauma of the lower lip. To avoid injury, most commonly during a chin implantation procedure, dissection should be done medial to the foramen.

CONCLUSION

Although permanent nerve injury occurring during facelift surgery is rare, it does occur in 0.8% to 1% of cases. The surgeon's keen understanding of the peripheral nerve anatomy can help to avoid such an injury. This chapter simply defines the critical regions where nerves are most susceptible to injury. To identify injuries, it is imperative for all surgeons, novice and experienced, to document facial nerve function after the patient awakes from facelift surgery.

SUGGESTED READING

Baker DC, Conley J. Avoiding facial nerve injuries in rhytidectomy: anatomical variations and pitfalls. *Plast Reconstr Surg*. 1979;64:781.

Barton FE. The aging face: rhytidectomy adjunctive procedures. *Selected Readings Plast Surg*. 1991;6:19.

Bernstein L, Nelson RH. Surgical anatomy of the extraparotid distribution of the facial nerve. *Arch Otolaryngol*. 1984; 110:177.

Hamra ST. *Composite Rhytidectomy*. St. Louis, MO: Quality Medical Publishing, 1993.

Hamra ST. The deep-plane rhytidectomy. *Plast Reconstr Surg*. 1990;86:53.

Hamra ST. The zygorbicular dissection in composite rhytidectomy: an ideal midface plane. *Plast Reconstr Surg*. 1998; 102:1658.

Larrabee WF, Makielski KH. *Surgical Anatomy of the Face*. New York, NY: Raven Press, 1993.

Liebman EP, Webster RC, Gaul JR, Griffin T. The marginal mandibular nerve in rhytidectomy and liposuction surgery. *Arch Otolaryngol Head Neck Surg*. 1988;114:179.

Marino H. The forehead lift: some hints to secure better results. *Aesthetic Plast Surg*. 1977;1:251.

McKinney P, Katrana DJ. Prevention of injury to the great auricular nerve during rhytidectomy. *Plast Reconstr Surg*. 1980;66:675.

Nelson DW, Gingrass RP. Anatomy of the mandibular branches of the facial nerve. *Plast Reconstr Surg*. 1979;64:479.

Pitanguy I, Ramos AS. The frontal branch of the facial nerve: the importance of its variations in face lifting. *Plast Reconstr Surg*. 1966;38:352.

Seckel BR. *Facial danger zones: avoiding nerve injury in facial plastic surgery*. St. Louis, MO: Quality Medical, 1994.

Chapter 8. Preoperative Evaluation in Aesthetic Head and Neck Surgery

Kenneth B. Hughes, MD; Samuel J. Lin, MD, FACS

ANATOMIC NORMS

A general recognition of facial norms and proportions has great relevance for the plastic surgeon during the preoperative assessment of aesthetic surgery. The face can be divided into roughly equal thirds consisting of the trichion to nasal root, the nasal root to nasal base, and the nasal base to inferior mandibular midline (gnathion).

The forehead comprises the area from the trichion to highest point of the brow. The average height is 7 cm in men and 6 cm in women. An aesthetic eyebrow has its apogee at the lateral limbus with the lateral extent positioned 3 mm superior to the medial. In women, the eyebrow rests up to 3 mm above the supraorbital rim. Conversely, in males, the eyebrow should lie at the level of the rim. The intercanthal distance should be roughly 34 mm in men and 32 mm in women. The youthful eye should exhibit a positive vector, with the lateral canthus 2 mm above the medial. Scleral show should not be present superiorly or inferiorly.

The nose is composed of 3 sections: root (radix), dorsum, and soft nose. The nose can be divided further into 9 total subunits: nasal dorsum, tip, columella, paired ala, paired sidewalls, and paired soft triangles. The soft nose is comprised of the nasal tip, columella, and ala. The width of the ala should roughly equal the intercanthal distance. The angle between columella and upper lip (nasolabial angle) is 100 degrees in men and 105 in women.

The upper incisor shown at rest should be approximately 2 mm. On lateral view of the face, the chin and upper lip should have similar projection.

It is important to realize that these proportions can vary subtly or dramatically based upon ethnicity. These norms have largely been developed based upon Caucasian models. Every effort should be made to preserve ethnic identity for any aesthetic facial surgery contemplated.

PHYSICAL EXAMINATION

All facial assessment should include a thorough examination of the patient's skin. The surgeon should note signs of poor skin elasticity, actinic damage, and deep facial wrinkles, as these factors can have dramatic implications upon any excisional or redraping procedure. Examinations of cranial nerves V and VII, in particular, should be performed and asymmetries noted. The relative amount of facial fat, as well as overall facial shape (eg, square or conical) should be documented. One should note the height of the trichion, the level of brow descent, and the amount of dermatochalasis. The surgeon should characterize the tear trough, the degree of malar fat pad descent, nasolabial fold prominence, degree of jowling, and relative laxity or banding of the platysma. A discussion of more specific anatomic considerations is addressed in specific chapters, but one should bear in mind general facial characteristics as no one feature exists in a vacuum. Operating on one aspect of the face inevitably alters perception of the remaining facial elements.

PREOPERATIVE PLANNING

The history should include a complete medical and surgical history. The family history should include inquiries about familial bleeding tendencies and problems with anesthesia. A social history should include use of tobacco (nicotine products), alcohol, and illegal drugs. Allergies (including adhesives, skin prep, and latex) and medications (including birth control pills, over the counter vitamins, and herbal preparations) should be documented. Later in this chapter, herbal medications, which may alter bleeding times, are highlighted.

The surgeon should be able to accurately determine and predict anatomic characteristics that may result in a difficult airway situation including poor cervical mobility, retrognathia, decreased cervicomental angle, and limited mandibular opening. Mallampati assessment of pharyngeal visualization is also a useful adjunct.

Patients with coronary artery disease, valvular disease, or congestive heart failure merit special consideration. A cardiologist should evaluate these patients to determine if their disease process is stable before one considers elective surgery for these patients. Patients with valvular disease should receive prophylaxis with amoxicillin or ampicillin. In penicillin-allergic patients, clindamycin or a macrolide is appropriate.

The surgeon should obtain an accurate smoking history and determine if the patient has restrictive or obstructive lung disease, as well as obstructive sleep apnea. Smoking should be discontinued for at least 4 weeks prior to and following elective surgery, and an aggressive smoking cessation program should be instituted. Serum and urine cotinine levels can be utilized to determine patient reliability.

Patients with chronic liver disease should receive liver function tests and may need a hepatology consult before considering elective surgery, as they can carry greater risk for bleeding, malnutrition, and metabolic derangements. Chronic alcohol use can alter metabolism of perioperative drugs.

Hypertension, a contributor to hematoma formation, should be meticulously controlled. The patient should be well managed on an outpatient regimen, and any blood pressure medication should be taken the day of surgery. Anxiolysis and pain control should be addressed as well.

Postoperative cough and vomiting should be controlled and may be preempted intraoperatively to prevent increased intraabdominal and intrathoracic pressures, which can lead to bleeding and hematoma formation. Propofol and a serotonin receptor antagonist such as ondansetron (Zofran) should be considered unless contraindicated. Deep extubation in the hands of an experienced anesthesiologist can be utilized to minimize pressure increases during extubation. Nasal and throat packing should be used to minimize swallowed blood. Acid-blocker prophylaxis should be considered in patients with a history of gastric esophageal reflux disease, hiatal hernia, and other diseases that may compromise gastrointestinal motility. Finally, patients should be free of ingestion of clear liquids for 2 to 3 hours and of solids for 6 to 8 hours prior to induction.

Diabetic patients should be well controlled to minimize wound-healing implications. Glucocorticoid-dependent patients should be given vitamin A in doses of 25,000 IU/day, to help reverse many of the adverse steroid effects.

Surgical weight-loss patients deserve special mention as nutritional deficiencies of vitamins A, C, and K may be present, which would impair normal wound healing. They may also have protein calorie malnutrition (serum albumin level of less than 3 g/dL may be indicative).

Vitamin supplementation and protein supplements should be instituted prior to surgery to minimize wound-healing issues.

To screen for bleeding diatheses, in addition to family history, a personal history of problematic bleeding with minor trauma (dental procedures), frequent nosebleeds, and history of blood transfusions suggest a clotting problem. Complete blood count (CBC), prothrombin time (PT), and partial thromboplastin time (PTT) tests should be ordered, and a hematology consult may be appropriate.

Aspirin and nonsteroidal antiinflammatory drugs (NSAIDs) should be discontinued at least a week prior to surgery. Patients should stop taking warfarin (Coumadin) and clopidogrel (Plavix) at least 5 days prior to surgery and may require a temporizing measure (eg, low-molecular-weight heparin [LMWH]).

Although the risk for postoperative deep venous thrombosis (DVT) and pulmonary embolism (PE) has not proven to be as high as for body-contouring procedures, perioperative prophylaxis should be considered for longer operations and patients with multiple risk factors or previous DVT/PE. Young and Watson's *The Need for Venous Thromboembolism (VTE) Prophylaxis in Plastic Surgery* provides a more detailed review and analysis.

High fever or prolonged ventilator requirements in patients or a family history thereof should raise suspicion for malignant hyperthermia and precautions should be taken if surgery is elected. With any perioral procedure, herpes prophylaxis should be considered based upon prior outbreaks. Isotretinoin use should be discontinued at least one year before considering any resurfacing procedure or operation.

Given the increasing popularity of the supplement market, the surgeon must have some familiarity with the more commonly ingested items. Echinacea may impair hepatic metabolism and should be discontinued well before surgery. Ephedra was used as an appetite suppressant that resulted in numerous deaths. The U.S. Food and Drug Administration (FDA) prohibited the sale of ephedra in 2004. Garlic, ginkgo, ginseng, and kava inhibit platelet aggregation and should be discontinued at least 7 days prior to surgery. St. John's wort should be discontinued at least 5 days prior to surgery and avoided postoperatively because of a host of drug–drug interactions. Valerian, a sedative, should be discontinued prior to surgery, but should be tapered due to a benzodiazepine-like withdrawal.

PREOPERATIVE LABORATORY TESTING

Routine labs do not need to be performed unless elements of the history and physical suggest their appropriateness. Despite this, surgeons continue to order CBC, chemistry, and PT/PTT routinely. A urine pregnancy test should be considered in all women of childbearing age. An electrocardiogram (EKG) may be ordered for the elderly and for those with a history of cardiopulmonary disease.

PATIENT SELECTION AND PREOPERATIVE COUNSELING

Many of the technical pitfalls for a particular operation are presented in their respective chapters, but patient selection and preoperative counseling are perhaps the 2 most critical elements to having satisfied patients and avoiding poor outcomes. When evaluating the aesthetic patient, the surgeon should be able to recognize a patient's motivations and expectations. Unrealistic expectations, obsession about appearance, incorrect perception of the surgery, or dismissal of criticism on the part of the patient should produce an uneasy feeling in the surgeon. These findings may merit a second or third meeting with the patient, a psychiatric evaluation, or, perhaps, an inability of the surgeon to perform the procedure.

SUGGESTED READING

Young VL, Watson ME. The need for venous thromboembolism (VTE) prophylaxis in plastic surgery. *Aesthet Surg J.* 2006;26(2):157-175.

Chapter 9. Photography in Aesthetic Head and Neck Surgery

Kenneth B. Hughes, MD

All plastic surgeons must acquire the ability to record their results as accurately and precisely as possible. Photography becomes a unique ally in this pursuit, and it is incumbent upon plastic surgeons to develop a relatively sophisticated understanding of photography and its components. Unfortunately, much of the art of photography must be self-taught.

With this is mind, this chapter represents a compendium of insights from several dozen amateur and professional photographers to help elucidate fundamental concepts in photography. The chapter also explores issues in photography singular to plastic surgery and reviews the plastic surgery literature as it relates to photography.

THE DIGITAL REVOLUTION

The advent of digital photography has rendered conventional film all but obsolete, as digital images can be manipulated, archived, and reconstituted with software to create 3-dimensional images. Digital imaging and manipulation have revolutionized preoperative planning as well as patient counseling.

The advantages of digital photography are manifold and include no film or processing costs, no need for physical storage of slides or negatives, elimination of scanning of slides, immediate viewing of image, ability to erase images instantly and reuse space, digital compression, and transmission for purposes of consultation or discussion.

DIGITAL IMAGE CAPTURE

The development of the charge-coupled device (CCD) in 1969 created an image sensor tuned to the visible spectrum of light, which was able to convert captured light to electrical charge. An image is projected onto a capacitor array, causing each capacitor to store an electric charge proportional to light intensity at that location. Ultimately, these charges are converted to binary representation stored digitally. Most cameras are CCD or CMOS (complementary metal–oxide–semiconductor), both of which are composed of silicon doped with other elements that allow light sensitivity. Red, green, and blue filter strips are placed before the sensor to enable digitization of the color components.

In common parlance, the digital image is captured across an array of pixels. Thus, the number of pixels becomes a determinant of picture resolution. However, the number of megapixels is only one factor. Pixel size relative to overall size of imaging area on the sensor is also important, but difficult to determine. Thus, technical reviews and your own observations can prove more reliable.

TYPES OF DIGITAL CAMERAS

Digital cameras can be classified as "point-and-shoot" cameras and digital single lens reflex (SLR). Digital SLRs are very much like film SLRs apart from image sensor and the liquid crystal display (LCD) screen. Point-and-shoot cameras have evolved tremendously over the last 5 years, many with manual controls that can produce very reliable, reproducible images with excellent resolution. Digital SLRs still have the advantages of greater aperture control, removable lenses, and better image quality secondary to larger pixel size. However, these SLR cameras are more expensive and require more maintenance (lens cleaning).

UNDERSTANDING THE FUNCTIONS OF THE DIGITAL CAMERA

Lens

In general, a lens in conventional film photography with a focal length from 90 to 110 mm is utilized for facial photography. Most digital cameras have a preset focal length for portraits ("portrait mode"). This represents the correlative focal length for the smaller sensors in the digital cameras.

Aperture

The lens aperture is the size of the opening that admits light to the sensor. A wider aperture allows more light, whereas a narrower aperture allows less light. There is usually an ample range of openings (f-stops) to allow for changing light conditions.

The larger the f-stop the more light admitted and the better suited to dim light situations. Most digital cameras, when using auto mode, perform these calculations to assure optimal aperture. The widest possible aperture characterizes the speed of the lens and refers to the ability of the lens to be used in low light without flash. The standard f/2 aperture is fast, whereas an f/16 aperture is slow.

Shutter Speed

The shutter speed represents the amount of time the shutter is open. There is a reciprocal relationship between shutter speed and f/stop. Thus, there exist multiple combinations of shutter speed and f/stop that can generate the same amount of light reaching the lens.

Without a flash, slower shutter speeds may lead to suboptimal image as a result of hand motion of the photographer if the camera is not mounted. With a flash, shutter speed can be slower than 1/250.

ISO

ISO (International Organization for Standards) is a measure of the sensor's sensitivity to light. One of the great advantages of digital cameras is that you can change the ISO settings, a characteristic that was film specific. However, as you increase ISO settings to compensate for lower light conditions, noise increases. Noise is the result of increased pixel sensitivity to light causing sensor misinterpretation. The lowest possible ISO setting should be used to maximize quality.

Changes in aperture, shutter speed, flash, and ISO settings all affect the exposure and ultimate image generation.

Image Compression and Storage

Image data from digital cameras can be saved in several different formats with RAW, TIFF, and JPEG being the most common. RAW files represent the full uncompressed image file. RAW is not a standardized file format. RAW file formats differ from one camera manufacturer to another and require special software peculiar to that manufacturer.

TIFF (Tagged Image File Format) uses lossless compression, which preserves image quality. This form of file compression creates a less compressed, larger file than that produced with JPEG. JPEG (Joint Photographic Experts Group) is the most common method of compression and can be done at different levels; more compression gives smaller files while simultaneously degrading the image. JPEG compression uses a compression algorithm that sacrifices image quality for smaller file sizes. In most of the available digital cameras, one can

select Fine or SuperFine image compression, which corresponds to a higher quality (less compressed) JPEG setting. More specifically, in most digital cameras, there is a choice of resolutions, which can be as low as 640 × 480 pixels and as high as the resolution of the camera allows (eg, 3024 × 2016 for a 6-MP camera).

FACIAL PHOTOGRAPHY STUDIO AND TECHNIQUE

To ensure reproducibility, a dedicated photography room should be used. With lighting for the background, the front, and both sides, one can create a good picture without shadows. This even lighting scheme is intuitive, simple to create (although not inexpensive), produces soft rather than harsh facial features, and does not require a flash. An alternative and comparable lighting scheme would consist of 2 front lights positioned at 45-degree obliquities and a background light (Fig. 9-1). These two oblique lights can also be used for patient alignment on oblique view acquisition. If a separate flash is used, it should be positioned in front of the patient so that the shadow develops behind the patient.

The patient should be devoid of all personal affects, and the background should be uniform. The background can be a single color sheet or wall, preferably black or blue. The patient's hair, if obtrusive, should be fixed behind the ears to allow visualization of all facial landmarks.

The camera can be positioned on a tripod, which is recommended, at the height of the patient's face. A frontal, 2 oblique, 2 lateral, and a worm's-eye view are the conventional views to be obtained, although other orientations and animated views may be useful for certain procedures. Floor markings for patient foot position enhance reproducibility. Uniform head alignment

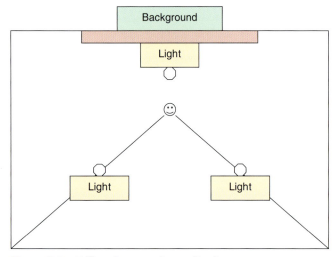

Figure 9-1 Office photography studio diagram.

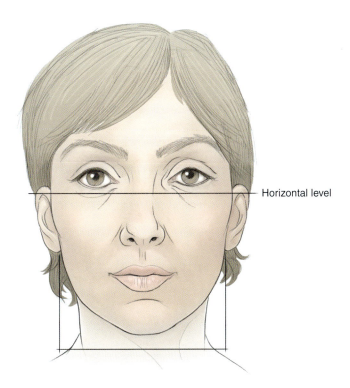

Horizontal level

Ear visualization prevents rotation

Figure 9-2 Facial reference points.

can be facilitated by placing marks along the wall to focus and orient the patient gaze. The midsagittal plane, by using a grid viewfinder, can be used to align head position. The Frankfort line, representing the infraorbital rim in continuity with the tragus, can be used as a reference for the horizontal level. In addition, the canthi or tragi position can serve the same purpose. To minimize rotation in the frontal view, reference the visibility of the ears (Fig. 9-2).

LEGAL ISSUES IN PHOTOGRAPHY

Consent should be obtained from the patient before photographs are taken. Consent should include mention of publication (journals or textbooks) or display (presentations, websites).

Chapter 10. The Complete Aesthetic Package

Renato Saltz, MD, FACS; Omid Adibnazari, BS; Alyssa Lolofie, BS

Modern aesthetic surgery practice offers patients a complete array of noninvasive treatments that will improve the visible signs of aging, with reduced morbidity, swift recovery, and minimal downtime. These services, which are often intended to enhance the results of aesthetic surgery, extend far beyond standard surgical procedures and include topical treatments, neurotoxins, tissue fillers, microdermabrasion, laser treatments, facials, makeup consultations, lymphatic drainage massage (LDM), and various spa services.

Such noninvasive treatments can make up an important portion of an aesthetic surgery practice because they appeal to different patient types:

- For young patients, as a preventive measure to avert the aging process;
- Among all patient ages, to battle photoaging of skin;
- Among aesthetic surgery patients, to enhance and maintain the results of surgical procedures
- For patients who are not ready for surgical procedures or who want to avoid aesthetic surgery.

As cosmetic medicine becomes increasingly competitive, the aesthetic surgeon needs to consider and address all stages of aging. To accommodate this need, the conventional aesthetic surgeon–nurse team must be expanded to include other professionals, such as master aestheticians, certified massage therapists, camouflage makeup specialists, and various business-related personnel.

We call this comprehensive approach to patient care the *Complete Aesthetic Package*. The ultimate goal is to provide a range of services that accommodates every patient, so that every consultation for rejuvenation results in identification of an appropriate treatment. Obviously, this package may differ immensely between individual practices, depending on the knowledge of the surgeon and the support staff. Incorporation of cosmetic medicine into a practice can help attract a wider assortment of patients, particularly if the variety of treatments and services provided appeals to many different types of patients and patient problems. Moreover, combining multiple treatments allows surgeons to offer patients superior results while improving patient safety and satisfaction.

The components of the Complete Aesthetic Package are as follows:

- Consultation
- Patient evaluation
- Skin care protocol
- Nonsurgical treatments for skin rejuvenation
- Facial rejuvenation and body-contouring surgery
- Lymphatic drainage massage
- Camouflage makeup
- Comprehensive maintenance program

CONSULTATION

Amid the goals of a plastic surgery, consultation is prospective patient education; patients should be informed of all the surgical and nonsurgical options available to them, along with details of the procedure, such as risks and complications, financial costs, and possible psychological issues. The master aesthetician at the practice should perform skin evaluation and preparation during the initial consultation, and should also inform the patient of treatments that will complement any surgery the patient may receive. The entire office staff, from the front desk personnel and office managers to aestheticians and massage therapists, must understand and commit to the philosophy of the Complete Aesthetic Package to ensure its success.

PATIENT EVALUATION

Meticulous evaluation of prospective patients is integral to selecting the best combination of treatments for patient rejuvenation. Again, the entire staff must be actively involved in selecting suitable treatments and to prime patients for facial rejuvenation and body contouring procedures. The Complete Aesthetic Package is individualized for each patient depending on the patient's specific needs and demands, concentrating on combining multiple therapies for enhanced rejuvenation.

Options for Rejuvenation

Numerous treatments, both surgical and nonsurgical, are available to rejuvenate the face and body. Surgical procedures generally address the excessive soft-tissue accumulation associated with aging, loss of facial volume, and tissue hypertrophy. Nonsurgical treatments are aimed at skin quality and deficiencies in the dermis. Unsurprisingly, the rejuvenating effects of various surgical and nonsurgical treatments frequently intersect.

SKIN CARE PROTOCOL

The Complete Aesthetic protocol includes an aggressive skin care program, aiming to improve skin quality and texture, as part of the preoperative protocol. Facial rejuvenation patients, for example, undergo a skin care regimen of skin bleaching, intense pulsed light (IPL), daily skin care, and peels in preparation for surgery. This regimen is resumed after the facial rejuvenation procedure to maintain and enhance the effects of the surgery.

Nonsurgical Treatments for Skin Quality

Microdermabrasion is a noninvasive, nonsurgical treatment that uses aluminum oxide (Al_2O_3) or sodium chloride (NaCl) crystals to resurface the superficial layer of the skin. This is a very safe procedure that needs no local anesthesia or preoperative medication. Treatments are usually administered every 2 weeks, and a series of 3 to 6 sessions is recommended to enhance skin quality before facial surgeries. Patients with oily skin, dilated pores, thick skin, mild acne scarring, melasma, and solar lentigines are fit candidates for microdermabrasion. The procedure is contraindicated in cases of severe rosacea, telangiectasias, uncontrolled diabetes, active acne, skin cancer, sunburned skin, or dermatitis. Microdermabrasion is also contraindicated for patients using isotretinoin (Accutane) or taking oral blood thinners.

Intense pulsed light (IPL), also known as photorejuvenation, is also a noninvasive, nonsurgical technique used to reverse the signs of photoaging. IPL is a no-coherent, no-laser, filtered flash lamp that emits polychromatic light in the wavelength range of 500 to 1200 nm. Altering the light spectrum, impulse length, impulse sequences, and fluencies allows adaptation to different skin types and indications. Topical anesthetics can be used 20 minutes before the treatment to make it more comfortable for patients. Treatment should consist of 3 to 6 sessions spaced 2 to 3 weeks apart. Superficial and deep localized vascular malformations, as well as irregular pigmentation, can be successfully treated with IPL. The high-intensity polychromatic pulsed-light source has also shown value in improving skin texture and grade I rhytid appearance. Absolute contraindications are abnormal response to sunlight, pregnancy, and presence of suspicious lesions. Relative contraindications include use of blood thinners, conditions that affect wound healing, and suntanned or artificially tanned skin.

Radiofrequency is yet another method for noninvasive facial rejuvenation. The treatment causes thermal injury to the dermis with stimulation of fibroblasts and production of abundant collagen, thereby promoting skin tightening. Radiofrequency is indicated for treatment of skin laxity of the face, neck, upper and lower extremities, and abdomen. Although results are not spectacular, the procedure can help restore a youthful appearance. Radiofrequency is a painful procedure and typically requires analgesic medication, meaning patients should be thoroughly evaluated and given detailed informed consent. Additionally, radiofrequency is not indicated for correction of jowling, nor is it a replacement for facelift surgery.

Nonsurgical Treatments for Facial Wrinkles

Nonsurgical rejuvenation treatments for facial wrinkles consist of one or several methods. Botox injections cause chemodenervation of the underlying muscles responsible for repetitive motion that result in wrinkles and thinning overlying skin. Lasers, chemical peels, and dermabrasion are useful for leveling the epidermis and for improving collagen in the dermis. Tissue fillers can effectively replace lacking dermal components or subcutaneous fat. Fillers can also augment areas of dermal atrophy by supporting the dermal matrix or volumetric enhancement. Fat grafting is also useful for filling, recontouring, and regenerating.

FACIAL REJUVENATION AND BODY-CONTOURING SURGERY

The surgical component of the Complete Aesthetic Package is integral to the overall aesthetic result. Modern, minimally invasive surgical techniques, such as endoscopy, have drastically decreased the incidence of complications, while providing results comparable to traditional open techniques. Tissue sealants also improve the results of surgery by reducing the rate of complications, promoting hemostasis, and improving patient comfort. These adhesives provide an excellent alternative to skin sutures, particularly in visible scar locations, such as the preauricular and submental areas.

In body-contouring surgery, the consistent use of tumescent solutions, preset limits for fat aspiration, and cautious use of mechanical and chemical prophylaxis for deep vein thrombosis (DVT) and pulmonary embolism (PE) keeps the procedure safe. Use of pain pumps makes body-contouring surgeries more tolerable for patients. Immediate compression and early lymphatic massage drainage help to decrease swelling, reduce bruising, and allow early return to daily activities.

POSTOPERATIVE CARE

The Complete Aesthetic Package strongly emphasizes the postoperative patient care. Patients are seen within 24 to 48 hours of surgery, and within 3 to 4 days patients are treated by a certified LDM specialist. LDM plays a vital role in postoperative care because of its ability to enhance skin quality and because of its comforting effects on the mind and body. This treatment reduces tension and stress, treats various forms of edema, diminishes scar tissue, improves cellulite, lowers blood pressure, reduces chronic fatigue and mild depression, supports the immune system, and improves skin tone and quality.

The lymphatic system functions primarily on the movement of muscle groups, which stimulate the pumping of lymph. After surgery, a patient's physical activity is limited, reducing lymphatic system function. LDM accelerates healing by reducing edema and swelling while concurrently relaxing the patient with a correlated effect on the sympathetic nervous system. Additionally, one of the most valuable effects of LDM is that it meets patients' needs for support and nurturing during the healing process.

Depending on the patient's state before surgery, a certified LDM therapist can determine how many treatments a patient may need after surgery. After surgery, it is generally best to wait at least one week before LDM treatments. To maximize the benefit of treatment, patients should receive treatments once or twice a week for the first 4 to 6 weeks. Following this period, LDM should be performed at least twice each month for maintenance purposes, to increase lymph flow, increase blood circulation to new tissue, and to reduce tension and stress.

PUTTING A PACKAGE TOGETHER

To develop the Complete Aesthetic Package, the surgeon must assess what components are needed in the practice. These elements should be carefully selected to that patient needs are attended to through every part of the process. Although noninvasive cosmetic treatments can improve skin conditions when used alone, their potential for enhancing the results of cosmetic surgical procedures cannot be overlooked. For the surgeon offering cosmetic medicine in his or her practice, products and services can be combined in numerous ways to enhance aesthetic surgery and provide matchless results.

Chapter 11. Local Anesthesia

Stephen L. Ratcliff, MD; Fred E. Shapiro, DO

INDICATIONS

Local anesthesia can be used as the sole anesthetic or as an adjunct to general or monitored anesthesia for multiple aesthetic head and neck procedures. Common methods of administration include local infiltration, topical application, and regional nerve blockade. Each route affords different benefits to the patient, but all are intended to reduce anesthetic requirements, postoperative opioid use and its associated side effects, and time to discharge in the recovery area. Additional benefits include having a patient maintain spontaneous ventilation with a patent airway, facilitation of tissue undermining, reduction of bleeding when a concurrent vasoconstrictor is used, and reduction in costs associated with the procedure.

Local anesthetics are not without their concerns. When given in excessive amounts, plasma concentrations can reach toxic levels and lead to a progression from simple numbness of the tongue or lightheadedness, to convulsions and coma, and, ultimately, to respiratory arrest and cardiovascular depression.

PREOPERATIVE PREPARATION

There are two main considerations to keep in mind when preparing for a procedure in which large amounts of local anesthetics will be given. Of utmost importance is the ability of the healthcare provider to respond to an emergency should one arise. In addition to having intravenous access, this entails having all the necessary resuscitation equipment immediately available, including an oxygen delivery system, resuscitation drugs, suction apparatus, monitoring equipment, and personnel (see Chapter 13 for full list of necessary equipment). The second consideration is to avoid high plasma concentrations that can lead to drug toxicity.

WHAT IS THE SAFEST DOSE OF LOCAL ANESTHETIC?

Recent advances in the use of local anesthetic solutions in surgery has led to much controversy regarding the absolute safe-dose limit of local anesthetic. Total dose, rate of administration, dilution, vascularity of the area injected, and coadministration of a vasoconstrictor can all affect blood levels. However, even though manufacturers publish maximum recommended doses, it is still difficult to predict blood levels from the dose that is given in the clinical setting.

When epinephrine is contained in a lidocaine solution, the published recommended doses do not exceed 7 mg/kg or a maximum of 500 mg. Plasma levels of lidocaine between 5 and 10 mcg/mL can lead to hypotension by cardiac suppression and vascular smooth muscle relaxation, and in concentrations greater than 20 to 30 mcg/mL cardiopulmonary arrest may occur. Recent studies have challenged these recommendations. A good example in practice is tumescent liposuction, whereby lidocaine doses in the range of 35 to 55 mg/kg have been used safely. Ramon et al found that for facelift surgery dilute lidocaine with epinephrine can be given at doses 3.1 times higher than the recommended dose with a plasma concentration 72% below the level that would lead to signs of toxicity. Although these studies show that greater doses of lidocaine than recommended have been given safely to patients without achieving toxic blood levels, there still remain reported incidents of toxicity with higher doses. This warrants further evaluation with larger prospective studies.

LOCAL ANESTHETICS: VARIOUS TYPES AND CHOICES

Although all local anesthetics can lead to local and systemic toxicity if given in excessive amounts, a more desirable goal is to avoid toxicity by judicious selection of the appropriate drug and by paying attention to concentration and volume used (Table 11-1). Commonly used drugs for ambulatory anesthesia include lidocaine, bupivacaine, ropivacaine, and levobupivacaine.

The benefit of lidocaine is its short duration of action and rapid onset. Bupivacaine is employed when a longer duration of action is desired, but care should be taken with this medication as it has a smaller therapeutic window. The main concern with bupivacaine is potential cardiac (bradycardia, arrhythmias, and/or cardiac arrest) and central nervous system (nervousness, seizures, respiratory depression) effects that are associated with unintentional intravascular injection. Concern for cardiotoxicity led to the development of ropivacaine and levobupivacaine, both of which are structurally similar to bupivacaine, but which have a greater safety profile.

Table 11-1   Local Anesthetics Used for Infiltration Anesthesia

Drug	Plain Solution		Epinephrine-Containing Solution	
	Maximum Dose (mg)	Duration (min)	Maximum Dose (mg)	Duration (min)
Short Duration				
Procaine	400	20 to 30	600	30
Chloroprocaine	800	15 to 30	1000	30
Moderate Duration				
Lidocaine	300	30 to 60	500	120
Mepivacaine	300	45 to 90	500	120
Prilocaine	300	30 to 90	600	120
Long Duration				
Bupivacaine	175	120 to 240	225	180
Etidocaine	300	120 to 180	400	180

Reproduced, with permission, from: Miller RD. *Miller's Anesthesia*. 6th ed. Elsevier Churchill Livingstone; 2005.

ADJUVANTS

Adjuvants are commonly added to the local anesthetic to either prolong the anesthetic effect or to speed the onset of the drug. A vasoconstrictor such as epinephrine is frequently added to reduce peak blood levels by delaying absorption and subsequently prolonging the anesthetic's duration. A good example, which is described below, is tumescent local anesthesia solution.

To speed the onset of the local anesthetic, 8.4% sodium bicarbonate can be added just before injection. Bicarbonate (makes the pH more alkaline), when added, affects the onset of lidocaine and mepivacaine more than it affects the onset of bupivacaine. The suggested dose is 1 mL of bicarbonate added for each 10 mL of lidocaine or mepivacaine; with larger doses, precipitation may occur within the solution.

PROCEDURES

Liposuction

In 2008, liposuction was the second-leading surgical cosmetic procedure in the United States. There are 2 similar techniques of liposuction, superwet and tumescent, that involve infiltrating the surgical area with a mixture of normal saline or lactated Ringer solution with lidocaine. Common lidocaine concentrations range from 0.025% to 0.5% and contain epinephrine, usually in a dilution of 1:200,000 to 1:1,000,000. In the context of aesthetic head and neck surgery, if closed (cervicofacial) liposuction is performed, local anesthesia and monitored sedation may be adequate. Infraorbital, mental, and cervical plexus nerve blocks are often used to supplement this technique. If liposuction is performed with another aesthetic procedure, such as rhytidectomy, general anesthesia with a laryngeal mask or endotracheal tube may be preferred by the surgeon. In all instances, close communication should be maintained among the healthcare team so as to avoid local anesthetic toxicity, particularly when more than one provider may be administering local anesthetic through various regional and infiltrative techniques.

Complications that can arise from liposuction include hypervolemia, hypovolemia, pulmonary embolism, hypothermia, and lidocaine toxicity. Although smaller volumes of tumescent injection are used for head and neck procedures, care should be taken as cervicofacial liposuction may be undertaken in the same setting as lower-extremity liposuction, where larger volumes of tumescent solution are employed. In this setting, complications may have a greater incidence, particularly with lidocaine toxicity. There is evidence to suggest that lidocaine toxicity may occur earlier than expected with head and neck liposuction. Although Ramon et al used total lidocaine doses in facelift procedures that amounted to 21 mg/kg without adverse events and with plasma levels 72% below the level considered as safe, other studies have shown higher plasma concentrations with liposuction.

Rubin et al prospectively studied 8 patients who underwent tumescent liposuction of the neck in 1 session and of the thighs in a subsequent session. Lidocaine 0.1%, $NaHCO_3$ 12.5 mEq/L, and epinephrine 1:1,000,000 in normal saline was used as the injected solution. Peak lidocaine concentrations occurred at 5.8 hours after neck injection and at 12 hours for thigh injection, with average peak concentrations 16% higher with neck injection. Although no adverse outcomes occurred, this study cautions the use of tumescent liposuction above the clavicles if injection is also planned of the lower extremities, as absorption curves would be superimposed.

Rhytidectomy

With increasing numbers of aesthetic procedures being performed annually it is becoming increasingly important to have anesthetic techniques that allow for quick,

Table 11-2   Guidelines for the Management of Severe Local Anesthetic Toxicity

THE ASSOCIATION OF ANAESTHETISTS
of Great Britain & Ireland
Guidelines for the Management of Severe Local Anaesthetic Toxicity

Signs of severe toxicity:
- Sudden loss of consciousness, with or without tonic-clonic convulsions
- Cardiovascular collapse: sinus bradycardia, conduction blocks, asystole and ventricular tachyarrhythmias may all occur
- Local anaesthetic (LA) toxicity may occur some time after the initial injection

Immediate management:
- Stop injecting the LA
- **Call for help**
- Maintain the airway and, if necessary, secure it with a tracheal tube
- Give 100% oxygen and ensure adequate lung ventilation (hyperventilation may help by increasing pH in the presence of metabolic acidosis)
- Confirm or establish intravenous access
- Control seizures: give a benzodiazepine, thiopental or propofol in small incremental doses
- Assess cardiovascular status throughout

Management of cardiac arrest associated with LA injection:
- Start cardiopulmonary resuscitation (CPR) using standard protocols
- Manage arrhythmias using the same protocols, recognising that they may be very refractory to treatment
- Prolonged resuscitation may be necessary; it may be appropriate to consider other options:
  - **Consider the use of cardiopulmonary bypass if available**
  - **Consider treatment with lipid emulsion**

Treatment of cardiac arrest with lipid emulsion: (approximate doses are given in red for a 70-kg patient)
- Give an intravenous bolus injection of Intralipid® 20% 1.5 mL.kg⁻¹ over 1 mm
  - Give a bolus of 100 mL
- Continue CPR
- Start an intravenous infusion of Intralipid® 20% at 0.25 mL.kg⁻¹.min⁻¹
  - Give at a rate of 400 mL over 20 min
- Repeat the bolus injection twice at 5 min intervals if an adequate circulation has not been restored
  - Give two further boluses of 100 mL at 5 min intervals
- After another 5 min, increase the rate to 0.5 mL.kg⁻¹.min⁻¹ if an adequate circulation has not been restored
  - Give at a rate of 400 mL over 10 min
- Continue infusion until a stable and adequate circulation has been restored

Remember:
- Continue CPR throughout treatment with lipid emulsion
- Recovery from LA-induced cardiac arrest may take >1 h
- Propofol is not a suitable substitute for Intralipid®
- Replace your supply of Intralipid® 20% after use

Follow-up action:
- Report cases from the United Kingdom to the National Patient Safety Agency (via *www.npsa.nhs.uk*). Cases from the Republic of Ireland should be reported to the Irish Medicines Board. Whether or not lipid emulsion is administered, please also report cases to the LipidRescue™ site: *www.lipidrescue.org*.
- If possible, take blood samples into a plain tube and a heparinised tube before and after lipid emulsion administration and at 1 h intervals afterwards. Ask your laboratory to measure LA and triglyceride levels (these have not yet been reported in a human case of LA intoxication treated with lipid).
- Please read the notes overleaf

Your nearest bag of Intralipid® is kept...

Reproduced, with permission, from the Association of Anaesthetists of Great Britain and Ireland.

safe recovery while providing optimal surgical conditions. Aesthetic facial surgery, which previously had been primarily done under general anesthesia, is now possible to be done under local anesthesia and a total intravenous anesthesia technique. Taghinia et al retrospectively reviewed 142 consecutive rhytidectomies with 2 different sedation/analgesia techniques. Both techniques included propofol, ketamine, fentanyl, and midazolam. However, one group employed the α_2-agonist dexmedetomidine. This short-acting medication allows the patient to breathe spontaneously on room air while providing sedation and analgesia and avoiding the risk of combustion with the combination of oxygen and electrocautery. In this study, patients encountered lowered blood pressure, decreased episodes of oxygen desaturations, a decreased requirement of supplemental oxygen, and reduced opioid, anxiolytic, and antiemetic use. This technique is largely made possible by the use of local infiltration of 0.5% lidocaine with 1:200,000 epinephrine as a background analgesic.

Blepharoplasty

Blepharoplasty under local anesthesia or with conscious sedation affords surgeons the ability to perform the procedure in multiple settings, including office-based settings, as well as the hospital. In a recent study, Harley and Collins examined 86 healthy patients who underwent blepharoplasty using oral medication and local anesthetic in an office-based setting. This retrospective review assessed patient satisfaction and determined that the procedure is well accepted and highly rated by patients. Patients were given propoxyphene with acetaminophen (100 mg/650 mg) and diazepam (10 mg) 30 minutes before slow injection of 2 mL of 1% lidocaine with 1:100,000 epinephrine per lid. An 83% response rate was obtained with 91% reporting an excellent experience. The authors believed the ability to choose local anesthesia and sedation in the office setting was a major factor in determining whether patients would have the procedure done. They concluded that this anesthetic approach to blepharoplasty is safe, convenient, and cost saving.

Rhinoplasty

Rhinoplasty can be performed both under general or local anesthesia depending on how extensive the operation is. In both settings, local anesthetics can provide analgesia while lowering opioid requirements. In one study, Demiraran et al compared 60 patients who were randomly assigned to be given preincisional lidocaine 2% with epinephrine or levobupivacaine 0.25% without epinephrine, and found that patients who received levobupivacaine required significantly less supplemental analgesics and had lower visual analog scale values. In a recent study evaluating the use of intravenous sedation, Cinella

et al compared 2 different fentanyl regimens in patients undergoing office-based aesthetic procedures under local anesthesia. In one group ($n = 50$) fentanyl was given in a bolus of 0.7 mcg/kg once prior to local anesthetic infiltration. The second group ($n = 50$), in addition to receiving a 0.7 mcg/kg fentanyl bolus as in the first group, also received a bolus of 0.6 mcg/kg every 45 minutes. Both groups also employed midazolam as their sedation technique. Results showed that the additional doses of opioid in the second group did not add to patient comfort or improve postoperative analgesia, but instead contributed to lower intraoperative blood pressure and arterial oxyhemoglobin saturation (SpO_2) values.

TREATMENT OF LOCAL ANESTHETIC TOXICITY

Along with local anesthetics becoming an invaluable part of head and neck aesthetic procedures come the concerns for increased risks of local anesthetic toxicity. To prevent toxicity, the healthcare provider should not only understand the current literature on dosing guidelines and on recognizing the signs and symptoms of toxicity, but also be well versed in managing adverse outcomes. Table 11-2 includes a plan for management of the airway, seizures, cardiopulmonary resuscitation, and administration of 20% intralipid emulsion if needed.

SUGGESTED READING

American Society of Aesthetic Plastic Surgery. Cosmetic surgery national databank. 2008. http://www.surgery.org/press/statistics-2008.php. Accessed April 21, 2009.

ASA Committee on Ambulatory Surgical Care and the SAMBA Committee on Office Based Anesthesia. *Office-Based Anesthesia: Considerations for Anesthesiologists in Setting Up and Maintaining a Safe Office Anesthesia Environment.* 2nd ed. American Society of Anesthesiologists, Park Ridge, IL; 2008.

Association of Anaesthetists of Great Britain and Ireland. Guidelines for the management of severe local anaesthetic toxicity. http://www.aagbi.org/publications/guidelines/docs/latoxicity07.pdf. Accessed April 21, 2009.

Bhananker SM, Posner KL, Cheney FW, et al. Injury and liability associated with monitored anesthesia care: a closed claims analysis. *Anesthesiology.* 2006;104:228-234.

Cinnella G, Meola S, Portincasa A, et al. Sedation analgesia during office-based plastic surgery procedures: a comparison of two opioid regimens. *Plast Reconstr Surg.* 2007;119(7): 2263-2270.

Demiraran Y, Ozturk O, Guclu E, et al. Vasoconstriction and analgesic efficacy of locally infiltrated levobupivacaine for nasal surgery. *Anesth Analg.* 2008;106(3):1008-1011.

Harley DH, Collins DR. Patient satisfaction after blepharoplasty as office surgery using oral medication with the patient under local anesthesia. *Aesthetic Plast Surg.* 2008;32: 77-81.

Iverson RE, Pao VS. MOC-PS(SM) CME article: liposuction. *Plast Reconstr Surg*. 2008;121(4 Suppl):1-11.

Ramon Y, Baak Y, Ullmann Y, et al. Pharmacokinetics of high-dose diluted lidocaine in local anesthesia for facelift procedures. *Ther Drug Monit*. 2007;29:644-647.

Rubin JP, Xie Z, Davidson C, et al. Rapid absorption of tumescent lidocaine above the clavicles: a prospective clinical study. *Plast Reconstr Surg*. 2005;115(6):1744-1751.

Shapiro FE. Anesthesia for outpatient cosmetic surgery. *Curr Opin Anaesthesiol*. 2008;21:704-710.

Strichartz GR, Berde CB. Local anesthetics. In: Miller RD, ed. *Miller's Anesthesia*. 6th ed. Philadelphia, PA: Elsevier; 2005: 573-603.

Taghinia AH, Shapiro FE, Slavin SA. Dexmedetomidine in aesthetic facial surgery: improving anesthetic safety and efficacy. *Plast Reconstr Surg*. 2008;121:269-271.

Urman RD, Shapiro FE. Choosing anesthetic agents. Which one? In: Shapiro FE, ed. *Manual of Office-Based Anesthesia Procedures*. Philadelphia, PA: Lippincott Williams & Wilkins; 2007:58-74.

Chapter 12. Conscious Sedation Techniques in Plastic Surgery

John B. Hijjawi, MD, FACS; Thomas A. Mustoe, MD

As operative techniques in plastic surgery become more refined and predictable, the ability of a surgeon to provide an overall pleasant patient experience is increasingly expected by patients. Providing a pleasant and safe "patient experience" is dependent not only on the surgeon's technical ability with the scalpel, but indeed on their ability to minimize perioperative and postoperative pain, anxiety, nausea, vomiting, and expense, all in the context of uncompromising patient safety.

The unique nature of most plastic surgery procedures, occurring largely in subcutaneous or submuscular planes, provides an ideal opportunity for the surgeon to exploit knowledge of cutaneous patterns of innervation, thus establishing very satisfactory regional sensory blockade. Combining techniques of regional blockade, which often involve local anesthesia delivery in the form of "tumescent anesthesia," with conscious sedation allows the surgeon to perform procedures safely without forcing the patient to submit to general anesthesia.

There has been an increasing trend toward outpatient surgery over the past two decades, whether done in the hospital or surgicenter setting. There have been substantial improvements in the techniques of general anesthesia that have allowed more rapid recovery, but there are still disadvantages to general anesthesia, including the risks inherent in induction, intubation, blood stasis in the extremities, and extubation, as well as the nausea and postanesthesia "hangover."

Achieving effective local anesthesia is the foundation of safe conscious sedation or deep sedation, making this anesthetic technique applicable to the full range of aesthetic surgery and breast surgery, as well as facilitating many reconstructive procedures. As suggested, such techniques do not rely on the use of sedative or analgesic medications to make painful surgical procedures tolerable. Rather, relatively moderate amounts of opioid and benzodiazepines are used to make the infiltration of high-volume, dilute lidocaine solution tolerable. The resultant surgical field anesthesia makes the ensuing procedure tolerable.

Plastic surgeons have accepted the dual responsibilities of providing both surgical and anesthesia care in office situations for some time. Despite the ready availability of dedicated anesthesia care, a large segment of plastic surgeons performing high-volume aesthetic surgery choose to combine local anesthesia with surgeon-directed conscious sedation about a third of the time. An American Society of Plastic Surgeons study found that in 2007 more than 80% of cosmetic surgery procedures did not occur in hospital settings. As a result, all plastic surgeons should be familiar with conscious sedation whether they pursue these techniques or opt for anesthesiologist-directed care in all cases.

Currently, in Illinois and Florida, deep sedation in an office setting is restricted without the presence of an anesthesiologist. Furthermore, in Illinois, conscious sedation in an office setting is restricted to those situations in which the surgeon is supervising a certified registered nurse anesthetist (CRNA). In a hospital or surgicenter setting where anesthesia support is readily available, surgeon-directed conscious sedation without a CRNA is permitted.

DISTINGUISHING CONSCIOUS SEDATION FROM DEEP SEDATION

Conscious sedation is routinely provided by nonanesthesiologists in situations such as colonoscopy, bronchoscopy, and dental, emergency room, and interventional radiology procedures. During conscious sedation, patients preserve the ability to maintain a patent airway independently and continuously, and remain capable of responding purposefully to verbal and tactile commands. This provides the added benefit of maintaining the patient's ability to cooperate with simple tasks, such as changing positions. This can be extremely beneficial in procedures such as liposuction where several position changes may be necessary. At no point is the patient's spontaneous ventilation or airway patency impaired. Sedation may or may not be combined with analgesic medications and local anesthesia depending on the nature of the procedure to be performed. Unlike deep-sedation protocols, no interventions are required to maintain airway patency, spontaneous ventilation, or hemodynamic stability. Accordingly, it is imperative that dedicated nursing personnel continuously monitor the patient's state of alertness and communicate that to the surgeon, along with the patient's vital signs, including oxygen saturation.

Recall of the procedure is generally limited or nonexistent. Hasen has compared surgeon-directed conscious-sedation techniques to anesthesiologist-directed deep-sedation techniques in patients undergoing aesthetic surgery procedures. That analysis revealed no difference in patient recall of painful events or anxiety during surgery. Significantly more fentanyl was required in the cases performed under a deep-sedation technique (typically with anesthesia-directed propofol infusion) relative to those performed under a surgeon-directed conscious-sedation technique. As would be expected in patients receiving more fentanyl, the deep-sedation group experienced significantly more postoperative nausea and vomiting.

A critical component of successful conscious sedation for surgical procedures is the ability to achieve adequate local anesthesia through a combination of wetting solutions (dilute preparations of lidocaine and epinephrine) and nerve blocks, thus limiting the amount of opioid analgesia required for a given procedure.

Deep Sedation

The spectrum continues into deep sedation where the patient experiences a partial loss of protective airway reflexes and becomes unable to respond purposefully to verbal stimulation. Some assistance may be needed to maintain airway patency and spontaneous ventilation. The patient's responses may be limited to reflex withdrawal from painful stimuli. Cardiopulmonary function may become depressed as the patient proceeds along the spectrum from deep sedation to general anesthesia.

"Overshooting" when attempting to achieve conscious sedation results in the patient progressing to deep sedation. As discussed, this means that the patient typically will require some verbal or tactile stimulation to continue breathing spontaneously. Additionally, the patient may require supplemental oxygen. We have been able to avoid giving reversal agents, although they are always immediately available as a backup maneuver.

In contrast, "overshooting" when a deep sedation protocol is being carried out typically results in complete cessation of any respiratory drive as the patient is already in a state of significantly depressed ventilation as part of the deep sedation state. This becomes especially problematic because deep sedation protocols are typically carried out with propofol, which, while metabolized in relatively short order, has no available reversal agent.

As a result, a significantly higher level of training is required of the individual delivering medications and monitoring the patient when a deep sedation protocol is pursued. Rather than a registered nurse with additional in-hospital training, a CRNA or anesthesiologist must be present for any deep-sedation protocol.

General Anesthesia

In general anesthesia there is a complete loss of protective reflexes accompanied by an inability to independently maintain a patent airway or spontaneous ventilation. Deeper states of general anesthesia are associated with depressed cardiovascular function. Conscious sedation, as noted, is routinely directed by nonanesthesiologists. However, deep sedation and general anesthesia is strictly limited to anesthesiologists or CRNAs under the direction of a surgeon or, more commonly, an anesthesiologist.

PROCEDURE SELECTION

A common misconception regarding the use of conscious sedation is that the technique is geared exclusively toward aesthetic surgery patients as a means to decrease the total cost of procedures. Consequently, many would assume that conscious-sedation techniques are not used for reconstructive procedures where insurance is involved. On the contrary, we routinely use conscious-sedation techniques in aesthetic, reconstructive, and combined procedures.

The most common reconstructive procedures for which we employ conscious sedation include contralateral symmetry procedures after unilateral breast reconstruction; secondary breast procedures, such as expander-implant exchanges; autologous fat grafting for contour refinement; and secondary recontouring of implant or autologous breast reconstructions. Expanding the application of this technique to include reconstructive procedures can be an invaluable opportunity for those gaining experience with conscious sedation.

Aesthetic procedures, including rhytidectomy, browlift, blepharoplasty, and limited liposuction, have routinely been performed under conscious sedation in office and hospital settings for years. In addition to these more traditional procedures, conscious sedation has evolved into our procedure of choice for abdominoplasty, liposuction, both submuscular and subglandular breast augmentation, and mastopexy or limited breast-reduction procedures.

The critical factor that makes the safe execution of all of these procedures possible under conscious sedation is the ability to achieve effective local anesthesia. Essentially, in healthy patients, conscious sedation can be safely utilized in any procedure or combination of procedures in which effective local anesthesia can be achieved with an upper-limit lidocaine dose of 35 mg/kg (delivered using a tumescent technique), given an operative duration of less than approximately 5 hours.

PATIENT SELECTION

Medical Status

It is a firm plastic surgery principle that properly selected patients with realistic expectations prior to surgery are patients who will most likely be satisfied with the results of plastic surgery procedures. The same holds true for the patient's anesthesia experience, an increasingly crucial factor in their overall satisfaction. Properly selecting the method of anesthesia for a given patient and clearly communicating to the patient what they can expect are important factors in a safe, successful, and pleasant surgical experience for the patient and surgeon alike.

Patients who are candidates for conscious sedation must be scored as American Society of Anesthesiology (ASA) Class I or II. More recently, Physical Status Classifications have been used to stratify patients into risk-based categories. Within the Physical Status (PS) Classification, conscious-sedation techniques are limited to those patients qualifying as a PS-1 or PS-2. This limits conscious sedation to either healthy patients or patients with mild systemic diseases resulting in no functional limitations (ie, well-controlled hypertension or diabetes, mild obesity). Particular attention is paid to preoperative electrocardiograms and cardiac status as indicated by a patient's functional status.

Relative contraindications to conscious sedation include either extremely young or old patients, a history of heavy smoking, or significant cardiopulmonary, hepatic, renal, or central nervous system (CNS) disease. This technique is not appropriate for those with a significant history of alcohol or illicit drug use, patients who are morbidly obese, have sleep apnea or atypical airway anatomy, or a prior history of complications related to sedation or general anesthesia.

Beyond Medical Issues

Simply meeting specific medical requirements does not make a given patient an optimal candidate for conscious sedation. Patients who are highly motivated to avoid a general anesthetic for any reason and are reasonably comfortable with the idea of undergoing a surgical procedure make ideal candidates for conscious sedation. In contrast, the patient who is extremely anxious about undergoing a procedure, is adamant that they want to be completely unaware of the procedure, or has had a negative experience with a previous sedation is probably best treated with a general anesthetic or anesthesiologist-monitored deep-sedation protocol.

Gottlieb has discussed the concept of the "comfort zone" in regard to a surgeon's comfort level not only with a particular procedure but also with a given patient. A procedure that is considered technically routine in one patient may be much more challenging in another patient. For example, a free deep inferior epigastric perforator (DIEP) breast reconstruction in a healthy patient may be a straightforward case for a given surgeon, well within that surgeon's "comfort zone." Add a significant smoking history, obesity, and small perforators to the picture, and that same surgeon may be entirely uncomfortable with the procedure.

This concept is equally important in assessing a patient's appropriateness for a conscious sedation approach to surgical anesthesia. Patients with high levels of anxiety or those undergoing relatively long procedures may make even a surgeon experienced with conscious sedation uncomfortable with anything short of a general anesthetic or deep sedation technique. It is particularly important to recognize this while gaining experience with conscious sedation. If a given patient pushes the limits of a surgeon's "comfort zone" with conscious sedation, it is safest to opt for anesthesiologist-directed care. As experience with conscious sedation is gained, each surgeon's "comfort zone" will subsequently grow in a broader range of patients and procedures.

PREOPERATIVE EVALUATION

Preoperative evaluation of conscious sedation candidates includes a thorough history and physical, age-appropriate lab testing, electrocardiography and radiographic evaluation, and consultation with appropriate medical specialists. Healthy patients younger than 40 years of age require no specific laboratory evaluation short of pregnancy testing in females uncertain of their pregnancy status. Between 40 and 65 years of age, a preoperative hemoglobin and electrocardiogram are obtained. Patients older than 65 years of age should also have a preoperative chest radiograph review.

Eliciting a thorough and complete medical history can be challenging. This can be particularly true for aesthetic surgery candidates who may believe that they need to give the "right" answers to questions regarding their medical history in order to be "accepted" for elective surgery. If clear, specific questions are not asked, information regarding significant medical history, problems with previous procedures requiring anesthesia or sedation, a history of drug or alcohol use, and the use of prescription medications can be altered or omitted entirely. Patients, frequently omit medical problems that are perceived as chronic but stable, such as asthma, unless specific questions are asked.

Clearly, a thorough knowledge of a patient's history of any alcohol or substance abuse, and any history of even chronic medical problems is critical when the surgeon is providing not only surgical care, but also responsible for directing conscious sedation. When problems do occur during a conscious-sedation procedure, there frequently has been a lack of appreciation for the seriousness of issues such as cardiac disease, epilepsy, and pulmonary problems such as chronic obstructive pulmonary disease (COPD).

SAFETY CONSIDERATIONS AND PREPARATION

Patient safety is of paramount importance when performing plastic surgery procedures under conscious sedation. To maximize the safety of our patients and the reproducibility of our techniques, we have instituted very specific protocols and standards in regard to conscious sedation.

Although our protocols have been designed to consistently keep patients in the state of conscious sedation, it is mandatory that the physician providing conscious sedation be prepared to manage those patients who will inevitably fall into the next level of sedation, deep sedation. Physicians providing conscious sedation must therefore be trained to manage a compromised airway, establish a patent airway, and provide adequate positive-pressure ventilation and oxygenation. To this end the Illinois Department of Professional Regulation requires nonanesthesiologist physicians providing conscious sedation to complete 8 hours of continuing medical education (CME) geared toward anesthesia delivery every 3 years.

At least one person trained in basic life support (BLS) must be with the patient in the operating room and in the recovery room. Finally, advanced cardiac life support (ACLS) services must be available within a reasonable amount of time. In most office settings, emergency medical services (EMS) responders provide these services when needed. It is important that any facility performing procedures under conscious sedation communicate with the directors of local emergency rooms so that they are aware that conscious sedation care is being provided in their community. Contact information for local EMS responders should be periodically verified. Our procedures are performed in a hospital setting with anesthesia backup immediately available. In an office situation, use of a nurse anesthetist adds an extra margin of safety with this technique, but each physician will have to make a decision regarding appropriate safety measures for their particular practice setting.

Any person ordering or delivering sedative and narcotic medications should be thoroughly familiar with their pharmacology and the potential interactions of any agents given on the day of surgery. To maximize our team's expertise with the medications used during these procedures, we strictly limit our intraoperative selection of sedative and analgesic drugs to 2 agents. A single benzodiazepine, midazolam, and a single opioid, fentanyl,

are available intraoperatively. These agents are discussed in detail in the next section. Both incremental and total doses as well as the exact time medications are given are charted on a large board that is visible to the entire operative team. A "medication-monitoring" nurse announces the total doses every 5 minutes.

The surgical team for conscious sedation procedures includes the surgeon and 3 nurses, none of whom is required to be a CRNA, but all of whom have specific roles. The surgeon is responsible for determining the dosing and frequency of medication delivery. The "medication-monitoring" nurse has very strictly defined responsibilities during the intraoperative period. These responsibilities include monitoring the patient's level of comfort and consciousness, monitoring and recording vital signs, delivering, charting, and announcing the total doses of medications, and, most importantly, communicating with the patient and surgeon. This nurse does not function as a circulating nurse at any point in the procedure, nor does this nurse need to be a CRNA. Additionally, there is a scrub nurse or technician and circulating nurse.

MONITORING AND SUPPORTIVE THERAPIES

Basic monitoring includes level of comfort and consciousness, pulse, blood pressure, and respirations measured at least every 5 minutes, and continuous electrocardiogram and oxygen saturation monitoring. Oxygen saturation is maintained at or above 92%. We consider oxygen saturation below this level to be indicative of a transition out of conscious sedation into deep sedation. Singer demonstrated that the level of oxygen saturation is the most sensitive objective indicator of a patient's level of consciousness during intravenous sedation procedures.

The corollary to monitoring the oxygen saturation level as an indicator of the patient's level of consciousness is *the avoidance* of routine supplemental oxygen. Although deep-sedation protocols routinely include supplemental oxygen to provide an added margin of safety in the event of apnea or airway obstruction, deep sedation techniques are, by definition, hindering the patient's ability to independently maintain a patent airway and breathe spontaneously. In conscious-sedation protocols, adding supplemental oxygen will elevate a patient's oxygen saturation at a given level of sedation, masking one of the most sensitive indicators of descent into deep sedation.

By eliminating oxygen supplementation we maintain the ability to detect the critical transition into oversedation or narcotization at a relatively early point. Thus, respiratory depression is detected at a point where it is more readily reversed with verbal stimulation and temporarily holding of any further sedative or analgesic medications.

Essential equipment in the operating room includes a source of continuous oxygen, equipment to provide positive-pressure ventilation (Ambu bag and facemasks), emergency airway equipment (oral airways, intubation equipment), suction, defibrillation equipment, reversal agents, and monitoring equipment with adequate emergency backup power. The equipment is only as good as the training of the surgeon and staff responsible for using it.

The training and equipping of staff in the recovery area is no less important than that in the operating room. A registered nurse trained in BLS should be directly responsible for patients in the recovery area. Appropriate equipment for the monitoring of vital signs, including oxygen saturation level, and a continuous supply of oxygen should be immediately available for each patient. Finally, emergency medications and airway equipment should be present.

PREOPERATIVE PROCEDURES AND MEDICATIONS

Preparation for the day of surgery begins the night before surgery. As with general anesthesia, patients are required to abstain from oral intake prior to procedures performed under conscious sedation. Solids and nonclear liquids are restricted for 6 to 8 hours prior to surgery. Clear liquids are restricted for 2 to 3 hours prior to surgery. Factors that traditionally increase the period of restriction, such as pregnancy, obesity, and significant diabetes mellitus, are not an issue as these patients are precluded from conscious-sedation techniques as previously discussed.

Ondansetron

One of the most unpleasant postoperative consequences of any surgery or opioid administration can be effectively dealt with in the preoperative period. Postoperative nausea and vomiting not only prolong recovery, but can also increase the incidence of hematoma following plastic surgery procedures (ie, rhytidectomy) and unintended admission following planned outpatient procedures. A prospective, randomized, double-blinded study has clearly demonstrated the efficacy of preoperative ondansetron (Zofran) in reducing the incidence of postoperative nausea and vomiting in patients undergoing surgical procedures performed under conscious sedation.

Risk factors for postoperative nausea and vomiting include female gender, facial rejuvenation procedures, procedures lasting longer than 90 minutes, and a history of opioid-induced emesis or of postoperative nausea and vomiting following a prior procedure. In these patients, preoperative ondansetron reduced the incidence of postoperative nausea and vomiting by 50% over placebo. Of note, in procedures less than 90 minutes, the risk of postoperative nausea and vomiting are virtually zero.

Therefore, the expense of ondansetron is probably not justified for procedures typically lasting less than 90 minutes.

Clonidine

It is extremely important to maintain stable blood pressure and heart rate in patients undergoing facial rhytidectomy. Even brief episodes of hypertension can have catastrophic results in these patients. Hematoma and seroma formation can potentially lead to skin flap necrosis or delayed wound healing. Even when hematomas are detected and drained expeditiously, the overall experience of the cosmetic surgery patient is made significantly less pleasant. Therefore, we routinely premedicate all patients undergoing facial rhytidectomy with 100 to 200 mcg of oral clonidine (Catapres) approximately 1 hour prior to surgery.

Clonidine is an α_2-adrenergic receptor agonist that acts centrally to inhibit sympathetic outflow. This inhibition of sympathetic outflow is responsible for many of the effects that make clonidine so useful perioperatively. Clonidine improves hemodynamic stability with reductions in both baseline heart rate and mean arterial pressure. Unlike many β-blockers, there is no significant "rebound hypertension" associated with clonidine; in fact, its effect lasts well into the recovery period. Additionally, there is a sedative effect associated with clonidine that serves as a useful adjunct in the conscious sedation technique.

Clonidine significantly reduces the use of sedative, analgesic, and anesthetic agents in a wide range of surgical procedures performed under both general anesthesia and sedation techniques. Within plastic surgery, it decreases propofol requirements in patients undergoing facial rhytidectomy. The shivering associated with recovery from anesthesia is also reduced by the preoperative administration of clonidine. It is important to note that patients should always have heart rate and blood pressure documented prior to the administration of clonidine, with doses adjusted accordingly.

INTRAOPERATIVE PROCEDURES AND MEDICATIONS

Opioids and Benzodiazepines

Multiple agents are available for use in conscious sedation protocols, including benzodiazepines, opioids, barbiturates, phenothiazines, and hypnotics. The agents selected for use in any conscious sedation protocol achieve the goals of anxiolysis, anesthesia, analgesia, and amnesia. Ideally, these goals are achieved using the most limited number of agents possible. We strictly limit our agents to diazepam (given only in the preoperative period), midazolam, fentanyl, and lidocaine. By limiting our protocol to 3 classes of agents, we maximize the familiarity of both physician and nursing staff with the appropriate doses, onset of action, and duration of action of a limited number of agents. Furthermore, we limit all agents to intravenous delivery routes. This eliminates the sometimes unpredictable onset of action of orally delivered agents (ie, diazepam). By maximizing the familiarity of all caregivers to fundamentally 3 agents (fentanyl, midazolam, and lidocaine), a "safe triangle" of conscious sedation is created.

Intraoperatively, this "safe triangle" is further limited with just lidocaine, fentanyl, and midazolam forming the arms of the triangle. Fentanyl and midazolam are ideal agents. Their rapid onset of action and short half-lives greatly facilitate the titration of drug delivery to a given effect. Small, incremental doses separated by at least 5 minutes are key because of the rather steep dose–response curve of both of these agents. Typical incremental doses of midazolam are in the range of 0.5 to 1 mg. Generally, once the total dose of midazolam reaches 15 mg, amnesia is complete.

Incremental fentanyl administration is limited to doses of 25 mcg. We limit the total administration of fentanyl to 250 mcg for a 2-hour case and 300 mcg for cases taking up to 4 hours. Patients older than 55 years of age are given relatively smaller doses, whereas younger adults or those with a significant history of alcohol consumption are given relatively higher doses. The successful use of midazolam infusions in aesthetic surgery has been reported, although it is our practice to limit midazolam administration to incremental doses.

Reversal Agents

Flumazenil and naloxone specifically antagonize benzodiazepines and opioids, respectively. Their use is reserved for situations in which clear oversedation or narcotization have occurred. These situations are indicated by a loss of patient-maintained ventilation that is refractory to verbal stimulation, hypoxemia refractory to oxygen supplementation, and the patient's inability to maintain a patent airway.

Reversal agents do have significant side effects. The sudden blockade of opioid receptors in a patient who has recently or is currently undergoing a surgical procedure can induce significant pain-mediated hypertension and tachycardia. Additionally, naloxone is known to cause nausea and vomiting, pulmonary edema, and ventricular dysrhythmias. Flumazenil is associated with dizziness, agitation, and seizures. Therefore, rather than administering these agents at the first hint of a potentially oversedated patient, supplemental oxygen should be administered and the patient should be verbally encouraged to breathe deeply. Next, a painful stimulus, such as injection of local anesthetic or a sternal rub, is applied. Basic airway maneuvers, such as jaw thrust and application of oxygen by nasal cannula, are simultaneously performed. Positive-pressure ventilation can be administered if these maneuvers fail. Only after these interventions have failed should reversal agents be considered. However, there should be no hesitation in administering these agents once it is clear that positive-pressure ventilation cannot be maintained.

These agents are given incrementally and titrated to effect. These reversal agents have durations of action that are significantly shorter than the agents they antagonize. Consequently, they may need to be readministered several times before the benzodiazepine or opioid has completely been cleared and the phenomenon of resedation ceases to be a concern. These agents need to be kept available and the patient closely monitored for up to 2 hours following the completion of surgery.

The endpoint of any conscious sedation protocol, whether applied to surgery, endoscopy, or radiology procedures, is a hemodynamically stable patient who remains cooperative and maintains the ability to verbally confirm comfort and relaxation. Indeed, a lack of cooperation by the patient is one of the earliest signs of oversedation and typically represents the disinhibition sometimes induced by benzodiazepines. Reflexively increasing sedation in an uncooperative patient must be avoided, as it will only make the situation more difficult to manage. The patient should be assessed for hypoxemia, signs of lidocaine toxicity, or oversedation. All of these factors may potentially contribute to agitation. Finally, the adequacy of local anesthesia in the surgical field is reassessed.

LOCAL ANESTHETICS

The first described clinical use of regional, or local, anesthesia in Western medicine was in 1884 in Vienna. Cocaine, originally isolated in 1860, was applied to the corneas first of lab animals then of ophthalmology patients by Carl Koller, at that point an ophthalmology resident. Although cocaine continues to be used by some surgeons and dentists today, other less-addictive substances, which are administratively less complex than cocaine, have gained favor.

Two major groups of local anesthetics exist. The *ester group* includes cocaine, procaine, tetracaine, and benzocaine. These agents are derived, in part, from para-aminobenzoic acid (PABA). Allergic reactions to these agents are known to occur and are largely thought to be reactions to the PABA component of the ester anesthetics. Because the ester anesthetics are metabolized by plasma pseudocholinesterase, impaired metabolism is rarely an issue.

The isolation of lidocaine in 1948 introduced the *amide group* of local anesthetics. Amide group anesthetics, such as lidocaine, mepivacaine, and bupivacaine, are virtually never associated with allergic reactions. They are metabolized via a hepatic route, however, and thus should be used cautiously in patients with significantly impaired liver function.

Ester and amide anesthetics both function by blocking sodium channels, inhibiting threshold potentials, and thereby reversibly blocking nerve conduction. Both anionic and cationic molecules exist in any preparation of local anesthetic. The anionic molecules penetrate nerve membranes and so it is the anionic portion of a given anesthetic preparation that provides the true effect of local anesthesia. Adding sodium bicarbonate to these agents achieves 2 goals. First, the acidity of commercial local anesthetics is decreased, thus diminishing the discomfort associated with infiltration in awake or sedated patients. Second, the proportion of local anesthetic existing in an anionic form is increased, maximizing the effect and onset of action of a given volume of agent. Ultimately, however, the single most important factor in potency and onset of action of any given local anesthetic is total dose delivered.

TUMESCENT ANESTHESIA

Tumescent anesthesia, familiar to any surgeon performing liposuction, is a fundamental component of the conscious sedation technique. No longer unique to liposuction procedures, tumescent anesthesia has been used throughout aesthetic surgery, oncologic breast surgery, and even pressure sore treatment. The tumescent technique provides the advantages of excellent local anesthesia delivered over a broad anatomic region, hemostasis and decreased intraoperative blood loss, a reduction in the need for intravenous fluid resuscitation, and an elimination of the need for more toxic long-acting local anesthetic agents like bupivacaine.

We have found the tumescent technique especially useful in rhytidectomy and aesthetic breast procedures. Not only are anesthesia and hemostasis facilitated, but hydrodissection of surgical, avascular planes expedites operative dissection in many cases.

Typical solutions consist of 100 mL 1% Xylocaine, 1 mL epinephrine (1:1000), and 250 mL of saline for facelifts, breast augmentations, and mastopexies. For abdominoplasties, breast reductions, mastopexies with liposuction, and liposuction, a standard mix of 50 mL 1% Xylocaine, 1 mL epinephrine in 1000 mL lactated Ringer solution or saline is used as a supplement to a more concentrated solution for the skin incisions. As with traditionally delivered lidocaine, the addition of sodium bicarbonate to more concentrated tumescent lidocaine solutions increases the proportion of anesthetic in the more functional anionic form. Additionally, sodium bicarbonate decreases the discomfort typically associated with the injection of acidic agents in awake or even sedated patients. Ideally, the normal saline or lactated Ringer solution is stored at 40°C (104°F). Warming fluids not only minimizes the potential for hypothermia associated with infiltration of relatively large volumes of room-temperature fluids, but also reduces the discomfort associated with infiltration.

Traditionally formulated preparations of lidocaine are not considered safe in doses greater than 5 mg/kg without epinephrine and 7 mg/kg with epinephrine. Lidocaine delivered in tumescent solution has been safely given in doses of approximately 5-fold these recommended maximum doses. Ostad reported delivering lidocaine doses as high as 55 mg/kg in tumescent solution without complications, although more typical maximum doses are 35 mg/kg. We adhere to the 35 mg/kg maximum, occasionally slightly exceeding that in combination procedures involving abdominoplasty, because much of the infusion is removed during the excision.

The safety of such high doses of lidocaine was initially thought to be a result of the evacuation of anesthetic agent along with tumescent fluid and aspirated fat during liposuction procedures. However, Klein has demonstrated that plasma levels of lidocaine are not significantly decreased by liposuction. In fact, peak plasma concentrations of lidocaine occur at approximately 12 hours after infiltration whether or not aspiration is performed. When higher doses are delivered more rapidly, peak plasma concentrations occur at approximately 6 hours after infiltration. Importantly, even with doses as high as 2600 mg of lidocaine, Ostad showed that plasma concentrations remain below 4 mcg/mL.

Currently, the safety of high-dose lidocaine delivered in wetting solution is thought to be largely a result of the massive dilution of anesthetic agent, the relatively slow rate of administration, the vasoconstriction attendant with the addition of epinephrine, and the relatively avascular spaces in which wetting solution is delivered.

LIDOCAINE TOXICITY

Recognition

Despite the documented safety of the tumescent technique, it is important to recognize the signs of lidocaine toxicity whenever delivering such high doses. At plasma concentrations of 3 to 5 mcg/mL dizziness and lightheadedness are seen, whereas levels of 5 to 9 mcg/mL are associated with muscle fasciculations and tinnitus. At levels of 9 to 12 mcg/mL seizure activity is manifested, and levels greater than 20 mcg/mL are accompanied by respiratory arrest and cardiovascular collapse. Of note, benzodiazepines significantly increase the seizure threshold for lidocaine, and may contribute in part to the safety record of high-dose lidocaine delivered via the tumescent technique.

Treatment

When lidocaine toxicity does occur, it is critical to act quickly to counteract the resulting CNS and cardiovascular sequelae. Seizure activity is treated initially with hyperventilation with 100% oxygen delivered by Ambu bag. This maneuver circumvents the deterioration in

CNS status seen with hypercarbia. If seizure activity continues, diazepam or thiopental can be given intravenously in doses of 0.1 mg/kg and 2 mg/kg, respectively. Hypotension is treated with aggressive IV fluids resuscitation and Trendelenburg positioning. The judicious use of peripheral vasoconstrictors may need to be considered. While inducing hypertension is certainly not desirable in a patient undergoing surgery in a wide or richly vascularized field (ie, abdominoplasty or rhytidectomy), maintenance of mean arterial pressure, and thus cardiac output, is always the first priority. Finally, if arrhythmias do develop, resuscitation may be prolonged as toxicity may not resolve until significant redistribution of local anesthetic can occur. As a footnote, in more than 3000 cases the senior author has not observed any cases of even mild lidocaine toxicity.

As noted earlier, the peak plasma concentration of tumescently delivered lidocaine occurs approximately 12 hours after infiltration. This sustained effect completely eliminates the need for longer-acting anesthetic agents such as bupivacaine to provide supplemental, immediate postoperative anesthesia. Bupivacaine and the longer-acting local anesthetics typically result in CNS depression and cardiovascular toxicity at significantly lower doses than lidocaine. This toxicity makes their use in broad surgical fields such as those encountered in abdominoplasty or liposuction impractical.

PRINCIPLES

- Limit the variety of sedative and analgesic agents used to maximize expertise and safety.
- Use small, incremental doses of fentanyl and midazolam.
- Limit the total allowable dose of fentanyl to 250 mcg.
- Clearly chart both incremental and total doses of intraoperative medications in plain view of the whole team.
- Be prepared to treat those patients who are progressing into deep sedation.
- Local anesthesia delivered by high-volume, dilute lidocaine solution is the foundation of this technique, *not* opioids or benzodiazepines.

SUGGESTED READING

Apfel CC, Roewer N. Risk assessment of postoperative nausea and vomiting. *Int Anesthesiol Clin.* 2003;41:13-32.

Bayat A, Arscott G. Continuous intravenous versus bolus parenteral midazolam: a safe technique for conscious sedation in plastic surgery. *Br J Plast Surg.* 2003;56:272-275.

Buck DW 2nd, Mustoe TA. An evidence-based approach to abdominoplasty. *Plast Reconstr Surg.* 2010;126:2189-2195.

Byrd HS, Barton FE, Orenstein HH, et al. Safety and efficacy in an accredited outpatient plastic surgery facility: a review of 5316 consecutive cases. *Plast Reconstr Surg.* 2003;112:636-641; discussion 642-646.

Carlson GW. Total mastectomy under local anesthesia: the tumescent technique. *Breast J.* 2005;11:100-102.

Cinella G, Meola S, Portincasa A, et al. Sedation analgesia during office-based plastic surgery procedures: comparison of two opioid regimens. *Plast Reconstr Surg.* 2007;119:2263-2270.

Courtiss EH, Goldwyn RM, Joffe JM, Hannenberg AA. Anesthetic practices in ambulatory aesthetic surgery. *Plast Reconstr Surg.* 1994;93:792-801.

De Jong RH, Heavner JE. Diazepam prevents local anesthetic seizures. *Anesthesiology.* 1971;34.

Friedberg BL, Sigl JC. Clonidine premedication decreases propofol consumption during bispectral index (BIS) monitored propofol-ketamine technique for office-based surgery. *Dermatol Surg.* 2000;26:848-852.

Gay GR, Inaba DS, Sheppard CW, Newmeyer JA. Cocaine: history, epidemiology, human pharmacology and treatment. Perspective on a new debut for an old girl. *Clin Toxicol.* 1975;8:149-178.

Gottlieb LJ, Gurley JM, Parsons RW. Patient selection and risk factors. In: Achauer BM, Erkisson E, Guyuron B, Coleman JJ, Russel RC, Vander Kolk CA, eds. *Plastic Surgery: Indication, Operations, and Outcomes.* St. Louis, MO: Mosby; 2000.

Han H, Few J, Fine NA. Use of the tumescent technique in pressure ulcer closure. *Plast Reconstr Surg.* 2002;110:711-712.

Hasen KV, Samartzis D, Casas LA, Mustoe TA. An outcome study comparing intravenous sedation with midazolam/fentanyl (conscious sedation) versus propofol infusion (deep sedation) for aesthetic surgery. *Plast Reconstr Surg.* 2003;112:1683-1689; discussion 1690-1681.

Horton JB, Reece EM, Broughton G 2nd, et al. Patient safety in the office-based setting. *Plast Reconstr Surg.* 2006;117:61e-80e.

Jabs D, Richards BG, Richards FD. Quantitative effects of tumescent infiltration and bupivicaine injection in decreasing postoperative pain in submuscular breast augmentation. *Aesthet Surg J.* 2008;28:528-533.

Jastak JT, Peskin RM. Major morbidity or mortality from office anesthetic procedures: a closed-claim analysis of 13 cases. *Anesth Prog.* 1991;38:39-44.

Klein JA. Tumescent technique for regional anesthesia permits lidocaine doses of 35 mg/kg for liposuction. *J Dermatol Surg Oncol.* 1990;16:248-263.

Kryger ZB, Fine NA, Mustoe TA. The outcome of abdominoplasty performed under conscious sedation: six-year experience in 153 consecutive cases. *Plast Reconstr Surg.* 2004;113:1807-1817; discussion 1818-1809.

Kucera IJ, Lambert TJ, Klein JA, et al. Liposuction: contemporary issues for the anesthesiologist. *J Clin Anesth.* 2006;18:379-387.

Lewis CM, Lavell S, Simpson MF. Patient selection and patient satisfaction. *Clin Plast Surg.* 1983;10:321-332.

Marcus JR, Few JW, Chao JD, et al. The prevention of emesis in plastic surgery: a randomized, prospective study. *Plast Reconstr Surg.* 2002;109:2487-2494.

Marcus JR, Tyrone JW, Few JW, et al. Optimization of conscious sedation in plastic surgery. *Plast Reconstr Surg.* 1999;104:1338-1345.

Mustoe TA, Buck DW 2nd, Lalonde DH. The safe management of anesthesia, sedation, and pain in plastic surgery. *Plast Reconstr Surg.* 2010;126:165e-176e.

Mustoe TA, Kim P, Schierle CF. Outpatient abdominoplasty under conscious sedation. *Aesthet Surg J*. 2007;27:442-449.

Ostad A, Kageyama N, Moy RL. Tumescent anesthesia with a lidocaine dose of 55 mg/kg is safe for liposuction. *Dermatol Surg*. 1996;22:921-927.

Practice guidelines for sedation and analgesia by non-anesthesiologists. *Anesthesiology*. 2002;96:1004-1017.

Reinisch JF, Bresnick SD, Walker JW, Rosso RF. Deep venous thrombosis and pulmonary embolus after face lift: a study of incidence and prophylaxis. *Plast Reconstr Surg*. 2001;107: 1570-1575; discussion 1576-1577.

Rohrich RJ, Parker TH 3rd, Broughton G 2nd, et al. The importance of advanced cardiac life support certification in office-based surgery. *Plast Reconstr Surg*. 2008;121:93e-101e.

Shapiro FE. Anesthesia for outpatient cosmetic surgery. *Curr Opin Anaesthesiol*. 2008;21:704-710.

Singer R, Thomas PE. Pulse oximeter in the ambulatory aesthetic surgical facility. *Plast Reconstr Surg*. 1988;82:111-115.

Zide BM, Swift R. How to block and tackle the face. *Plast Reconstr Surg*. 1998;101:840-851.

Chapter 13. A Comprehensive Approach to Sedation, Analgesia and General Anesthesia

Stephen L. Ratcliff, MD; Fred E. Shapiro, DO

INDICATIONS

More than 10 million surgical and nonsurgical cosmetic procedures were performed in the United States in 2008. Of these, 53% were performed in the office facility, 19% were performed in the hospital, and 26% were performed in a freestanding surgical center. Newer anesthetic and surgical techniques have allowed the total number of cosmetic surgeries to increase more than 162% since 1997. With the increase in environments in which anesthesia is provided, it is imperative that both the anesthesiologist and nonanesthesiologist administering anesthesia adhere to evidence-based standards and safe practices. This is done while continuing to offer patients lower costs, increased efficiency, faster recovery times, fewer infections, and a more streamlined and comfortable experience.

GENERAL ANESTHESIA

Accompanying the increase in number of aesthetic procedures being performed in office and ambulatory surgicenters is an increase in the number of patients with major medical problems and risk factors undergoing these procedures. Therefore, there is great concern to ensure patient safety, particularly as the number of healthcare providers who administer sedation in the office-based setting continues to grow.

The importance of maintaining quality and safety can be understood by examining levels of sedation on a continuum. The American Society of Anesthesiology (ASA) has outlined various guidelines and issued related statements regarding patients, policies, and personnel involved in the perioperative management of patients. Introduced in 1999 and revised in 2008, the ASA House of Delegates approved the Continuum of Depth of Sedation—Definition of General Anesthesia and Levels of Sedation/Analgesia (Table 13-1).

For aesthetic head and neck surgery, the desired level of sedation may range from minimal sedation or moderate sedation ("conscious sedation") to deep sedation or general anesthesia. The location of the surgery and patient characteristics often dictate the appropriate level of anesthesia. Regardless of the plan, the levels of sedation that are defined in Table 13-1 are not absolute and one must

Table 13-1 Continuum of Depth of Sedation

	Minimal Sedation (Anxiolysis)	Moderate Sedation/Analgesia ("Conscious Sedation")	Deep Sedation/ Analgesia	General Anesthesia
Responsiveness	Normal response to verbal stimulation	Purposeful response to verbal or tactile stimulation	Purposeful response following repeated or painful stimulation	Unarousable even with painful stimulation
Airway	Unaffected	No intervention required	Intervention may be required	Intervention often required
Spontaneous Ventilation	Unaffected	Adequate	May be inadequate	Frequently inadequate
Cardiovascular Function	Unaffected	Usually maintained	Usually maintained	May be impaired

plan for an unintended deeper level of sedation. This concept of "rescue" has an impact upon the clinical training of the personnel involved in administering the anesthesia. "Rescue" of a patient implies that the practitioner must be proficient in airway management and advanced life support, and be able to correct adverse physiologic consequences of the deeper-than-intended level of sedation (eg, hypoventilation, hypoxia, hypotension) in order to return the patient to the originally intended level.

MONITORED ANESTHESIA CARE VERSUS CONSCIOUS SEDATION

It is important to clarify the difference between monitored anesthesia care (MAC) and conscious sedation.

In October 2003, the ASA position on MAC stated that MAC is a specific anesthesia service for a diagnostic or therapeutic procedure. It encompasses all aspects of pre-, intra-, and postoperative anesthesia management. The services include diagnosis and treatment of clinical problems, support of vital functions, administration of sedatives, hypnotics, analgesics as necessary for patient safety, psychological support and physical comfort, and preparation to convert to a general anesthetic when necessary.

In October 2004, the ASA issued a related statement delineating the difference between MAC and conscious sedation. In addition to the definitions previously stated, a provider's ability to intervene to rescue a patient's airway from any sedation-induced compromise is a prerequisite to the qualifications to provide MAC. By contrast, moderate sedation is not expected to induce depths of sedation that would impair the patients own ability to maintain the integrity of his or her airway.

MAC allows for the safe administration of a maximal depth of sedation in excess of that provided during moderate sedation. The ability to adjust the sedation level from full consciousness to general anesthesia during the course of a procedure provides maximal flexibility in matching sedation level to patient needs and procedural requirements. In situations where the procedure is more invasive, or when the patient is especially fragile, optimizing sedation level is necessary to achieve ideal procedural conditions.

Like all anesthesia services, MAC includes an array of postprocedure responsibilities, including assuring a return to full consciousness, pain relief, and management of side effects of medications administered during the procedure, as well as diagnosis and treatment of coexisting medical problems. These components of MAC are unique aspects of an anesthesia service that are not part of moderate sedation.

MAC is a service that is clearly distinct from moderate sedation because of the expectations and qualifications of the provider who must be able to utilize all anesthesia resources to support life and to provide

Box 13-1   Clinical Care Patient and Procedure Selection

- The anesthesiologist should be satisfied that the procedure to be undertaken is within the scope of practice of the healthcare practitioners and the capabilities of the facility.
- The procedure should be of a duration and degree of complexity that will permit the patient to recover and be discharged from the facility.
- Patients who, by reason of preexisting medical or other conditions, may be at undue risk for complications, should be referred to an appropriate facility for performance of the procedure and the administration of anesthesia.

patient comfort and safety during a diagnostic or therapeutic procedure.

THE CHOICE OF ANESTHESIA

There are 4 broad types of anesthesia employed for aesthetic head and neck procedures: local anesthesia, MAC, regional anesthesia, and general anesthesia. The technique employed may comprise 2 or more types of anesthesia and is determined by taking several factors into consideration, such as type and length of the procedure, level of sedation required, whether the procedure is in a hospital or an office-based setting, the patient's physical and psychological status, and the qualifications of the anesthesia provider.

The ASA has published guidelines for patient and procedure selection (Box 13-1) and has emphasized the importance of proper qualifications for administering anesthesia, particularly in an office-based setting (Box 13-2). Regardless of the anesthetic technique chosen for a particular patient or procedure, the standard for patient selection, monitors, equipment, and drugs is the same. Please refer to specific chapters within the atlas for common anesthetic techniques employed for particular procedures.

PREOPERATIVE PREPARATION

Before undergoing anesthesia for aesthetic surgery of the head or neck, a complete preoperative history and physical examination should be performed and an ASA class assigned. Patients who are healthy or who have mild systemic disease (ASA 1 and 2) are generally appropriate candidates for a procedure in an office-based setting. If

Box 13-2   Statement on Qualifications of Anesthesia Providers in the Office-Based Setting (Excerpt)

The American Society of Anesthesiologists believes that specific anesthesia training for supervising operating practitioners or other licensed physicians, while important in all anesthetizing locations, is especially critical in connection with office-based surgery where normal institutional backup or emergency facilities and capacities are often not available.

Box 13-3   Anesthesia in the Office-Based Setting

The following is a partial list of specific factors that should be taken into consideration when deciding whether anesthesia in the office setting is appropriate:

- Abnormalities of major organ systems, and stability and optimization of any medical illness.
- Difficult airway, morbid obesity, and/or obstructive sleep apnea.
- Previous adverse experience with anesthesia and surgery, including malignant hyperthermia.
- Current medications and drug allergies, including latex allergy.
- Time and nature of the last oral intake.
- History of alcohol or substance use or abuse.
- Presence of a vested adult who assumes responsibility specifically for accompanying the patient from the office.

Box 13-4   Guidelines for Monitoring and Equipment

- At a minimum, all facilities should have a reliable source of oxygen, suction, resuscitation equipment, and emergency drugs.
- There should be sufficient space to accommodate all necessary equipment and personnel, and to allow for expeditious access to the patient, anesthesia machine (when present), and all monitoring equipment.
- All equipment should be maintained, tested, and inspected according to the manufacturer's specifications.
- Backup power sufficient to ensure patient protection in the event of an emergency should be available.
- In any location in which anesthesia is administered, there should be appropriate anesthesia apparatus and equipment that allow monitoring consistent with ASA "Standards for Basic Anesthetic Monitoring" and documentation of regular preventive maintenance as recommended by the manufacturer.

the patient has a higher severity of underlying medical disease (ASA 3 or 4), further direct consultation with an anesthesiologist is necessary and the decision to undergo the procedure at a hospital or surgical center can be made so that resource risks can be minimized.

Preoperative testing, such as laboratory tests, electrocardiogram (EKG), and chest radiography, should be guided by preexisting medical conditions and whether the anesthetic plan will be changed by the outcome of such tests. In addition to testing, it is imperative that patient evaluation and selection take specific factors into consideration, particularly in the office-based setting (Box 13-3).

ASA MONITORING AND EQUIPMENT

Standard monitoring of any patient undergoing surgery includes continual assessment of oxygenation, circulation, ventilation, and temperature. The use of such monitors allows the anesthesia provider to recognize and detect potential adverse events. Although it is not possible to eliminate all risk associated with a given patient or procedure, the goal is to avoid complications and minimize morbidity. Consequently, it is imperative that all anesthetics, whether sedation, MAC, or general anesthesia, be provided with the same level of monitoring and with the necessary equipment to respond to any potential adverse outcome that may result (Box 13-4).

In addition to their fundamental importance, the specific implications in aesthetic facial surgery of the ASA "Standards for Basic Anesthetic Monitoring" include:

- Oxygenation (prevention of fires in the operating room; see Appendix A)
- Circulation (deep venous thrombosis prophylaxis)
- Ventilation (airway management)
- Temperature (detection of malignant hyperthermia)

For a detailed explanation of the above, please refer to the American Society of Anesthesiologists (ASA)/ Society for Ambulatory Anesthesia (SAMBA) *Office-Based Anesthesia Task Force Manual, Considerations for Setting Up and Maintaining a Safe Office Environment.*

DRUG DESCRIPTIONS

Table 13-2 outlines common dosing regimens for various anesthetics. Selecting the appropriate drug depends on the operation planned, patient profile, and consideration of the need for anxiolysis, amnesia, sedation, analgesia, and prevention of side effects, such as postoperative nausea and vomiting. At this time, no single agent has all of these properties. Consequently, it is necessary to use a combination of drugs to achieve the desired effect. The benefit of drug combinations is the synergy and decreased potential for side effects. Appendix B lists commonly used drug combinations. For this to be most effective, a thorough knowledge of the pharmacology and drug interactions is essential.

LOCAL ANESTHETICS

Local anesthetics used in aesthetic head and neck procedures include lidocaine, bupivacaine, ropivacaine, and levobupivacaine. These anesthetics can be administered a variety of routes, including local infiltration within the area of the wound, topical administration, or through peripheral nerve block. The use of local anesthetics can reduce the use of opioids and their associated side effects and allow patients to proceed through recovery with reduced delays caused by sedation, respiratory depression, nausea/vomiting, and urinary retention. Because toxicity concerns must be addressed, dosing must be weight-based (see Chapter 12).

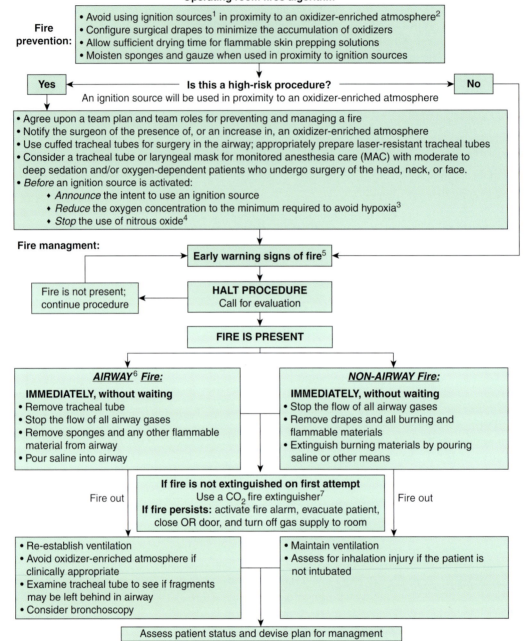

Operating room fires algorithm

Fire prevention:
- Avoid using ignition sources[1] in proximity to an oxidizer-enriched atmosphere[2]
- Configure surgical drapes to minimize the accumulation of oxidizers
- Allow sufficient drying time for flammable skin prepping solutions
- Moisten sponges and gauze when used in proximity to ignition sources

Yes ← **Is this a high-risk procedure?** → **No**
An ignition source will be used in proximity to an oxidizer-enriched atmosphere

- Agree upon a team plan and team roles for preventing and managing a fire
- Notify the surgeon of the presence of, or an increase in, an oxidizer-enriched atmosphere
- Use cuffed tracheal tubes for surgery in the airway; appropriately prepare laser-resistant tracheal tubes
- Consider a tracheal tube or laryngeal mask for monitored anesthesia care (MAC) with moderate to deep sedation and/or oxygen-dependent patients who undergo surgery of the head, neck, or face.
- *Before* an ignition source is activated:
    - *Announce* the intent to use an ignition source
    - *Reduce* the oxygen concentration to the minimum required to avoid hypoxia[3]
    - *Stop* the use of nitrous oxide[4]

Fire managment:

Early warning signs of fire[5]

Fire is not present; continue procedure ← **HALT PROCEDURE** Call for evaluation

FIRE IS PRESENT

AIRWAY[6] Fire:
IMMEDIATELY, without waiting
- Remove tracheal tube
- Stop the flow of all airway gases
- Remove sponges and any other flammable material from airway
- Pour saline into airway

NON-AIRWAY Fire:
IMMEDIATELY, without waiting
- Stop the flow of all airway gases
- Remove drapes and all burning and flammable materials
- Extinguish burning materials by pouring saline or other means

Fire out

If fire is not extinguished on first attempt
Use a CO_2 fire extinguisher[7]
If fire persists: activate fire alarm, evacuate patient, close OR door, and turn off gas supply to room

Fire out

- Re-establish ventilation
- Avoid oxidizer-enriched atmosphere if clinically appropriate
- Examine tracheal tube to see if fragments may be left behind in airway
- Consider bronchoscopy

- Maintain ventilation
- Assess for inhalation injury if the patient is not intubated

Assess patient status and devise plan for managment

[1] Ignition sources include but are not limited to electrosurgery or electrocautery units and lasers.

[2] An oxidizer-enriched atmosphere occurs when there is any increase in oxygen concentration above room air level, and/or the presence of any concentration of nitrous oxide.

[3] After minimizing delivered oxygen, wait a period of time (*eg*, 1–3 min) before using an ignition source. For oxygen dependent patients, *reduce* supplemental oxygen delivery to the minimum required to avoid hypoxia. Monitor oxygenation with pulse oximetry, and if feasible, inspired, exhaled, and/or delivered oxygen concentration.

[4] After stopping the delivery of nitrous oxide, wait a period of time (*eg*, 1–3 min) before using an ignition source.

[5] Unexpected flash, flame, smoke or heat, unusual sounds (*eg*, a "pop," snap or "foomp") or odors, unexpected movement of drapes, discoloration of drapes or breathing circuit, unexpected patient movement or complaint.

[6] In this algorithm, airway fire refers to a fire in the airway or breathing circuit.

[7] A CO_2 fire extinguisher may be used on the patient if necessary.

Appendix A   Operating Room Fires Algorithm

Table 13-2   Recommended Doses of Commonly Used Drugs in the Operating Room

Drug	Bolus Dose	Infusion Rate
Sedatives/Anxiolytics/Amnestics		
Lorazepam	0.02 to 0.08 mg/kg IV	
	0.05 mg/kg PO	
Valium		
Midazolam	0.02 to 0.1 mg/kg IV	
	0.5 to 0.75 mg/kg PO	
Dexmedetomidine (α_2 agonist)	1 mcg/kg IV over 10 to 15 min	0.2 to 1.0 mcg/kg/h
Intravenous Anesthetics		
Propofol	2 to 2.5 mg/kg IV	25 to 200 mcg/kg/min
Etomidate	0.2 to 0.6 mg/kg IV	
Methohexital	1 to 1.5 mg/kg IV (induction)	20 to 60 mcg/kg/min
	0.2 to 0.4 mg/kg IV (sedation)	
Thiopental	3 to 5 mg/kg IV (induction)	30 to 200 mcg/kg/min
	0.5 to 1.5 mg/kg IV (sedation)	
Ketamine	1 to 4 mg/kg IV (induction)	10 to 75 mcg/kg/min
	0.2 to 1 mg/kg IV (sedation)	
Opiate Analgesics		
Fentanyl	0.25 to 1 mcg/kg IV	
	(25 to 100 mcg/dose IV PRN)	
Remifentanil	0.5 to 1 mcg/kg IV	0.025 to 2 mcg/kg/min
Morphine	0.05 to 0.1 mg/kg IV	
Nonopiate Analgesics		
Ketorolac	15 to 30 mg IV	
Inhaled Anesthetics		
Nitrous oxide (inspired concentration)	30 to 70%	
Desflurane (MAC)	6.0	
Sevoflurane (MAC)	2.05	
Muscle Relaxants		
Succinylcholine	1 to 1.5 mg/kg IV (intubation)	
Rocuronium	0.6 to 1.2 mg/kg IV (RSI)	
Vecuronium	0.1 mg/kg IV (intubation)	
	0.01 to 0.02 mg/kg IV (maintenance)	
Reversal Agents		
Edrophonium (with atropine)	0.5 to 1.0 mg/kg IV	
Neostigmine (with glycopyrrolate)	0.07 mg/kg IV, 5 mg max	
Anticholinergics		
Atropine	10 to 15 mcg/kg	
Glycopyrrolate	7 to 10 mcg/kg	
Antiemetics		
Dolasetron	12.5 mg IV	
Ondansetron	0.1 mg/kg IV, 4 mg max	

Reproduced, with permission, from Shapiro FE. *Manual of Office-Based Anesthesia Procedures*. Philadelphia, Penn: Lippincott Williams & Wilkins.

Midazolam

Midazolam is a benzodiazepine that acts within the central nervous system to inhibit tone of γ-aminobutyric (GABA) receptors. It has a rapid onset and is short acting, making it ideal for ambulatory procedures. When used alone under MAC, intravenous doses within the range of 2.5 to 7.5 mg can cause marked anxiolysis, amnesia, and sedation. If used preoperatively, doses in the range of 1 to 2 mg are usually adequate for anxiolysis. Caution should be used in elderly patients because of a reduction in requirements to produce the desired effect. Typical elimination half-life is approximately 2 hours.

Ketamine

Ketamine is a phencyclidine (PCP) derivative that acts as an antagonist of N-methyl-D-aspartate receptors. The

General Anesthesia	MAC Anesthesia

Premedication
    Midazolam 2 mg IV (in holding area)
	Midazolam 2 mg IV (in holding area) *and* 0.25 to
	    1 mg IV during procedure titrated to effect

Induction
    Propofol 2.0 to 2.5 mg/kg IV *or*
    Thiopental 3 to 5 mg/kg IV *or*
    ± Fentanyl 1 mcg/kg IV
	O₂ 3 to 4 L/min by nasal cannula *or* 6 to 8 L/min by
	    face mask with capnograph

Muscle Relaxation
    Succinylcholine 1 mg/kg IV (for intubation)
    Vecuronium 0.1 mg/kg IV *or*
    Cisatracurium 0.2 mg/kg IV *or*
    Rocuronium 0.6-1.2 mg/kg IV *or*
	Propofol 1 to 1.5 mg/kg IV then 50 to 100 mcg/kg/min *or*
	Dexmedetomidine 1 mcg/kg for 15 to 20 min then 0.2
	    to 0.7 mcg/kg/h *or*
	Remifentanil 0.25 to 0.75 mcg/kg/min
	Fentanyl 12.5 to 25 mcg IV can be titrated to effect
	    and monitor for respiratory depression

Maintenance of Anesthesia
    O₂ 30% to 100%
    ± N₂O 0% to 70% *plus*
    Desflurane or Sevoflurane	

Reversal of muscle relaxation
    Neostigmine 0.07 mg/kg IV *plus*
    Glycopyrrolate 0.01 mg/kg IV	

Analgesia
    Fentanyl 25 mcg IV titrated to effect up to 100 mcg total
    Morphine 1 to 4 mg IV titrated to effect up to 8 mg total
    (monitor for respiratory depression)	

Nausea Prophylaxis
    Dolasetron 12.5 mg IV
    ± Metoclopramide 10 mg IV
    Consider orogastric tube placement and suction for patients
       at risk for postoperative nausea and vomiting (PONV)	

O₂ 100% Suction oropharynx Extubate (based on standard extubation criteria)	

Appendix B   Examples of Typical General and MAC Anesthetics

effect is a dissociative state that is accompanied by amnesia and analgesia. Ketamine administration results in sympathetic nervous system stimulation, which, in contrast with other anesthetics, can cause an increase in heart rate and blood pressure. For this reason it is generally avoided in patients with coronary artery disease, uncontrolled hypertension, congestive heart failure, and arterial aneurysms. An advantage of ketamine is its minimal respiratory depressant effects, with airway reflexes remaining overall intact. Because of the potential for psychomimetic effects (eg, hallucinations and unpleasant dreams) that can occur, it is suggested that propofol or midazolam be used concurrently.

Inhalational Agents

Desflurane and sevoflurane are often used in the ambulatory setting because they provide a smooth induction, optimal operating conditions, rapid recovery, and minimal side effects. Postoperative nausea and vomiting is significantly more common with the inhaled agents compared with propofol, but there has not been a difference shown between the two when oral intake and home readiness are taken into account.

Nitrous Oxide (N₂O)

Nitrous oxide is routinely used in aesthetic head and neck surgery as part of a balanced anesthesia technique. It has both anesthetic and analgesic properties and, when substituted for a portion of a volatile anesthetic, produces less decrease in systemic blood pressure than the same dose of volatile anesthetic alone.

The large concern regarding nitrous oxide has been related to postoperative nausea and vomiting (PONV). In a metaanalysis of randomized controlled trials, it was determined that removing nitrous oxide from the general anesthetic decreases vomiting significantly, but only if the baseline risk of vomiting is high. Furthermore, it was found that not using nitrous oxide does not affect nausea or complete control of vomiting.

The use of multiple antiemetics may be considered if the patient has multiple risk factors and the benefit of using nitrous oxide is clear. Established risk factors for

PONV include female gender postpuberty, nonsmoking status, history of PONV or motion sickness, childhood (after infancy) and younger adulthood, increasing duration of surgery, and use of volatile anesthetics, nitrous oxide, a large-dose of neostigmine, or intraoperative or postoperative opioids.

Propofol

Propofol is the most widely used agent for induction of general anesthesia and for maintenance of anesthesia during MAC cases. The ease of administration, rapid onset, short half-life, and low incidence of PONV make it ideal for ambulatory anesthesia and sedation.

The primary mechanism by which propofol works is through potentiation of GABA-A receptor activity, resulting in sedation, hypnosis, amnesia, anxiolysis, and muscle relaxation. Adverse effects include respiratory depression, hypotension, myocardial depression, and potential for infection. When used with midazolam and/or opioids, care must be taken as the respiratory depressant effects will be exacerbated, particularly in patients who are at risk for airway obstruction. The ASA issued a "Statement on the Safe Use of Propofol" in recognition that the response of each patient to the effects of propofol is different, with varying levels of sedation being experienced at similar infusion rates (Box 13-5).

Moreover, with the recent introduction of newer agents, the Food and Drug Administration (FDA) has maintained its warning on the safe administration of both propofol and fospropofol (Box 13-6).

Opioids

Opioids are used to reduce the pain of surgical incisions, pain from local anesthetic injection, and back pain that can occur from positioning on the operating room table. To reduce the side effects of opioids, such as PONV, pruritus, and respiratory depression, shorter-acting opioids, such as fentanyl and remifentanil, are often employed. Other anesthetic agents that have analgesic properties, such as ketamine and dexmedetomidine, are also used with local anesthetics to reduce the amount of opioids given.

Box 13-5   ASA Statement on Safe Use of Propofol

- During the administration of propofol, patients should be monitored without interruption to assess level of consciousness, and to identify early signs of hypotension, bradycardia, apnea, airway obstruction, and/or oxygen desaturation.

- Ventilation, oxygen saturation, heart rate, and blood pressure should be monitored at regular and frequent intervals.

- Monitoring for the presence of exhaled carbon dioxide should be utilized when possible, because movement of the chest will not dependably identify airway obstruction or apnea.

Box 13-6   Propofol Administration Warning

"Whenever propofol is used for sedation/anesthesia, it should be administered only by persons trained in the administration of general anesthesia, who are not simultaneously involved in these surgical or diagnostic procedures. This restriction is concordant with specific language in the propofol package insert, and failure to follow these recommendations could put patients at increased risk of significant injury or death."

Fentanyl is the most commonly encountered opioid as a result of its fast onset (3 to 5 minutes) and short duration of action when given in low doses (45 to 60 minutes). Remifentanil is currently the shortest-acting opioid (3 to 5 minutes) and is often given as an infusion for this reason. Metabolism of remifentanil is by a nonspecific plasma and tissue esterase, which means that accumulation does not occur even after long infusions.

Nonopioid Analgesics

Nonopioid analgesics include ketorolac, acetaminophen, ibuprofen, indomethacin, and celecoxib. Ketorolac is a commonly used nonsteroidal antiinflammatory drug (NSAID) that acts by decreasing the synthesis of prostaglandin. It is a parental agent and has less associated nausea, vomiting, and pruritus when compared to opioids. As with all NSAIDs, ketorolac should be used with caution in patients with gastrointestinal problems, renal dysfunction, and bleeding disorders.

α_2-Agonists

Clonidine and dexmedetomidine are α_2-adrenergic receptor agonists that act centrally to induce sedation, hypnosis, analgesia, and anxiolysis. Peripherally they have sympatholytic properties while preserving respiratory drive. Dexmedetomidine has higher selectivity of the two for the receptor and has a quicker onset of action, shorter half-life, and is much easier to titrate to effect. In October 2008, the FDA approved the use of dexmedetomidine for procedural sedation in nonintubated patients.

SUGGESTED READING

American Society of Aesthetic Plastic Surgery. Cosmetic surgery national databank. 2008. http://www.surgery.org/press/statistics-2008.php. Accessed August 8, 2009.

American Society of Anesthesiologists (ASA). Office-based anesthesia: considerations for anesthesiologists in setting up and maintaining a safe office anesthesia environment, 2nd edition, November 2008. URL: http://www2.asahq.org/publications/p-319-office-based-anesthesia-considerations-for-anesthesiologists-in-setting-up-and-maintaining-a-safe-office-anesthesia-environment-2nd-edition-november-2008.aspx. Accessed April, 2009.

American Society of Anesthesiologists Task Force on Operating Room Fires, Caplan RA, Barker SJ, Connis RT, et al. Practice advisory for the prevention and management of operating room fires. *Anesthesiology*. 2008;108:786-801. http://www.asahq.org/publicationsAndServices/orFiresPA.pdf. Accessed on August 8, 2009.

American Society of Anesthesiologists. Continuum of depth of sedation, definitions of general anesthesia and levels of sedation/analgesia. (Approved by ASA House of Delegates on October 13, 1999, amended October 27, 2004). http://www.asahq.org/publicationsAndServices/standards/20.pdf. Accessed August 8, 2009.

American Society of Anesthesiologists. Distinguishing monitored anesthesia care ("MAC") from moderate sedation/analgesia-conscious sedation. (Approved by the ASA House of Delegates; on October 27, 2004). www.asahq.org/publicationsAndServices/standards/35.pdf. 2004. Accessed August 8, 2009.

American Society of Anesthesiologists. Guidelines for office-based anesthesia. Statement on qualifications of anesthesia providers in the office-based setting. (Approved by ASA House of Delegates on October 13, 1999, last affirmed October 27, 2004). http://www.asahq.org/publicationsAndServices/standards/29.pdf. Accessed August 8, 2009.

American Society of Anesthesiologists. Position on monitored anesthesia care. (Approved by House of Delegates on October 21, 1986, amended on October 25, 2005, and last updated on September 2, 2008). www.asahq.org/publicationsAndServices/standards/23.pdf. 2004. Accessed August 8, 2009.

American Society of Anesthesiologists. Standards for basic anesthetic monitoring. (Approved by ASA House of Delegates on October 21, 1986, last affirmed October 25, 2005).

http://www.asahq.org/publicationsAndServices/standards/02.pdf. Accessed August 8, 2009.

American Society of Anesthesiologists. Statement on qualifications of anesthesia providers in the office-based setting. (Approved by ASA House of Delegates on October 13, 1999, last affirmed October 27, 2004). http://www.asahq.org/publicationsAndServices/standards/12.pdf. Accessed August 8, 2009.

American Society of Anesthesiologists. Statement on safe use of propofol. (Approved by the ASA House of Delegates on October 27, 2004). http://www.asahq.org/publications-AndServices/standards/37.pdf. Accessed August 8, 2009.

Bernardini DJ, Shapiro FE. Surgical procedures in the office-based setting. In: Shapiro FE, ed. *Manual of Office-Based Anesthesia Procedures*. Philadelphia, PA: Lippincott Williams & Wilkins; 2007:89-110.

Byrd HS, Barton FE, Orenstein HH, et al. Safety and efficacy in an accredited outpatient plastic surgery facility: a review of 5316 consecutive cases. *Plast Reconstr Surg*. 2003;112(2);636-641.

Gan T. Risk factors for postoperative nausea and vomiting. *Anesth Analg*. 2006;102:1884-1898.

Gupta A. Comparison of recovery profile after ambulatory anesthesia with propofol, isoflurane, sevoflurane, and desflurane: a systematic review. *Anesth Analg*. 2004;98(3):632-641.

Song D, Joshi GP, White PF, et al. Fast-track eligibility after ambulatory anesthesia: a comparison of desflurane, sevoflurane, and Propofol. *Anesth Analg*. 1998;86:267-273.

Tramèr M, Moore A, McQuay H. Omitting nitrous oxide in general anesthesia: meta-analysis of intraoperative awareness and postoperative emesis in randomized control trials. *Br J Anaesth*. 1996;76:186-193.

Chapter 14. Deep Plane Rhytidectomy

Samuel J. Lin, MD, FACS; Olubimpe A. Ayeni, MD, MPH, FRCSC; Thomas A. Mustoe, MD

INDICATIONS

The indications for this method of rhytidectomy include the patient with adequate expectations and anatomy for facial and neck rejuvenation. The advantages of this procedure are the ability to rejuvenate the midface and mouth area, as well as the neck.

PREOPERATIVE PREPARATION

Adequate time in consultation and preoperative planning is essential. The patient's expectations must be explored. An older patient with significant laxity will have an incomplete correction at one year as a result of inevitable tissue relaxation. A history of prior rhytidectomy is important for technical planning prior to performing revision rhytidectomy.

ANESTHESIA

Either monitored conscious sedation or general anesthesia is suitable for this procedure.

POSITION/MARKINGS

The patient is placed in the supine position, prepped and draped in the usual sterile fashion for head and neck surgery. The patient's head may be placed on a doughnut.

The blue outline signifies the extent of the superficial musculoaponeurotic system (SMAS) layer (Fig. 14-1A). Although variations may be present, standard rhytidectomy incisions (Fig. 14-1B) include a preauricular component with an anterior incision that borders the sideburn, with a V shape to allow correction of unequal incision length without a dog-ear. If more skin excision is anticipated, it useful to extend the incision up into the temporal scalp as well, which allows some posterior movement of the upper midface skin. The preauricular incision may be selected in a natural appearing crease; alternatively, the incision may extend behind the tragal cartilage. The latter is generally preferable except in secondary facelifts.

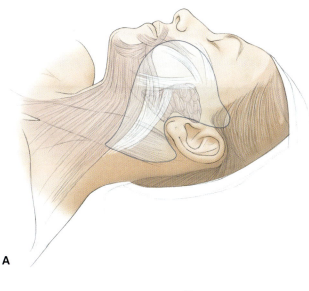

A

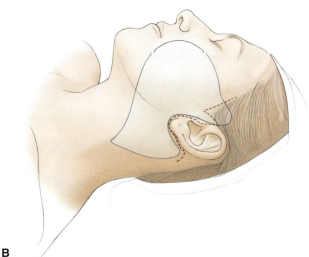

B

Figure 14-1 A. Outline of SMAS. B. Standard rhytidectomy incision.

INCISION AND EXPOSURE

A large volume of dilute local anesthesia is useful (100 mL 1% Xylocaine, 250 mL saline), which helps in defining the tissue planes. Following the injection of local vaso-constrictive/anesthetic agents, the incision is made with a no. 15 blade. Using sharp dissection, the incision is deepened through the subcutaneous tissues. Above the zygomatic arch, a superficial dissection is carried out. The SMAS is incised at the level of the arch, and 1 cm anterior to the ear. Above the arch, gentle blunt dissection with a peanut sponge may be used sparingly to separate the subcutaneous tissue from the temporoparietal fascia.

DETAILS OF THE PROCEDURE

The preauricular dissection separates the overlying SMAS from the parotid fascia. Once the anterior border of the parotid is reached, blunt dissection can be utilized except when incising the retaining ligaments (Fig. 14-2). The postauricular incision is also deepened and dissection is performed sharply with a knife to raise the superficial layer of the deep cervical fascia off the sternocleidomastoid fascia from a superior to inferior direction. A zone of adherence exists at the posterior border of the SMAS, which is just anterior to the greater auricular nerve (it is routinely seen and identified in this dissection), and so dissection proceeds carefully in this critical area to join the posterior dissection and the anterior dissection.

The SMAS is incised 1 to 2 cm anterior to the pretragal skin incision, along the superior border of the zygomatic arch, just below the ear lobule, and back toward the sternocleidomastoid (SCM). A sub-SMAS dissection plane is created around the ear lobule and traced inferiorly and posteriorly. The SMAS is elevated inferiorly to the level where the greater auricular nerve crosses the SCM, which allows mobilization of the lax neck skin all the way down to the sternal notch. In the preauricular

region, buccal branches of the facial nerve may be seen as the dissection progresses anteriorly. The marginal mandibular branch can be seen often under the masseteric fascia but is well protected by this thin fascia. The SMAS-platysma layer is dissected anterior and inferior to the submandibular gland, releasing the retaining ligaments around the parotid gland. In the neck, the cervical branch of the facial nerve exits the anterior inferior portion of the parotid gland, but can be avoided by releasing retaining ligaments in this area while not extending the dissection beyond the zone of adherence. The superior extent of dissection is the zygomatic arch. The inferior extent of the dissection is where the greater auricular nerve crosses the posterior border of the SCM.

The midface sub-SMAS dissection involves release of the zygomatic retaining ligaments, exposure of the zygomatic muscle, and extension of the dissection superior to the zygomatic muscle under the inferior edge of the orbicularis muscle.

Retaining Ligaments

The release of the retaining ligaments in each region of the face determines the extent of dissection necessary to allow adequate mobilization and advancement. The retaining ligaments found in the masseteric and zygomatic regions are addressed by extended SMAS rhytidectomy, deep plane rhytidectomy, or their variants, and in a different way by SMASectomy. The extent of elevation of masseteric and zygomatic retaining ligaments must be tailored to each patient's unique anatomy.

It is important to understand the restraints on platysmal mobility to determine the extent of necessary subplatysmal dissection. The platysma is attached firmly along its posterior border, and also down the inferior pole of parotid. The concept of retaining ligaments in the neck has not been clearly elucidated previously, but is as useful a concept in the neck as it is in the face. The posterior border of the SMAS is an anatomically constant structure, just anterior to the greater auricular nerve, while the posterior extent of the platysma (contained within the SMAS) can vary by 3 to 4 cm from patient to patient.

View of Completed Dissection

The concept of the lateral approach to the deep plane rhytidectomy is to fully release tissue where it is fixed so as to allow tissue to slide where it is not fixed. This technique results in even tension across the entire dissection plane and across the composite facial flap, achieving a "natural" result. This composite movement of tissue in which a large sheet of tissue is repositioned allows firm adherence without permanent sutures, and is long lasting. Additionally, this technique allows dissection to be done in the same plane in revisional procedures. It is important to treat the neck and the face as a single unit; the SMAS-platysma sheet in the neck and the face are continuous. Techniques in which the SMAS is pulled superiorly and posteriorly above

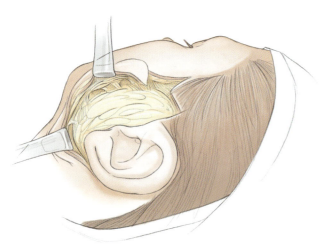

Figure 14-2 Visualization of the anterior border of the parotid gland.

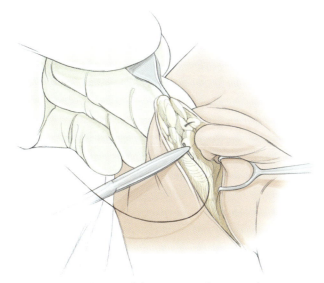

Figure 14-3 Anchoring of the SMAS to the mastoid periosteum.

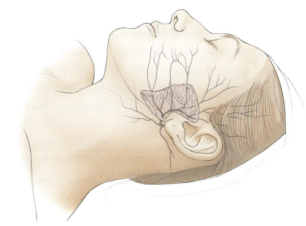

Figure 14-4 Branches of the facial nerve.

the jawline, and pulled anteriorly in the neck potentially create a line of tension in the lower face that can create an operated look, particularly in secondary facelifts.

Placement of Sutures

With the ear retracted superiorly, 3-0 PDS (polydioxanone) sutures are used to anchor the structural SMAS layer of the composite facial flap to the mastoid periosteum posterior to the ear (Fig. 14-3). Three or 4 sutures are used to spread tension, and relieve all tension on the skin sutures. Anteriorly, sutures are from the SMAS to the temporal fascia, and from the midface soft tissues over the cheek back to the temporal fascia. Following the placement of anchoring sutures, the excess skin is trimmed anteriorly first at the preauricular area. Following the placement of the anterior facial flap, the skin is trimmed at the lobule and in the postauricular area. Care is taken to have the incisions be closed with no tension.

PITFALLS

As with any facial procedure, branches of the facial nerve may be at risk (Fig. 14-4). In the deep plane rhytidectomy, the cervical branch is at risk with this dissection. This branch of the facial nerve exits anterior and inferior to the tail of the parotid. Nonetheless, it is still possible to release retaining ligaments in neck while preserving this nerve. Depending on the degree of injury, however, the morbidity should be mild and temporary. With experience, the risk of neurapraxia is less than 1%, and the permanent injury has been nonexistent. Other branches of the facial nerve at particular risk include buccal branches and the temporal branch. A key technical point is to stop the dissection at any time when the surgeon is not absolutely certain of tissue planes, and in effect adopt a more conservative

approach. With experience, the dissection can be completed in all patients.

The closure of the rhytidectomy incision is performed with no tension. All the tension is placed on the anchoring sutures that reset the position of the SMAS layer.

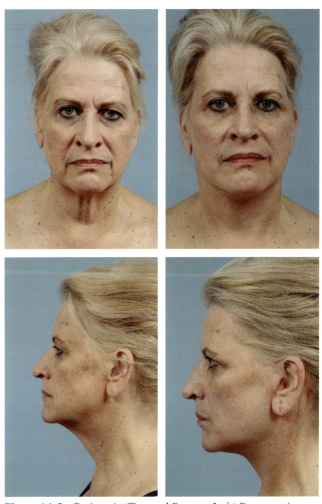

Figure 14-5 Patient 1. (Top and Bottom Left) Preoperative photographs. (Top and Bottom Right) Postoperative photographs taken following rhytidectomy.

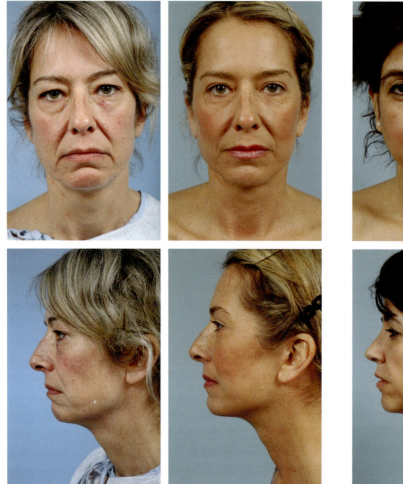

Figure 14-6   Patient 2. (Top and Bottom Left) Preoperative photographs. (Top and Bottom Right) Postoperative photographs taken following rhytidectomy.

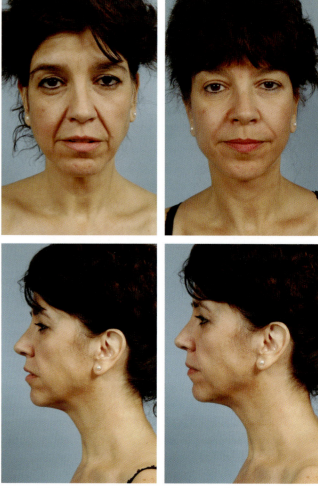

Figure 14-7   Patient 3. (Top and Bottom Left) Preoperative photographs. (Top and Bottom Right) Postoperative photographs taken following rhytidectomy.

Additionally, there should be no tension on the perilobular closure in order to avoid a "pixie" ear deformity (Figs. 14-5 to 14-7).

PEARLS

There are various technical points for safety that are relevant in this method of rhytidectomy. It is important to pay close attention to retraction during the procedure and to judiciously use local anesthetic to allow clear delineation of tissue planes. Sharp dissection allows for the most accuracy when dissecting the composite facial skin/SMAS flap. As described, it is safe to identify the SMAS-platysma

layer anterior to lobule, and this technique allows capture of the entire SMAS-platysma layer. Mobilization beyond "retaining ligaments" to area of mobile platysma allows the fixed points to be released prior to resetting of the facial flap. Close attention to detail must be maintained when performing cervical liposuction so as not to injure branches of the facial nerve.

SUGGESTED READING

Mustoe TA, Rawlani V, Zimmerman H. Modified deep plane rhytidectomy with a lateral approach to the neck: an alternative to submental incision and dissection. *Plast Reconstr Surg*. 2011;127:357.

Chapter 15. Short-Scar Facelift I

Hamid Massiha, MD

INDICATIONS

The technique of short-scar facelift is indicated in the entire spectrum of face and neck aging. Exceptions are uncommon and are limited to extreme aging and deformities unrelated to aging. In younger individuals, dissection is less extensive and could be more extensive as aging deformity is more advanced.

PREOPERATIVE PREPARATION

Patients are checked thoroughly for preexisting medical conditions. Standard, age-appropriate laboratory tests are done. If needed, medical clearance from their treating physicians is obtained. Anticoagulants are discontinued 10 days prior to surgery. Smokers are advised to discontinue smoking and use of all nicotine-containing substances, including gum and patches, at least 2 to 3 weeks preoperatively.

ANESTHESIA

Typically, general endotracheal anesthesia is recommended. However, this procedure could easily be done under local anesthesia with sedation especially in cases in patients with minimal skin ptosis. Local anesthesia with epinephrine is also injected (see details of procedure), allowing adequate time for the epinephrine to work. Because this maneuver minimizes bleeding, often, no hemostasis is required and no drains are needed.

POSITIONS AND MARKING

Markings are made at the preoperative holding area with the patient in a sitting position. This gives us one last chance to evaluate the patient's individual needs. Technical variances are made to accommodate each patient's case (Fig. 15-1).

The operation is done with the patient in the supine position. We usually do not use a headrest unless the patient has a neck problem. An extended neck may help in the judgment of the effectiveness and the efficiency of the vectors of traction.

DETAILS OF PROCEDURE

With the patient under appropriate anesthesia and in the supine position, the face and neck area is prepped and draped by the surgeon. The endotracheal tube is marked at the level of the front teeth and is held up until the sterile drape is placed under it. Next, the endotracheal tube is placed over an open blue cloth towel, which is then wrapped around the tube and fixed with a clamp to hold it on the patient's chest, thus holding the tube at the midline, out of the way of the surgeon yet readily available to the anesthesia personnel. This detail in draping gives direct access to the neck area. The endotracheal tube can be moved from one side to the other if central neck intervention is needed.

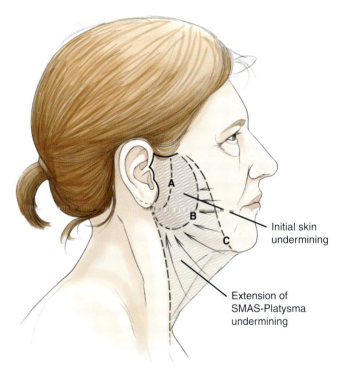

Figure 15-1 Preoperative markings. *Line A:* Initially some skin is removed. *Line B:* Skin dissection. *Line C:* SMAS-platysma dissection.

The operation is started by first infusing a total of 100 mL of a mixture of 0.5% lidocaine with epinephrine and 0.25% bupivacaine hydrochloride with epinephrine (50 mL per side). Adequate time should be allowed for the epinephrine to be effective (a minimum of 20 minutes). This minimizes bleeding to a level that makes the need for hemostasis rare. Suction drains are not usually necessary.

After deciding which side to do first (see Pearls section), the incision is made at the preauricular area. The incision travels in a manner that it follows the anatomical curves and it passes right at the top of the tragus (not inside of it) and is turned around the ear lobule. Usually, the identification of the superficial musculoaponeurotic system (SMAS) is facilitated if a strip of skin and fibrofatty tissue is removed initially from the preauricular area.

Skin dissection is done anteriorly toward the nose and nasolabial fold. As dissection turns toward the inferior aspect, it is limited to approximately 4 to 5 cm and very limited as dissection approaches the area under the ear lobule (Fig. 15-2).

SMAS dissection starts at the preauricular area and extends anteriorly to approximately 5 to 6 cm from the tragus and continues toward the jaw line. As soon as dissection reaches the platysma area it gets easy, and blunt spreading by just opening the blades of the scissors will suffice. If a surgeon has problems with blunt dissection using scissors, any blunt spreading instrument will be effective for the dissection. Dissection is complete whenever the traction on SMAS-platysma toward the ear pulls the vertical neck and jaw line adequately (see Fig. 15-2). It is an important step to release the platysma connection from the anterior border of the sternocleidomastoid muscle so as to gain mobility of SMAS-platysma flap. In less advanced cases, lesser dissection of both the skin and SMAS-platysma may suffice. In more advanced cases, dissection of SMAS-platysma may be extended to the midline of the neck. Usually, we do not use the midline incisions and midneck manipulation through this incision under the chin. Our observation is that a good lift with semivertical vectors will solve midneck problems adequately. Ultimately, the traction test mentioned above will dictate how much more dissection is needed.

The repair phase starts by fixing the SMAS in a higher position, usually vertical (close to 70 to 80 degrees vertical) to the superior preauricular area. Fixation continues with interrupted sutures (3-0 PDS [polydioxanone] sutures on an SH needle) toward and over the zygomatic arch. Often a dog ear of SMAS tissue is created over the zygomatic area that if left in place will enhance the cheeks, and in many patients may be desirable. If not so, it can be excised. SMAS is also fixed to deep fascia around the ear lobule (Fig. 15-3). As soon as SMAS is fixed in its new position, you will notice that skin has traveled upward, riding over the SMAS with no tension on it (because of connecting bands between skin and SMAS). At this stage,

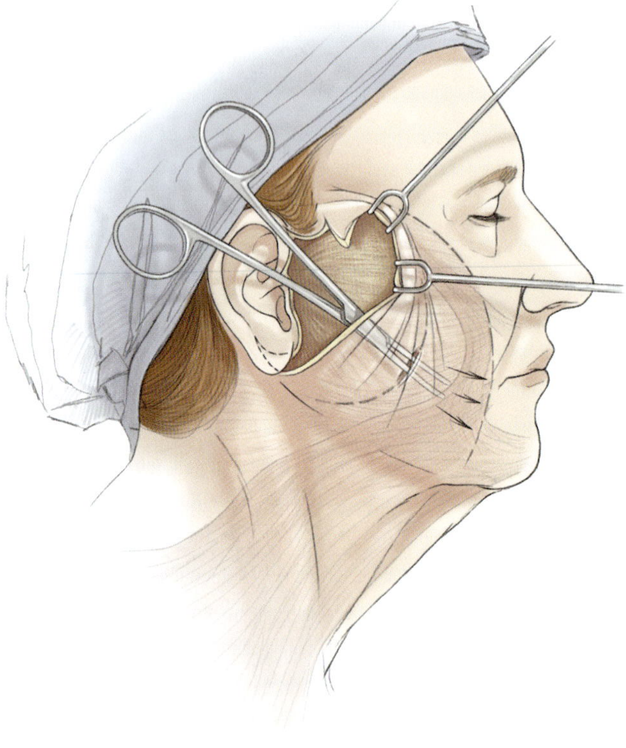

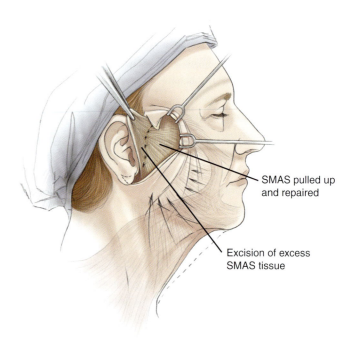

SMAS pulled up and repaired

Excision of excess SMAS tissue

Figure 15-2 Skin dissection completed. Scissors are under SMAS dissecting. SMAS-platysma layer.

Figure 15-3 SMAS is fixed in desired position with interrupted sutures. Excess is excised. Notice the different vectors for SMAS and skin. Also notice the posterior and anterior vectors.

skin is draped over and excess skin is removed with moderate tension. The only difficulty in this method of facelift is how to combat the bunching of skin (dog ear) at the temple and especially around the ear lobule area. The first facelift reported in 1910 by Lexer was a short, scar-type facelift with limited undermining. I have theorized that the reason the temple and occipital area incisions were added to the facelift procedures in the past was that surgeons were chasing the dog ears and adding incisions. This is a compelling reason to believe that a short-scar facelift is quite adequate for correction of aging problems. The dog ear at the temple area is dealt with by wedge excisions at the sideburn area and extended further, following the temporal hairline, if needed. The incision in this area should be vertical to the hair shafts; hair growth through the scar tissue may conceal the incision line.

LIMITING THE INCISION

There are several points that help minimize the size of dog ears in the postauricular area. Perhaps the most important point is not extending the incision around or behind the ear lobule until the very end of the procedure. It is true for all dog ears that the shorter the initial incision, the less prominent the dog ear will eventually be (eg, lateral eyelid incisions in blepharoplasty).

After excision of the dog ear, the skin at the post auricular area will still bulge. To decrease this bulge, the following maneuvers will help:

1. Defatting of the dermis.
2. Tucking the dermis down to the mastoid fascia and deep fascia under the ear lobule (thus there will be no tension on the ear lobule and it will be independent from the skin under it).
3. Further suturing between the sutures and on top of the small arching points of the skin edges to press it down to the deep fascia will further smooth out the suture line.
4. Posterior-anterior vector: This concept of pulling the skin from behind the ear anteriorly toward the postauricular crease is very helpful in reducing skin excess and correction of the posterior neck in advanced cases.

At completion, the incisions are closed with a running subcuticular suture of 4-0 PDS on a PS2 needle with buried knots. All guide sutures are then removed. The face and neck are bandaged with Kerlix and a 3-inch ace bandage. We do not use drains (Figs. 15-4 to 15-7).

PITFALLS

- After the SMAS lift is completed, skin may show dimples and unnatural pull. Simple dissection of distorted skin from the underlying SMAS will correct the problem.

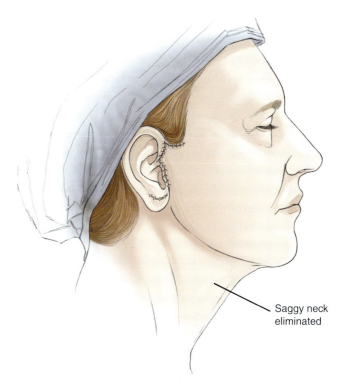

Figure 15-4 Short incision line follows natural lines of preauricular area. Neck laxity is eliminated.

- Difficulty may be encountered at the postauricular area in regard to the excess dog ear. You can extend the incision at the post auricular crease upward and pull the excess skin toward the crease then suture deep dermis to mastoid fascia with posterior anterior vectors.
- On the first attempt, performing a short-scar facelift and dealing with postauricular dog ears may be frustrating. I encourage the less-experienced surgeon not to give up. If needed, extend the incision at the postauricular area as high as is required. If redundant skin still exists, make a short, horizontal incision to eliminate the excess skin. You may consider using incisions horizontally behind the cartilaginous part of the ear lobe instead of the mastoid area.

PEARLS

- If in preoperative evaluation it is noticed that one side is more advanced than the other (a relatively common occurrence), the advanced side should be done first and more aggressively.
- Do not incise skin behind the ear lobe until the very end of the surgery. This will reduce dog ears immensely.
- In the area of the cheek, skin dissection is carried further than the SMAS toward the nasolabial fold. The SMAS is not very mobile in this area, so adequate skin dissection must be done to accomplish correction in this area.

- Vectors are more horizontal anterior posterior in the cheek area.
- Suturing the dermis down to the mastoid and deep fascia will reduce dog ears and prevent descent of skin downward resulting in a deformity of the ear lobule. Also this will re-create the normal depression between the mastoid bone and the angle of the mandible.
- Dividing the excess skin of dog ears to equal sections and suturing the dermis to the deep fascia is very helpful in tucking the skin down and flattening the dog ears.
- SMAS dissection should be started in the preauricular area close to the skin incision line.

- Excess SMAS should be removed after it is adequately lifted.
- Triangulating excess skin and placing guide sutures first below the tragus and then above the tragus are helpful. A third suture is placed in the ear lobule area.
- An important point concerning suctioning of the neck area is that it should be conservative. I believe a layer of fat under the dermis is a good cover for the platysma bands and irregularities of the neck anatomy. Also important in the issue of suction is not overdoing it at the region of the jaw line. After lifting the flap, the thin skin may end up at the jaw line and give it a skeletonized appearance.

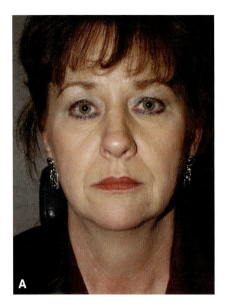
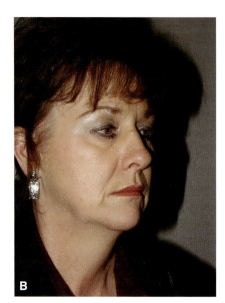
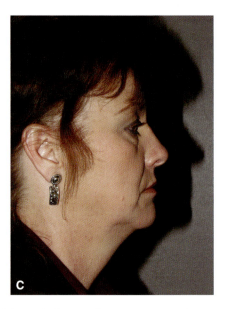

Figure 15-5   Before photo of a 50-year-old short-scar facelift patient. Suction lipectomy of the neck done at the same time. Patient also had simultaneous upper and lower blepharoplasty.

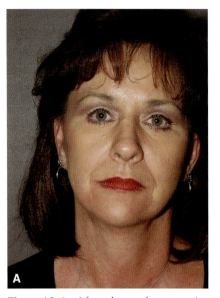
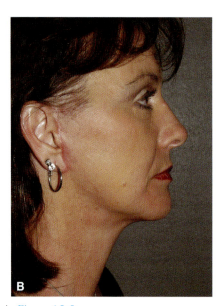
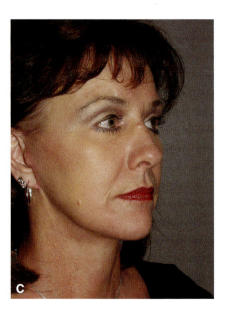

Figure 15-6   After photo of same patient as in Figure 15-5.

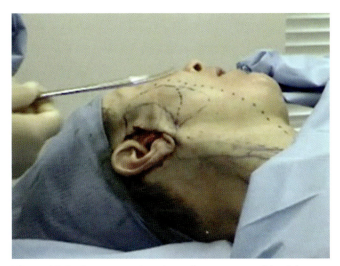

Figure 15-7 Intraoperative photo demonstrates skin tightening result because of SMAS-platysma fixation.

- All suturing in this procedure is done with 4-0 PDS sutures on PS2 needles. The only exception is for SMAS repair, which is done using a 3-0 PDS suture on an SH needle.

SUGGESTED READING

Massiha H. Combined skin and skin-muscle flap technique in lower blepharoplasty: a 10-year experience. *Ann Plast Surg.* 1990;25:467.

Massiha H. Short scar face lift with extended SMAS platysma dissection and lifting and limited skin undermining. *Plast Reconstr Surg.* 2003;112:663.

Mitz V, Peyronie M. The superficial musculo-apo-neurotic system (SMAS) in the parotid and cheek area. *Plast Reconstr Surg.* 1976;58:50.

Stuzin J, Baker T, Gordon H. The relationship of superficial and deep facial fascias: relevance to rhytidectomy and aging. *Plast Reconstr Surg.* 1992;89:441.

Chapter 16. Short-Scar II: Short-Scar Facelift with Barbed Suture and Fibrin Sealant

Alan Matarasso, MD; David Shafer, MD, FACS

INDICATIONS

The indications for the short-scar facelift with fibrin sealant and barbed suture include the patient with the appropriate anatomy desiring facial rejuvenation classically addressed via a traditional facelift incision.

PREOPERATIVE PREPARATION

Careful preoperative planning, consultation, and communication with the patient are essential. For instance, patients with midface, jowl, and neck laxity are candidates for this procedure. With experience, even patients with excessive, thin, loose neck tissue or massive weight loss can achieve excellent results. Patients are counseled to stop all medications affecting coagulation and herbal supplements, cease smoke exposure, and use antimicrobials topically and orally. Furthermore, patients must be appropriately evaluated and approved medically, have surgery performed in an accredited facility, and be carefully monitored postoperatively.

ANESTHESIA

Anesthesia may be administered by either monitored conscious sedation or general anesthesia (including laryngeal mask anesthesia). A local anesthetic solution of 200 mL of normal saline (NS), 100 mL of 1% lidocaine and 1 mL of 1:1000 epinephrine is infiltrated with 20 mL syringes through 20-gauge spinal needles into the operative field.

POSITION AND MARKINGS

Patients are marked in the seated position prior to the induction of anesthesia. Areas for fat removal, replacement, or repositioning are determined. Incisions are demarcated inferior to the submental crease, and in a continuous line beginning horizontally below the sideburn (according to their hair pattern), then continuing around the ear (pre- or posttragal) to the lobule into the postauricular fold stopping at the mastoid bone or at the first crease formed when retracting the ear laterally (Fig. 16-1). The patient is then placed on the operating table in the supine position, with minimal flexion and with his or her head resting on a doughnut cushion prior to induction of anesthesia.

OPERATIVE PREPARATION

Sequential pneumatic compression devices are placed and the anesthesiologist administers systemic anesthesia. The local anesthetic solution is injected widely in the subcutaneous plane. Broad-spectrum intravenous antibiotics, antiemetics, and corticosteroids are administered and the patient is prepped and draped in a sterile fashion. A cotton pledget soaked in povidone-iodine (Betadine) is

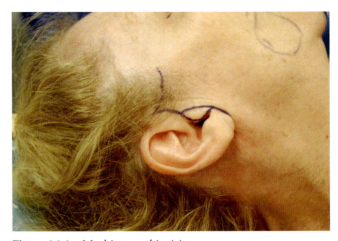

Figure 16-1 Markings and incision.

placed in the ear prior to the initial incision. During the procedure, the patient's head position is rotated to the degree that they are able to tolerate as indicated, and the anesthesia tube is mobilized accordingly.

DETAILS OF THE PROCEDURE

The operation begins with a submental incision and liposuction of the subcutaneous fat of the neck with a 2.4-mm Mercedes cannula. Any additional sites of the face, nasolabial folds, and jowls are liposuctioned with a 1.8-mm Mercedes cannula as indicated. Wide submental subcutaneous dissection is then carried out exposing the medial edges of the platysma. A wide strip of platysma is excised in the midline to reduce redundant platysma muscle (Fig. 16-2). When indicated, submuscular fat is excised or melted by electrocautery under direct vision using a ball-tipped cautery. The medial edges of the platysma are placed on traction and the muscle is backcut laterally at the level of the hyoid bone. A midline plication is then performed with a 3-0 Mersilene suture continuously running from the level of the hyoid bone to the chin. A second layer of interrupted sutures is then placed as reinforcement and to help contour any irregularities. The medial plication assists in defining the cervicomental angle and this deepening recruits excess skin into the submental hollow similar to the concept of skin needed after fat removal in a blepharoplasty. The submental incision is packed with gauze and left open until the remainder of the facelift procedure is complete to allow for final hemostasis.

The premarked incision is then made with a no. 10 blade beginning at the horizontal sideburn cut and ending in the postauricular sulcus. Wide subcutaneous dissection is performed under direct vision sharply with facelift scissors. The dissection extends posteriorly beyond the sternocleidomastoid muscle, anteriorly

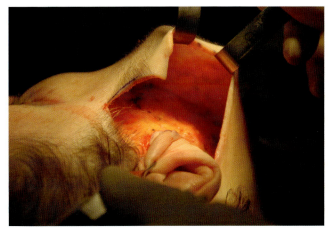

Figure 16-3   Wide subcutaneous dissection.

across the cheek and along the jowl, and inferiorly in the neck. Submental dissection is done in continuity to both sides (Fig. 16-3). Appropriate retaining ligaments are undermined or preserved according to the patient's anatomy and the desired result. The superficial musculoaponeurotic system (SMAS) layer is identified and a plication or imbrication is outlined so that the vector of pull is oriented in inverted 'L' -type pattern with the apex of the 2 limbs at the angle of the zygoma and parallel to the nasolabial fold. Plication is performed with a 2-0 PDO bidirectional, barbed (Quill) suture (Angiotech, Vancouver, BC, Canada), beginning at the angle of the zygoma (horizontal limb) and parallel to the nasolabial fold and running it across the zygoma with one end of the suture (Fig. 16-4). The second end of the suture (vertical limb) is run preauricularly completing the SMAS and around the earlobe to the lateral edge of the platysma 3 to 4 cm below the angle of the mandible and securing it to the mastoid fascia

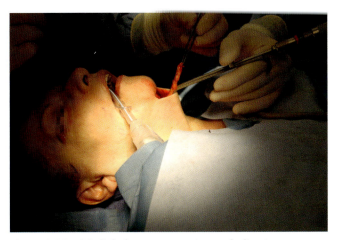

Figure 16-2   Medial platysma resection and plication.

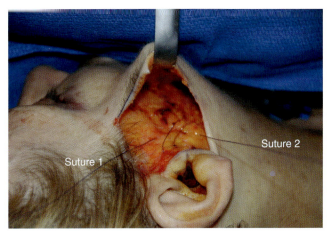

Figure 16-4   Superolateral platysma plication with barbed suture.

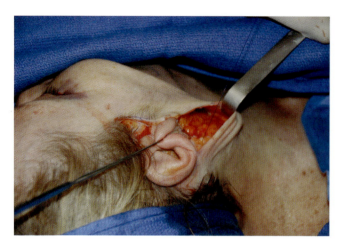

Figure 16-5 Posterolateral platysma plication with barbed suture.

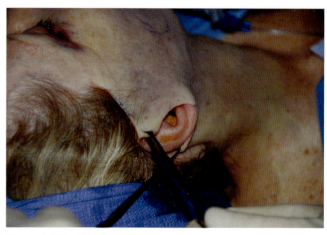

Figure 16-7 Skin flap vector.

(Fig. 16-5). At either end, the suture is repeatedly imbricated to secure it. The ball-tip electrocautery is then used for aggressive subcutaneous tissue contouring and hemostasis (Fig. 16-6).

The skin flaps are then grasped by the assistant at the level of the ear helix with an Allis clamp and posteriorly with a skin hook; these instruments are then crisscrossed. The Allis clamp is then retracted in an oblique and cephalic direction, assuring adequate skin removal while adjusting the wound edge to manage dog-ear formation at the medial end of the incision. Posteriorly, the skin hook is retracted vertically, making frequent adjustments, so that the mandible no longer represents a "border" to the advancement of the neck skin (Fig. 16-7). The skin is incised 5-0 nylon sutures are placed at the root of the helix and the tragus. Excess skin is then trimmed. Dog-ear formation can be managed in the horizontal sideburn cut by adjustment of the orientation of

the skin flap, blunt undermining at the end of the incision, or by removal of a wedge in the form of an inverted V in the midpoint of the sideburn hair. Posteriorly, after skin trimming despite a wide gap between the edge of the ear and the skin flap, a dog ear is often avoided by (a) first insetting the lobe appropriately, and then (b) progressively walking out the disparity in wound edges by purse-stringing the skin flap to the cuff of ear skin (Fig. 16-8) closing the wound.

The fibrin sealant is then sprayed in an even, thin layer on the undersurface of the flap and the raw dissected surfaces within 1 minute (3 to 5 mL for the face, brow) (Fig. 16-9). The assistant then applies uniform external pressure to the flaps with 2 moist gauzes for 3 minutes. While pressure is applied, the surgeon finishes closing the preauricular incision with running 5-0 nylon and the postlobule incision with staples (Fig. 16-10). Of note, no deep sutures or drains are placed in this procedure. The

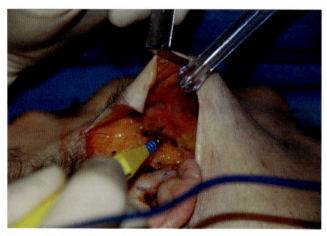

Figure 16-6 Ball-tip electrocautery subcutaneous contouring and hemostasis.

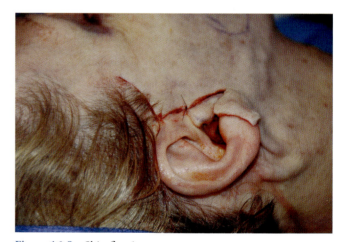

Figure 16-8 Skin flap inset.

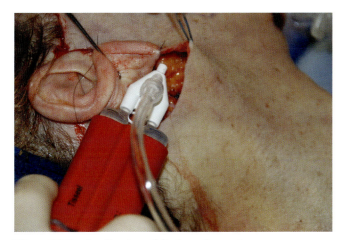

Figure 16-9 Application of fibrin sealant using a spray.

purpose of the sealant is to eliminate the routine use of drains; we have found that drains exacerbate any postauricular skin bunching. There are often technical issues with drains (eg, leaking, premature removal), potential for infection, and, generally, patients often prefer not to have them.

At the completion of the first side, the patient is turned and the opposite side is completed in a similar fashion. Attention then returns to the submental region. The area is inspected for hemostasis and the remaining sealant is sprayed into the submental pocket. Excess sealant is milked out and pressure is accomplished by a lap pad that slings under the neck and is pulled cephalically. The submental incision is closed with a subcuticular Prolene and interrupted 5-0 nylon sutures. The dressing consists of opened 4 × 8 gauze pads that are folded in half length-wise; one is placed postauricularly and the other preauricularly, with an open gauze layer covering both of these. Over these we place a surginct to secure the gauze.

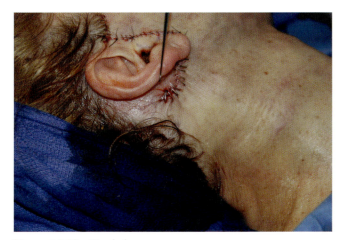

Figure 16-10 Final closure.

Patents are observed overnight and follow up in the office for routine sutures removed (Figs. 16-11 and 12) at 5-7 days.

POTENTIAL PITFALLS

- The short incision narrows the operative field and limits access to the orbicularis oculi muscle and the temporalis muscle (unless a sideburn flap is elevated or a counter incision is used to expose the temporalis fascia).
- The short-scar technique may cause temporary bunching in the temporal and postauricular regions (dog ears). This should be minimized intraoperatively as described. Small residual bunching in the postauricular area quickly resolves in the postoperative period.
- Performing a short-scar facelift requires a learning curve for appropriate redraping and removal of skin.
- Smaller incisions are utilized with traditional wide dissection and this necessitates adjustment in flap rotation.
- Barbed sutures provide a secure SMAS-platysma plication, and they are not easily "backed out." Additionally, excessive tension in the mastoid region may lead to "slip" of the suture and so the sutures should be locked in multiple dissections.
- Fibrin sealant is ideal for use over small areas of oozing and over large raw surfaces (ie, used for predominantly for flap apposition and in avoiding drains); fibrin sealant is not primarily used for hemostasis and is not indicated for arterial bleeding.
- Application of the glue without the aerosolized sprayer may cause clumping and deposition of too much glue, which can lead to improper coaptation of the flaps.

PEARLS

- Medial platysma muscle excision assists in removing neck redundancy not solely attributed to excess skin or muscle that cannot be tightened laterally.
- Furthermore, maximizing the medial plication of the platysma allows redundant skin to fill the submental hollow.
- Reduced incision length may ultimately shorten operative time and may reduce the postoperative recovery period. It avoids any hair loss or hairline displacement. It eliminates the most frequent area of scar revision over the mastoid bone encountered with the traditional incision.
- Barbed sutures (Quill, Angiotech, Vancouver, BC, Canada) allow a secure, running, knotless advancement of the SMAS-platysma layer.
- Fibrin sealant reduces dead space in coapting the flaps, which purportedly decreases postoperative bleeding,

PHOTOGRAPHY

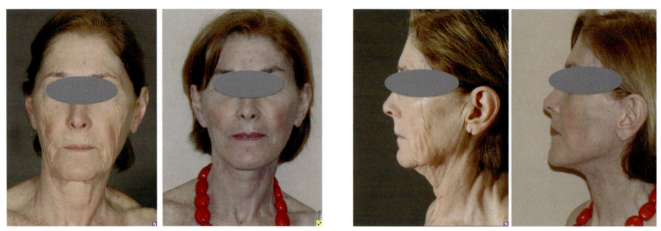

Figure 16-11   The patient is shown before and 2 months after short-scar facelift and lateral temporal brow lift.

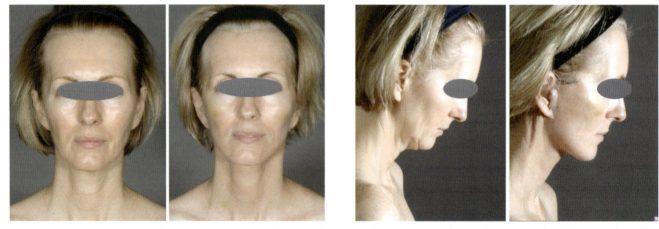

Figure 16-12   Preoperative and postoperative views of a second patient. She is shown before and 2 weeks after short-scar facelift.

edema, and pain. It eliminates the routine use of suction drains.

• Use of the spray applicator for the fibrin sealant facilitates mixing of the product and the atomizer helps to evenly distribute the sealant.

SUGGESTED READING

Marchac D, Sandor G. Face lifts and sprayed fibrin glue: an outcome analysis of 200 patients. *Br J Plast Surg.* 1994;47: 306-309.

Matarasso A, Elkwood A, Rankin M, Elkowitz M. National plastic surgery survey: face lift techniques and complications. *Plast Reconstr Surg.* 2000;106(5):1185-1195.

Matarasso A, Rizk S, Markowitz J. Short scar face-lift with the use of fibrin sealant. *Dermatol Clin.* 2005;23:495-504.

Matarasso A, Rizk S. Use of fibrin sealant in short scar facelift. In: Saltz R, ed. *Tissue Glues in Cosmetic Surgery.* St. Louis, MO: Quality Medical; 2003:133-147.

Pitanguy I, Radwanski H, Matarasso A. Approach to face and neck after weight loss. In: Rubin P, Matarasso A, eds. *Aesthetic Surgery after Massive Weight Loss.* Edinburgh, UK: Elsevier; 2007.

Chapter 17

Extended SMAS Rhytidectomy

Bruce F. Connell, MD, FACS; Scott R. Miller, MD, FACS

INDICATIONS

The indications for this method of rhytidectomy include patients with moderate to advanced facial aging, reflective of laxity of the soft tissues and their musculofascial support system, who desire top-quality, definitive facial rejuvenation with thoughtful tissue repositioning and discrete incisions (Fig. 17-1). The following is a basic technique, which is modified for each patient and for each side of the face, according to the specific anatomical problem.

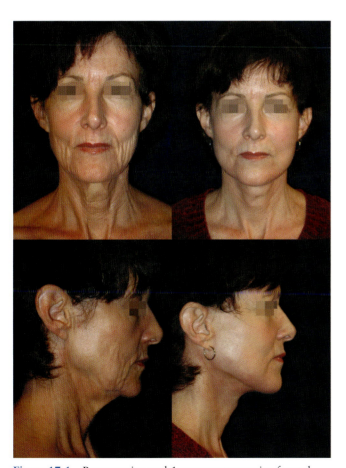

Figure 17-1 Preoperative and 1-year postoperative frontal and lateral views following extended SMAS rhytidectomy. Proper use of the SMAS allows volume redistribution and restoration to a more youthful appearance. This procedure elevates the tissue as a unit, thereby providing sling support from the malar to the submental regions.

PREOPERATIVE PREPARATION

The patient's medical status, prior operations and procedures, and results anticipated by both patient and surgeon should be reviewed. Each patient presents individual problems that require precise anatomical diagnosis, appropriate architectural planning, and skillfully executed repair. Without a thorough history, evaluation, and discussion of goals and expectations, surgery is ill-advised.

ANESTHESIA

Local infiltration, in combination with either full general anesthesia, total intravenous anesthesia (TIVA), or conscious sedation is appropriate for this procedure.

POSITION AND MARKINGS

The entire face and neck should be evaluated at rest and in animation. It is important to assess the skin redundancy with the shoulders down and with regard to quantity and vector of necessary removal. Abnormal fat accumulations, platysma laxity, and salivary gland and digastric muscle abnormalities are also marked.

DETAILS OF THE PROCEDURE

Incisions

The incisions are marked with attention to natural contour, texture, and skin tones. Respecting the hairline relative to the planned quantity and vector of skin shift determines incision at the sideburn margin versus in the temporal hair. The incision is then carried caudally at the anterior edge of the helical cartilage along the natural color change. It is passed deep into the depression superior to the tragus and then along the edge of the tragus. The V-shaped flap this creates upon inset and closure prevents scar contracture. The incision at the lower end of the tragus must be perpendicular to the long axis, thus defining the tragal height and preventing a subtragal skin fold. A planned incision 2 to 3 mm below the ear-cheek junction preserves the natural transition and avoids beard growth in an area difficult to shave.

With proper shift vectors, the postauricular scar does not descend. Consequently, the incision should be in the crease, not on the posterior surface of the ear. Extension posteriorly above or at the hairline depends on preoperative assessment of the amount and direction of neck skin to be removed. This is determined by pinching excessive skin with the patient seated during the preoperative examination. If incision at the hairline is chosen, a return behind the hairline at the fine hair at the nape of the neck with recipient site cut out and flap inset is necessary to maintain natural hair progression and prevent scar visibility. The submental incision, when necessary, is made posterior to the osseocutaneous adherence/crease. This allows release and redrape anteriorly, as well as mobility for exposure of fat, muscle, and/or glandular modifications.

Undermining

Skin flap elevation is to the malar eminence, more limited in the buccal region, and more extensive in the cervical region, and is based on skin laxity and crease release needs (Fig. 17-2).

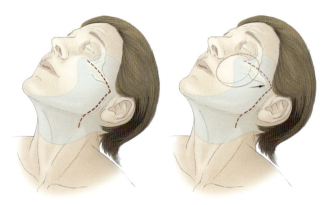

Figure 17-3 High transverse SMAS incision enables improvement of the midface and perioral region not available with a lower approach.

Deep-Tissue Modifications

In all except those rare patients with only excessive skin, a superior facelift result is not possible without modification of the deep-layer support composed of superficial musculoaponeurotic system (SMAS) and platysma. When utilized appropriately, the SMAS can provide support for the submental area, hyoid area, jowls, angle of the mouth, nasolabial fold, lower orbicularis oculi, and orbital septum. Although the choice of deep-layer modification is dependent on the patient's deformities, almost all patients will benefit from a posterior-superior rotation of the cheek SMAS about a pivot point situated over the malar eminence (Fig. 17-3).

The transverse incision of the SMAS is made over the upper part of the zygomatic arch and high onto the malar bone. This is done with careful elevation on each side as the incision is made with scissors, moving anteriorly. The same technique is used for the vertical portion, moving caudally over the parotid fasciae, 1 cm anterior to the tragus and along the anterior border of the sternocleidomastoid muscle (Fig. 17-4).

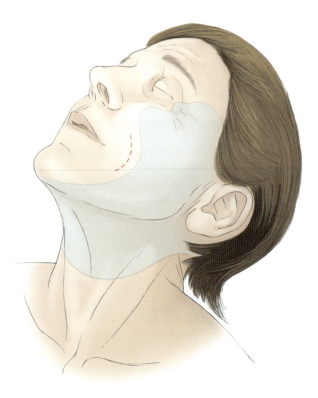

Figure 17-2 Limited skin-flap elevation in buccal region maintains SMAS connections and vascular supply, allowing deep-layer support structurally and nutritionally.

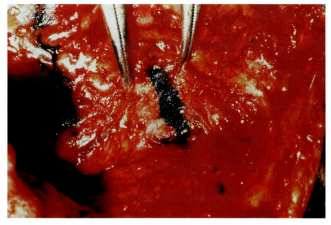

Figure 17-4 Two-clamp elevation method for SMAS incision provides protection for the underlying tissues.

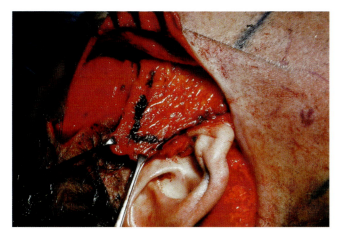

Figure 17-5 Posterior-superior retraction of the SMAS achieves desired clinical endpoints.

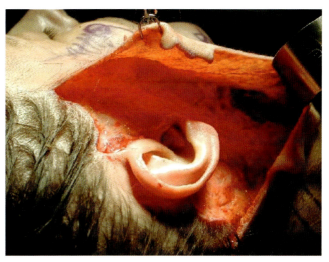

Figure 17-6 Transilluminated skin-flap technique allows even cutaneous elevation with preservation of SMAS, as well as subcutaneous vascular arcade.

Using Allis forceps on the edge, gently holding up and proximally, the SMAS is elevated distally. The endpoint is determined by the achievement of the desired movement and support to the orbicularis oculi and orbital septum, the upper nasolabial fold, the angle of the mouth, and the lateral upper lip. Commonly, this involves liberation to the origin of the zygomaticus major muscle cephalad and the anterior edge of the parotid fasciae inferior to this level.

Retraction posterosuperiorly is followed by a pilot cut and insetting with 4-0 nylon (Fig. 17-5). Often, a transposition flap approximately 1 cm wide is fashioned from the excess SMAS anterior to the ear and rotated posteriorly. Mild tension on this flap should show visible support at the level of the hyoid. It is then secured to the mastoid fasciae. The remainder of the SMAS is then inset, trimming or folding it upon itself, depending on the volumetric needs. Subsequent to this, submental platysmaplasty is performed as necessary, followed by submandibular contouring.

In regard to the dissection technique for performing a primary or secondary SMAS support facelift surgery, it is essential to be able to elevate the skin without damaging the underlying SMAS. The dissection is greatly aided by using transillumination instead of direct light (Fig. 17-6). When the skin is elevated in the proper plane, which is just below the hair bulbs in men, and for other patients, the flap should have the appearance of cobblestones and the subdermal vessels are visible and not damaged. With transillumination, if the dissection becomes too superficial, the skin flap loses the appearance of the cobblestones and appears brighter. If the dissection goes deeper, the skin flap appears to be darker. Sharp dissection avoids the occasional damage to the SMAS. For almost all patients who have secondary facelifts, a sufficient amount of strong SMAS tissue can be found to enhance and make the best deep-layer support. With primary patients, we have never encountered a patient who did not have an adequate SMAS to provide proper submental support,

elevation of the depressed angle of the mouth, flattening of the upper and lower nasolabial folds, and changing the nasojugal groove from the diagonal of old age closer to the horizontal direction of youth. If the SMAS flap is designed to accomplish the required factors, the upper transection of the SMAS is at the top of the zygomatic arch or sometimes higher. Otherwise the periorbital effect and the effect on the angle of the mouth and upper nasolabial fold would be lost and a lower transection would permit only improvement of the anterior cheek and around the mouth. In addition, the skin should not be separated from the SMAS in the anterior cheek because there are connections that would give support to the skin and remove the tension from the incisions along the temporal hairline and the ear.

Closure

The D'Assumpcão facelift clamp is used for skin redraping in a superoposterior vector. Primary tension points are at the scalp-helical junction and the occipital-mastoid hairline. Tragal borders are inset with no tension as is the earlobe, which is set at 12 to 15 degrees posterior to the long axis of the ear for an unoperated appearance. In other areas, skin is trimmed with 2 to 3 mm of excess, avoiding any unwarranted and noncontributory tension. To facilitate precise tensionless skin tailoring in the tragal closure, a finger is pressed in the pretragal concavity. This avoids any possibility of anterior tragal distortion. To avoid the shift of beard onto hairless areas in males, excision and electrocoagulation of beard hair bulbs are used (Fig. 17-7).

Final closure is routinely done with 6-0 nylon in an interrupted fashion anteriorly. Along hairlines, 4-0 nylon half-buried mattress sutures are used.

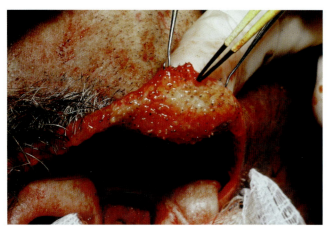

Figure 17-7　Electrocoagulation and excision of beard hair bulbs avoids tragal hair growth.

Dressings

Dressings can place pressure on delicate skin flaps. This factor can decrease venous return, contributing to edema or skin compromise. Dressings can conceal an incipient or full-blown problem. Most are tight, confining, obstruct hearing, complicate hygiene, and attract undue attention. A small, loose wrap that confines the hair is appreciated by most patients and is removed the next day.

PITFALLS

Surgeons are misled regarding the amount and direction of skin removal required by only examining the neck skin excess with the patient lying on the operating table. This position elevates the shoulders and creates the appearance of excessive skin perpendicular to the sternocleidomastoid muscle. This is a frequent cause of excessive skin removal, resulting in postauricular wide scars and scar descent.

An incision in the submental crease contributes to a double chin on downward gaze and to "a witch's chin." This also accentuates the crease and does not allow for the needed mobility and exposure without excessive traction.

Securing the submental platysmaplasty before superolateral support can limit utility of the SMAS in cephalad volumetric rejuvenation and restoration of youthful facial proportion.

If the shift of the deep layers is not visible at the time of surgery, it means the SMAS liberation was inadequate.

PEARLS

It is helpful to review the patient's youthful photographs when planning a pleasing and natural-appearing surgical rejuvenation.

All people have, to some degree or another, a larger side of their face, including soft tissue and bone structure.

Often, the smaller side appears older than the larger side. Making this observation clear to patients prior to surgery helps in precise diagnosis and planning. It also eliminates postoperative misinterpretation by the patient, whose face will be subjected to closer scrutiny.

The technique chosen for one area of improvement should not destroy the full potential of the SMAS support and movement of the tissues or create unbalanced tightening.

Patients with vertically short platysma muscles or tight bands are best treated by some form of localized muscle interruption and release.

If the patient smiles and suddenly looks much older because of deep orbital smile creases ("crow's feet"), then this problem needs to be corrected. Separation of dermal attachments and transection obliquely of the orbicularis muscle corresponding to a natural skin crease address this issue. Transection must begin 3 mm anterior to the lateral orbicularis oculi muscle edge and be beveled.

Despite the application of conventional techniques, when bulging persists just lateral to the midline in the

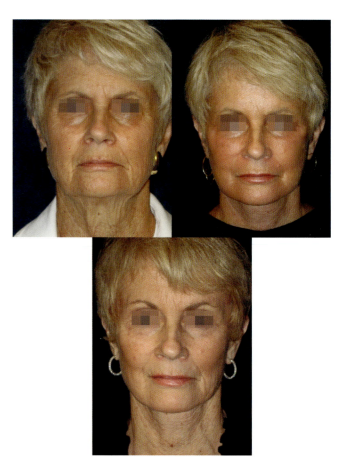

Figure 17-8　Preoperative, 6-month, and 10-year postoperative frontal views following extended SMAS rhytidectomy. The SMAS deep-layer support provides lasting contour to the anterior cheek, corners of the mouth, jowl/jawline, and neck over time.

submental region and is accentuated when the neck is flexed, a large bulky anterior belly of the digastric muscle should be considered as the etiology. In such cases, tangential excision with closed suction draining of the subplatysmal space can prevent residual fullness.

The proper direction of flap shift is perpendicular to the targeted skin folds.

SUMMARY

Public sophistication and expectations have forced surgeons to rethink accepted concepts. The basic deep-layer support technique presented can be utilized for most patients. With accurate diagnosis, appropriately conceived and executed procedures, and thoughtful postoperative care, complications are rare and patient and surgeon satisfaction are high (Fig. 17-8).

SUGGESTED READING

Connell BF, Marten TJ. Facelift. In: Cohen M, ed. *Mastery in Plastic Surgery*. Boston, MA: Little Brown; 1994:1873-1902.

Connell BF, Miller SR, Gonzalez-Miramontes H. Skin and SMAS flaps for facial rejuvenation. In: Achauer BM, Eriksson E, Guyuron B, et al, eds. *Plastic Surgery: Indications, Operations, and Outcomes*. St. Louis, MO: Mosby; 2000:2583-2607.

Connell BF, Semlacher RA. Contemporary deep layer facial rejuvenation. *Plast Reconstr Surg*. 1997;100:1513-1523.

Rees TD, Aston SJ. Clinical evaluation of results of submusculoaponeurotic dissection and fixation in facelift. *Plast Reconstr Surg*. 1977;60:851.

Stuzin JM, Baker HL. The relationship of superficial and deep fascias relevance to rhytidectomy and aging. *Plast Reconstr Surg*. 1989;83:265-271.

Chapter 18

The MACS-Lift Rhytidectomy

Lee E. Edstrom, MD

INDICATIONS

The short-scar technique is ideal for the younger patient, generally between 45 and 65 years of age, who still has some skin elasticity and does not have a lot of redundant neck skin. The suspension technique for superficial musculoaponeurotic system (SMAS) elevation is used whether or not a short scar is used. As described by Tonnard and Verpaele, an ellipse of skin can be excised from the posterior hairline to treat the patient with more neck redundancy.

PREOPERATIVE PREPARATION

Preoperative consultation should determine the patient's suitability for facial rejuvenation, whether they are adequately healthy and with realistic expectations. Prior facial surgeries, a history of bleeding problems or smoking are necessary to ascertain. Nonsteroidal antiinflammatory drugs (NSAIDs) should be discontinued 2 weeks prior to surgery.

ANESTHESIA

General anesthesia or MAC (monitored anesthesia care, or local with sedation) are suitable for this procedure. Generally patients are sent home after this procedure and MAC facilitates and expedites the recovery. The neck is infiltrated with 30 mL of 0.5% Xylocaine and epinephrine 1:500,000, and 40 mL of the same is used on each side of the face, using a 22-gauge spinal needle to infiltrate and hydrodissect the subcutaneous plane.

POSITION AND MARKINGS

The patient is marked in the preop holding area, where he or she can cooperate in the sitting position. I mark the extent of the cervicomental fat excess, and identify the spot on the malar prominence where the most effective midface lift would be achieved (Fig. 18-1). Marking for ancillary procedures such as fillers is done at this time as well.

INCISION AND EXPOSURE

The incision is carried through the sideburn from the anterior hairline to the preauricular skin in a curvilinear fashion (Fig. 18-2), and from there in standard fashion along the preauricular skin crease onto the tragal edge and back out and down to the base of the lobule. It is not necessary to extend the incision behind the ear. Access to the cervicomental fat is done through a single stab wound in the submental skin crease.

DETAILS OF THE PROCEDURE

Suction-assisted lipectomy (SAL) of the neck is done through a submental stab wound, using a 2.7-mm canula, and a variable amount is taken, depending on the patient. All fat taken is preplatysmal.

Flap Elevation

I prefer to elevate the cheek with the tips of my scissors up, holding tension on the skin edge, and not under direct

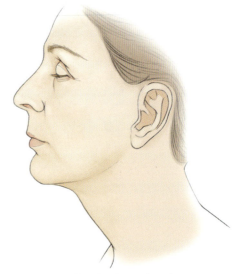

Figure 18-1   Maximal malar fat pad mobility.

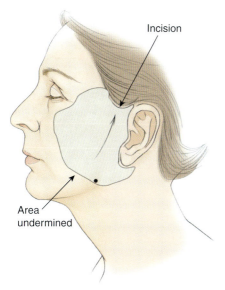

Figure 18-2 Extent of curvilinear incision from the sideburn at the anterior hairline to the preauricular skin.

vision, but this is a surgeon's preference. Flap elevation is carried out to include the angle of the mandible, the central cheek to within a centimeter of the nasolabial crease, and the malar prominence.

Suspension Sutures

With the skin flap elevated and hemostasis obtained, a hemostat is used to spread down to the deep temporal fascia in the immediate preauricular hollow above the zygomatic arch. The superficial temporal vessels are usually encountered here and preserved if possible.

A 2-0 PDS (polydioxanone) suture on a large-taper needle is then passed through the fascia, and threaded through the substance of the SMAS caudad to the angle of the jaw, where a forceps is used to determine the spot of maximum effect, at which traction upward on the SMAS provides the most effective lift of neck and jowl. At that point the stitch is turned back and threaded back through the SMAS cephalad to the preauricular start.

Another 2-0 PDS suture is started in the same fascia, but directed this time to the oral commissure, where once again a toothed forceps is used to identify the point of maximal effect on the jowl and oral commissure when elevated up and back. This stitch is then threaded back through the SMAS and tied, using a smooth-jawed needle holder to grasp the knot.

A hemostat is now used to spread vertically through the orbicularis oculi just lateral to the lateral orbital rim at the level of the lateral canthus, down to the deep temporal fascia. A third 2-0 PDS is placed in the fascia and threaded through the malar fat pad to the point previously marked, and then brought back, and tied at the level of the fascia. This effectively lifts the malar fat pad, resulting in a midface lift.

SKIN CLOSURE

The key to closure is upward rotation of the skin flap, excising the sideburn skin on the flap, and then carefully fitting the flap into the preauricular incision. The resultant tightness at the base of the lobule is dealt with by excising a crescent of skin below the lobule to allow the lobule to fit without tension into the elevated skin flap (Figs. 18-3 and 18-4). If bleeding has been a problem during the procedure, a Penrose drain is placed under the flap at the lobule; otherwise no drains are used.

LOWER-EYELID PINCH BLEPHAROPLASTY

A routine part of the MACS-lift is the correction of lower-eyelid redundancy encountered when the malar fat pad is elevated. The correction is done using the pinch technique, with suture line just under the lash line. Because of the strong midface lift directly supporting the lower lid, lateral canthal suspension or tightening is seldom necessary.

THE NECK AND PLATYSMA

The neck is very effectively dealt with using this technique. In most cases, the liposuction is a key element in the improvement, and the 2 lateral suspension sutures lift the SMAS up and back, correcting the skin and platysmal redundancy in the neck. The platysma is purposely not brought together in the midline, as that would work against the superior-lateral suspension in the opposite direction. A joining in the midline, however, is reserved as an effective secondary procedure at a later time.

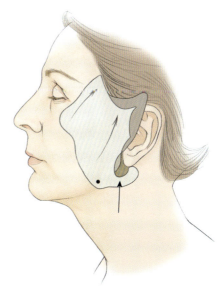

Figure 18-3 Excision of a crescent of skin below the ear lobule to reduce tightness at the base of the lobule and fit without tension into the elevated skin flap; skin excision after elevation.

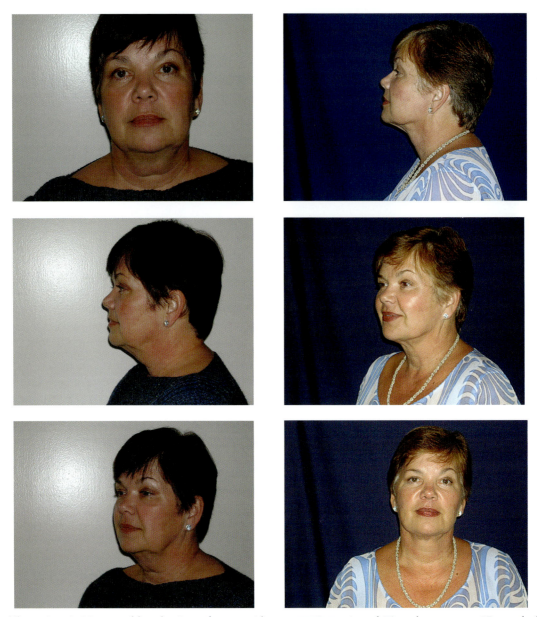

Figure 18-4   The patient is 58 years old at the time of surgery (the pre op pictures), and 59 at the post ops, 17 months later. She had the operation described in the text.

PITFALLS

- Risk to the facial nerve branches is less using this technique, because the SMAS is not elevated.
- The preauricular skin flap should be inset with no tension, and the lobule set into the crescent excision without tension to avoid lobular distortion.
- The usual care must be taken to avoid overdoing skin excision in the lower eyelid, even though the strong midface elevation provides considerable protection against lid retraction.
- Take care that the dressing does not put too much pressure on the preauricular flaps.

PEARLS

When the SMAS has been suspended with the 2-0 PDS loops, there may be surface irregularities, which should be carefully trimmed with the convex surface of the scissors so that the skin rests on a smooth SMAS layer.

SUGGESTED READING

Tonnard P, Verpaele A, Monstrey S, et al. Minimal access cranial suspension lift: a modified S-lift. *Plast Reconstr Surg.* 2002;109(6):2074-2086.

Tonnard P, Verpaele A. The MACS-lift short scar rhytidectomy. *Aesthet Surg J.* 2007;27(2):188-198.

Chapter 19. Short-Scar Facelift with Round-Block SMAS Treatment

Ithamar Nogueira Stocchero, MD

INDICATIONS

This technique is a superficial musculoaponeurotic system (SMAS) suspension method, and although a small undermining is usually done, it may be useful in any rhytidectomy involving subcutaneous undermining. Considering that this technique is essentially a purse-string suture, a great reduction in the surgical wound diameter will occur, thus allowing an easier execution and safer short-scar facelift, even in smokers and patients with significant alopecia.

PREOPERATIVE PREPARATION

In a survey of patients who were candidates for facelifts, most individuals expected procedures with minimal surgical stigmata, less-visible scars, a quick and comfortable recovery, low risk from surgery, early return to work, and fewer restrictions (considering themselves unable to give up habits). They also noted that they would accept good results rather than excellent ones, if possible, at lower costs. Expectations about long-lasting results were not present, especially if a painless postoperative course could be offered. The plastic surgeon must elucidate expectations before suggesting a technique to the patient. The facelift must reflect the patient's own expression.

ANESTHESIA

General anesthesia or monitored conscious sedation is suitable for the procedure. Patients' degree of anxiety will determine the best option.

POSITION AND MARKINGS

With the patient sitting on the operating table, the surgeon slides the facial skin toward the ear using his index finger, thus simulating the desired result. At the nearest point of the sideburn hair implantation, where the finger still maintains the intended result, an ink dot is drawn. This maneuver is repeated 4 or 5 times until a dotted line is drawn around the ear. This determines the minimum undermining needed to achieve the result.

The patient's hair, head, and face are washed in a basin. The hair remains wet with antiseptic solution, and the head is prepped into the sterile field, allowing the surgeon to move it right and left, and to extend the neck.

If the procedure is done under general anesthesia, a 1:250,000 epinephrine-saline solution is injected into the marked area, around the ear, and in the submental and neck areas. If the procedure is done under local anesthesia, a 0.5% lidocaine solution is used together with the vasoconstrictive agent.

DETAILS OF PROCEDURE

It is usually recommended to perform liposuction of the submental region and neck prior to the facelift, using a 3-mm incision made behind the chin. After liposuction is completed, an inverted-omega beveled incision is made, starting approximately 3 mm above the border of the sideburn, so as to protect hair follicles, and then contoured around the ear and finishing transversally behind it, above a projected line that passes above the tragus.

The previously marked area is undermined at the subcutaneous plane by sharp dissection. Pinch tests pulling the SMAS are executed to confirm that the tissues will allow for good traction by bringing the skin together (if that is not possible, additional undermining may be required). After that, accurate hemostasis is done. The risorius-masseterian zone is exposed, as well as the cranial portion and the mandibular insertion of the platysma muscle, leaving the muscle prepared to be plicated (Fig. 19-1). Regardless of the technique used, there will be an overlapping of muscles in this area; it is, indeed, convenient to restore volume.

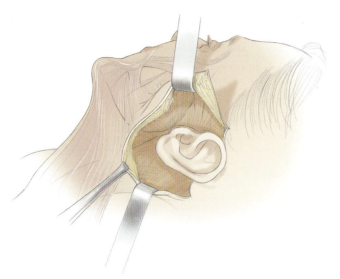

Figure 19-1   Minimal undermining to perform the running plication in the face.

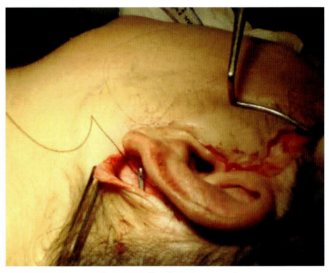

Figure 19-2   Stocchero needle already passed.

It is easier to begin the continuous suture from behind the ear toward the neck and face. There will be no tissue ascension in the mastoid fascia, because it is a strong and fixed area. The traction will begin to raise the tissues as soon as the platysma muscle is reached. The space between suture bites must be approximately 2 cm so as to permit the imbrications of tissues. Before passing the needle, it is important to choose the best traction by pulling the SMAS and then evaluating the changes that occur in the patient's face. A 45-degree insertion of the needle provides a stronger and safer suture, assuring better traction. The plication ends at the border of the sideburn. It is convenient to pull up this semicircular suture to confirm that the intended result was achieved, and that an effective vertical volume reposition was obtained.

With the Stocchero needle, a simulation of the best trajectory is done above the head, at least 2.5 cm higher than the ear. After choosing the ideal path, the needle is passed deeply, entering the anterior limit of the sideburn incision and being directed toward the limit of the retro-auricular incision. The needle must be passed in the galeal and deep muscular planes (Fig. 19-2). After arriving in the posterior area, the thread is passed in the needle hole and the needle is pulled toward the front (Fig. 19-3); after tying, the knot is complete (Fig. 19-4). For those who prefer not to use the Stocchero needle, it is perfectly feasible to achieve the same results by performing a 2- or 3-step suture in the hairy area (Figs. 19-5 and 19-6). Regardless, this circular suture must be able to anchor the soft tissues of the face to the strong tissues around and above the ear.

To offer a natural expression to the patient, with a smooth and progressive adaptation, the thread that sus-tains the SMAS-platysma must allow muscular action along the stitch. It is desirable to leave this suture without additional stitches in its anterior area so that the facial muscles may act in a dynamic fashion and adapt to the movements of the face. A sliding pseudoligament may be seen around the thread for several years after a round-block SMAS treatment (RBST) facelift has been done, which reflects its self-sustained condition (Fig. 19-7).

After this procedure, the excess amount of skin around the ear is ready to be resected, leaving minimal dead space (Fig. 19-8). It is important to avoid excessive tension in the skin suture. Drains are usually unnecessary.

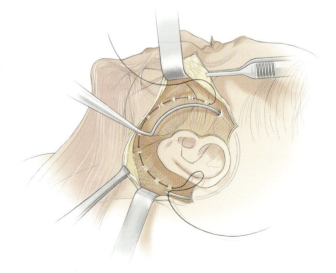

Figure 19-3   The running suture already done in the face, and the needle bringing the thread from behind to front.

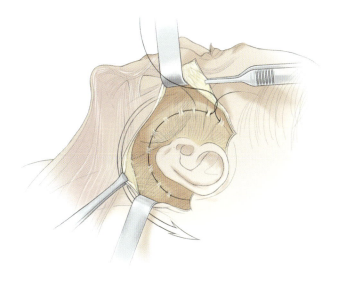

Figure 19-4   The completed circular suture will be stretched and tied.

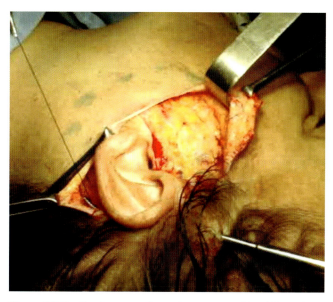

Figure 19-6   Option to perform the surgery with a Hagerdon or Reverdin needle (posterior).

PITFALLS

By observing the rules in performing this procedure and taking care regarding the depth of the stitches, it is almost impossible to damage a branch of the facial nerve. Regardless, it is always important to pay attention to the well-known danger zones.

There is a low possibility regarding the occurrence of hematomas. Although they may occur in a very limited area, they are mostly caused by a high blood pressure peak.

PEARLS

The quality of the result depends on the choice of good traction points. The more lax the patient's skin, the more traction that is needed. The final loop, after being tied, tends to resemble the shape of a circle. Sometimes it is necessary to perform a second plication (double stitch), or even a third one, mostly in cases where the patient has undergone massive weight loss. The second suture overlaps the first one.

In patients with a specific point of laxity, it may be necessary to perform additional suture passes to correct certain folds and undertractioned areas. With this

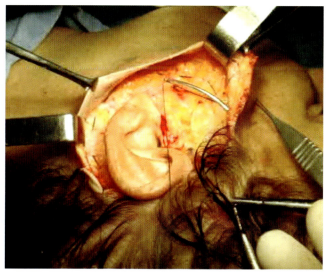

Figure 19-5   Option to perform the surgery with a Hagerdon or Reverdin needle (anterior).

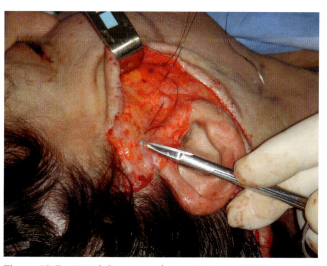

Figure 19-7   Pseudoligament after an RBST 6 years previously.

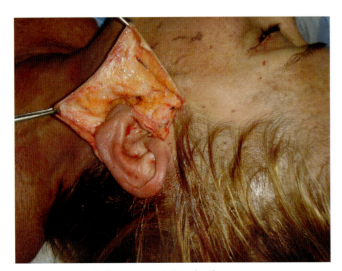

Figure 19-8   Minimum remaining dead space.

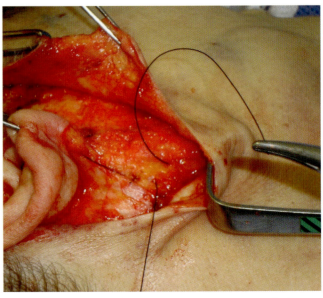

Figure 19-10   Pursestring suture to create a new cervical angle, anchoring the platysma to the Loré fascia.

purpose, it is very useful to execute a maneuver described as "fish and tie," by using a blunt Hagerdon Bayonet Modified needle. With this maneuver, it is possible to reach a desired location by pulling the insufficiently treated area (Fig. 19-9). Another helpful maneuver is fixing the platysma to the fascia of Loré, using it as a cervical brace (Fig. 19-10). It is recommended that all additional braces be done before the round-block stitch, allowing free adaptation of tissues according to facial expressions.

In selected cases, it is possible to perform the RBST in a "closed approach," that is, the circle stitch is made through 2 incisions: one at the sideburn, the other retroauricular, without any dissection or classic rhytidectomy incision. After tying the knot, it may be necessary to perform a small skin resection at the sideburn area. This is an alternative for patients who desire a quicker recovery and treatment, or when associated with endoscopic lift, or as a secondary facelift.

ACKNOWLEDGEMENTS

To my sons, Guilherme F. Stocchero and Gustavo F. Stocchero, and my son-in-law, Alexandre S. F. Fonseca, who have always helped me prepare my papers.

PHOTOGRAPHY

Case presentation of a 61-year-old insulin-dependent patient seen preoperatively and seven months after the aforementioned procedure (Photographs 19-1 to 19-6).

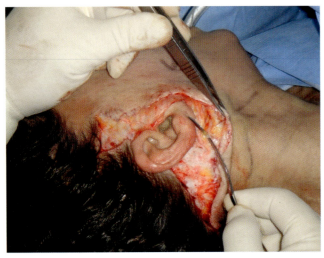

Figure 19-9   "Fish and tie"—creating a "new ligament" without undermining.

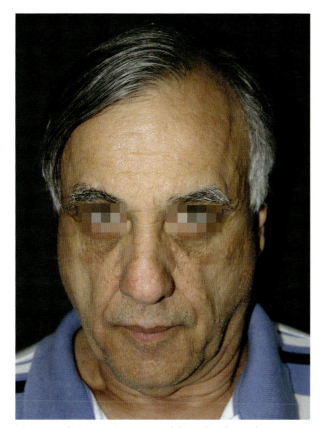

Photograph 19-1 A 61-year-old insulin-dependent patient seen preoperatively.

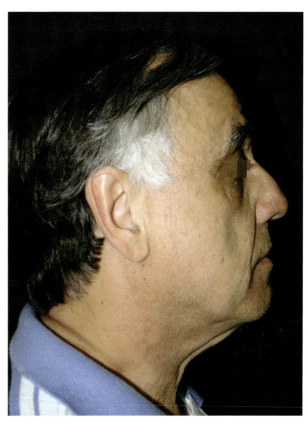

Photograph 19-3 A preoperative lateral image of a 61-year-old insulin-dependent patient.

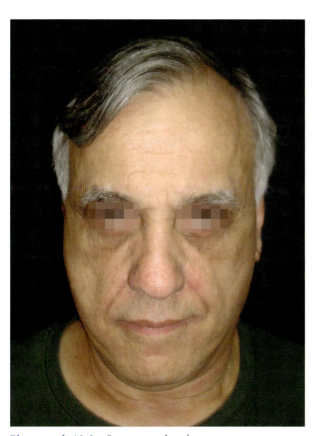

Photograph 19-2 Seven months after surgery.

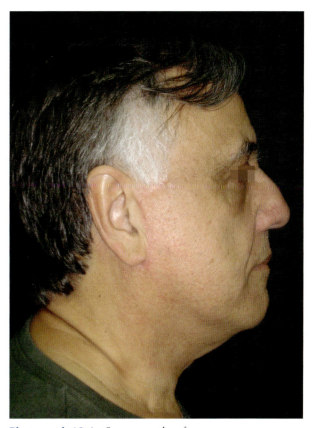

Photograph 19-4 Seven months after surgery.

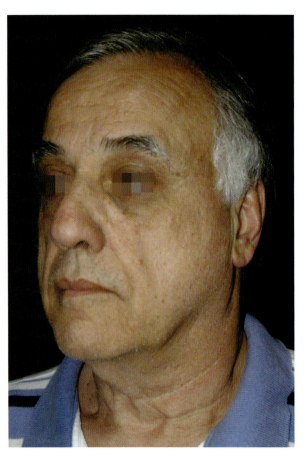

Photograph 19-5   A preoperative oblique image of a 61-year-old insulin-dependent patient.

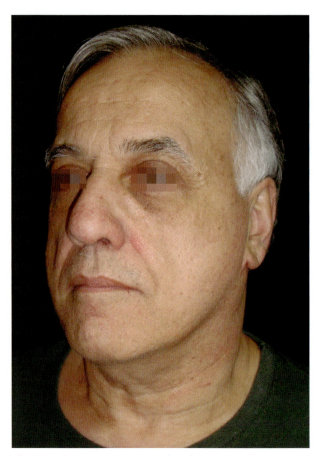

Photograph 19-6   Seven months after surgery.

SUGGESTED READING

Labbé D, Franco RG, Nicolas J. Platysma suspension and platysmaplasty during neck lift: anatomical study and analysis of 30 cases. *Plast Reconstr Surg.* 2006;117:2001-2007.

Marchac D. Against the "visible" short scar face lift. *Aesthetic Surg J.* 2008;28(2):200-208.

Marchac D, Nask MN. Avoiding the operated on look in multiple face lifts. *J Plast Reconstr Aesthet Surg.* 2008;61:1449-1458.

Stocchero IN. Shortscar face-lift with the round block SMAS treatment: a younger face for all. *Aesthetic Plast Surg.* 2007;31:275-278.

Stocchero IN. The roundblock SMAS treatment. *Plast Reconstr Surg.* 2001;107:1921-1923.

Chapter 20

Open Minimal Access Midface Lift

Malcolm D. Paul, MD

INDICATIONS

The indications for this approach to midface rejuvenation include younger patients with descent of the lid-cheek junction who would not be a candidate for an extended superficial musculoaponeurotic system (SMAS) facelift and older patients in whom an extended SMAS procedure will not give adequate vertical vector correction of midface soft-tissue ptosis.

PREOPERATIVE PREPARATION

Preoperative consultation and computer imaging with the ability to demonstrate the effect of shortening of the lid-cheek junction on midface rejuvenation. Patients must understand that this procedure may require several weeks for resolution of edema, typically occurring at 3 to 6 weeks postoperatively.

ANESTHESIA

General anesthesia supplemented with local infiltrative anesthesia is required when the dissection plane is sub-periosteal and to provide the hemostatic effect of epinephrine. At the conclusion of the procedure, infiltration of 0.25% bupivacaine with epinephrine along the incision line, and as an infraorbital nerve block, significantly diminishes postoperative discomfort.

POSITION AND MARKINGS

Preoperative markings include the proposed behind the hairline temporal access incision, typically approximately 3 cm in length and determined by passing a line from the nasal ala through the lateral canthus. The incision begins lateral to the line and ends at the anterior temporal crest.

The planned exit points for the barbed sutures are marked approximately 1.5 cm apart and 1 cm lateral to the nasolabial crease (Fig. 20-1).

Patients are positioned on a narrow headrest with head elevation of 30 degrees.

INCISION AND EXPOSURE

After the incision line is infiltrated with 1% lidocaine with epinephrine 1:100,000, the patient is prepped and draped, and the periorbital soft tissue and malar area are infiltrated with a tumescent infiltration of 0.06% lidocaine with 1:500,000 epinephrine and 10 mg triamcinolone/500 mL lactated Ringer solution delivered by a liposuction infusion pump and a 25-gauge needle. The tumescent infiltration provides for hydrodissection as well as vasoconstriction. The temporal incision is made down to the deep temporal fascia.

DETAILS OF THE PROCEDURE

Blind dissection continues with a periosteal elevator until the lateral orbital rim is reached. If the lateral brow requires elevation, the dissection is performed under direct vision with either a lighted retractor or a retractor and headlight, and the orbital ligament and periosteum are released along the superior orbital rim. The dissection continues along the lateral orbital rim and continues on

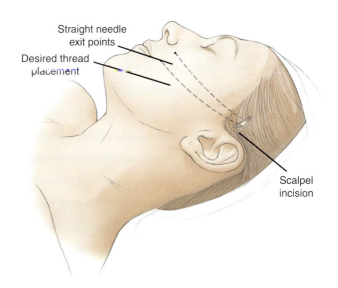

Straight needle exit points

Desired thread placement

Scalpel incision

Figure 20-1 Site of temporal incision.

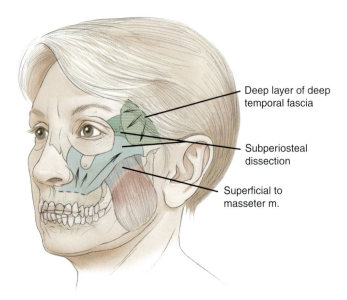

Figure 20-2   Communication of subperiosteal dissection with the temporal access incision.

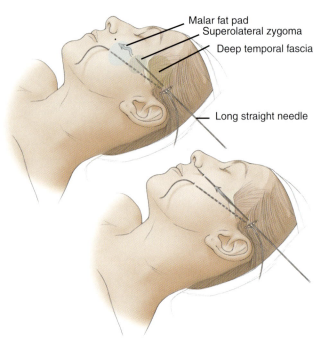

Figure 20-3   Sites of barbed suture placement.

top of the deep layer of the deep temporal fascia until the periosteum of the zygoma is reached. The periosteum is elevated off of the anterior surface of the zygoma and the dissection continues inferiorly. Typically, a counter 1-cm incision is made intraorally over the canine fossa after cleansing with an iodine solution and infiltrating 1% lidocaine with epinephrine 1:100,000 for hemostatis. Subperiosteal dissection continues over the anterior surface of the maxilla and communicates with the temporal access incision (Fig. 20-2). The medial fibers of the masseter tendon are released from the intraoral approach. Absorbable barbed sutures that are joined at the half point with a nonbarbed segment are utilized. The first half is anchored to the deep temporal fascia and is passed parallel to the deep temporal fascia, continues lateral to the lateral orbital rim, and then engages all layers from the periosteum to the subcutaneous fat, exiting the skin 1 cm lateral to the nasolabial crease to avoid deepening of the crease. The second half of the suture is passed parallel to the first suture and exits the skin approximately 1.5 cm on either side of the first suture (Fig. 20-3). If tension on the proximal end of the suture does not cause the cheek to elevate, either the deep temporal fascia has been engaged in the temporal pocket or the soft-tissue release is inadequate. A shish kebob effect occurs by engaging all layers of the cheek flap onto the barbed sutures and sequentially elevating the cheek flap (Fig. 20-4). The distal ends of the sutures may be left outside of the skin at a length of 1 cm. They can be covered by an antibacterial ointment and a Telfa pad (Kendall Lab, Mansfield, MA). The elevation of the midface flap can be checked at 72 hours postoperatively and further adjustment can be made before the distal ends of the sutures are cut flush with the skin.

The temporal and intraoral pockets are irrigated with a dilute iodine solution before closure (the intraoral

incision is closed with a 4-0 plain catgut running suture; the temporal incision is closed with skin staples). If the lateral brow requires elevation, it may be suspended with barbed sutures or by anchoring the temporoparietal fascia to the deep temporal fascia with a 3-0 PDS (polydioxanone) suture (Ethicon, Summerville, N.J.).

PITFALLS

There is little danger to branches of the facial nerve as the dissection is deep to the nerve branches. The dissection over the medial one-third of the zygomatic arch is medial to the pathway of the temporal branch of the facial nerve.

Intraoral infection can be avoided by careful intraoral cleansing, a small access incision, nonwatertight closure to allow for drainage, antibiotic coverage intraoperative and postoperatively for 6 days, and the use of oral antiseptic mouthwash after each meal.

Intraoperative and postoperative steroids seem to help with edema.

Overcorrection of midface ptosis can be adjusted by releasing the soft tissue over the barbs by gently squeezing the skin where the barbs are connected. Patients with a wide interzygomatic distance may look too wide with a subperiosteal midface lift.

PEARLS

Be certain to pass the barbed sutures parallel to the deep temporal fascia until the lateral orbital rim is approached. Engaging the deep temporal fascia in the temporal pocket will prevent lifting of the midface.

Sit the patient up to check symmetry of suture suspension before closing the incisions.

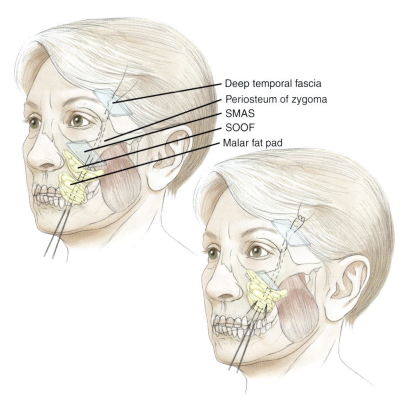

Deep temporal fascia
Periosteum of zygoma
SMAS
SOOF
Malar fat pad

Figure 20-4   Engagement of all layers of the cheek flap onto the barbed sutures and sequentially elevating the cheek flap resulting in a shish kebob effect.

Allow 2 to 3 weeks for the edema to subside. Typically, at that time, the tissue has relaxed and is rarely seen as overcorrected. If there appears to be excess lower eyelid skin after the cheek has been elevated, there arc 2 options: (a) a skin-pinch blepharoplasty or (b) delay any lower-lid procedure for 6 weeks to be certain that there is excess lower-eyelid skin to excise (especially important in secondary cases).

LATERAL BROWLIFT WITH BARBED SUTURES TECHNIQUE

The appropriate brow vector is determined by drawing a line from the nasal ala through the tail of the eyebrow, continuing behind the temporal hairline (Photographs 20-1 to 20-5). A 4-cm incision is marked obliquely beginning medial to the skin marking, ending just medial to the anterior temporal crest. The incision line and the lateral forehead ending medial to the anterior temporal crest are infiltrated with local anesthesia. The incision is made down to the deep temporal fascia. Using a periosteal elevator, the soft tissue is elevated to the orbital rim. A scissors cuts the orbital ligament blindly and the periosteum is released over the superior orbital rim. Hemostasis occurs from the epinephrine in the local anesthesia and direct pressure for 3 to 5 minutes over the superior orbital rim. A no. 0 or no. 2-0 Quill PDO suture measuring 7×7 cm or 14×14 cm, depending upon the distance from the

incision to the orbital rim, is used for brow suspension. One-half of the suture is passed through the deep temporal fascia, continuing until the barbs catch from the other direction, stopping the advancement of the suture, then both needles are cut off and replaced with Keith needles of appropriate length to reach the orbital rim from the incision. Each half of the suture is passed over the deep temporal fascia and enters the flap approximately 1 cm above the rim. The suture passes through the galeal glide plane and exits the brow just below the lowest brow hairs. The soft tissue is advanced over the barbs to raise the brow. The end of the suture may be cut flush with the skin or left approximately 1 cm in length, covered with an antibacterial ointment and a nonadherent dressing. If indicated, the brow height may be further adjusted 3 days later in the clinic. This is valuable in cases of brow asymmetry wherein the high side is adjusted during surgery, the suture is cut flush with the skin, and the low side is adjusted during surgery, left long, and further adjusted as needed 3 days later.

The temporal flap is sutured with a 2-0 PDS suture (Ethicon, Summerville, NJ) between the superficial and the deep temporal fascias for additional brow advancement and stabilization. The temporal scalp incision is closed with skin staples, which are removed at 1 week. A snug forehead dressing is applied for 3 days. Patients routinely receive intraoperative steroids and postoperative antibiotics for one week.

PHOTOGRAPHS

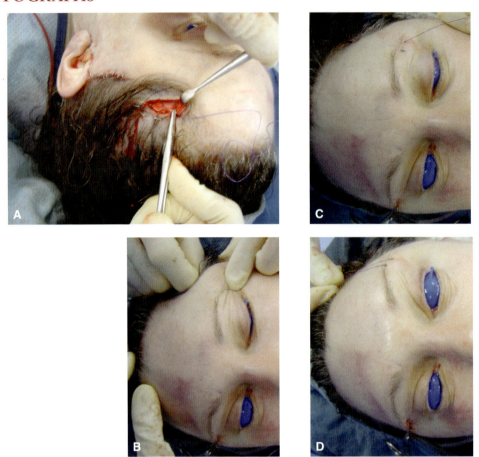

Photograph 20-1   Sequence of surgical steps in lateral browlifting. **A.** Suture placement in deep temporal fascia. **B.** Suture passed through brow soft tissue, exiting the skin over the lowest brow hairs. The end of the suture is returned through the same hole and exits at right angles at the point where the second half of the suture will exit the skin. The reverse occurs with the second half of the suture creating a U-shaped lock on the brow insuring a stable brow lift. **C.** Sutures passed on both sides. **D.** Adjustment of brow position.

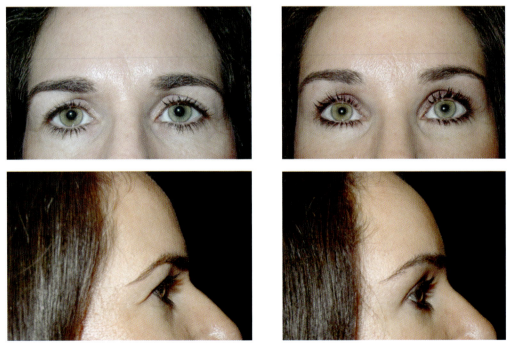

Photograph 20-2   Pre and post-op lateral browlift.

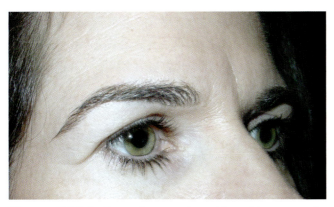
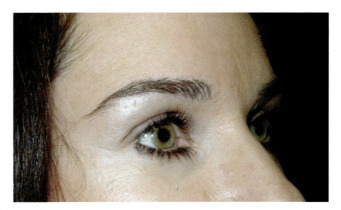

Photograph 20-3   Pre and post-op lateral browlift, same patient oblique view.

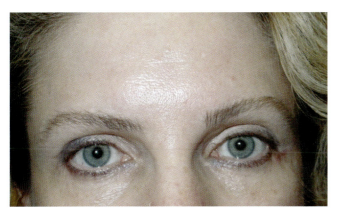
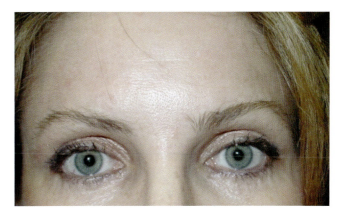

Photograph 20-4   Pre and post-op lateral browlift and midface lift.

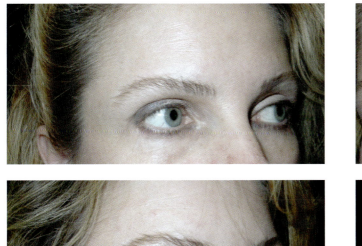
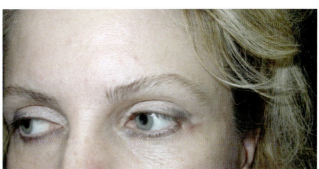
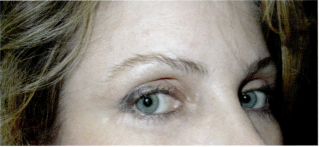
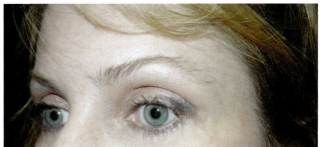

Photograph 20-5   Pre and post-op lateral browlift and midface lift, same patient oblique view.

Chapter 21. Neck Lift

Olubimpe A. Ayeni, MD, MPH, FRCSC;
Samuel J. Lin, MD, FACS; Thomas A. Mustoe, MD

INDICATIONS

The stigmata of an aging face manifest in the neck as lipodystrophy, medial or lateral platysmal bands, and jowls. These changes can occur as a result of skin laxity, attenuation of the masseteric cutaneous ligaments, accumulation of fat below the mandibular border or under the platysma, and ptosis of the platysma. Prominent submandibular glands or digastric muscles can also contribute to the appearance of an aged neck. In some individuals, a recessed chin and a prominent, low-set hyoid can accentuate this aged appearance.

Neck rejuvenation is usually performed in conjunction with facial rejuvenation, but this procedure can be performed by itself. Nonsurgical options for neck rejuvenation include injections (injectable fillers and botulinum toxin type A), chemical peels, and laser ablation. Surgical options include facelifting, submental liposuction, plastysmaplasty, neck sling/cervical suspension, and anterior cervicoplasty. More specifically, surgery on the neck can consist of a skin lift only, reapproximation of the medial borders of the platysma muscle, transection of the platysma muscle, or division of medial platysmal bands with superolateral elevation of the muscle.

PREOPERATIVE EVALUATION

The preoperative examination of the patient begins with a global assessment of skin quality and the degree of skin laxity (Fig. 21-1). Both static and dynamic evaluation of the neck should be performed. The amount of preplatysmal submental and submandibular fat deposits should be palpated, and the presence of malpositioned or ptotic submandibular glands should be noted. According to Ellenbogen and Karlin, there are 5 criteria for a youthful neck: (a) a distinct inferior mandibular border from mentum to angle with no jowl overhang; (b) subhyoid depression; (c) visible thyroid cartilage bulge; (d) visible anterior border of the sternocleidomastoid muscle; and (e) cervicomental angle between 105 and 120 degrees, or a sternocleidomastoid to submental line with an angle of 90 degrees. The relationship between the neck and the chin must also be assessed. The nose-chin-lip plane is defined as a line extending from a point half the distance of the ideal nasal length through the upper and lower lip vermilion. The ideal chin projection is 3 mm posterior to the nose-lip-chin plane.

Dynamic evaluation consists of watching the patient while talking. The patient is then asked to animate to accentuate potential medial or lateral platysmal banding. If the patient has jowls, the contribution of the skin, subcutaneous fat, platysma, and the submandibular gland to this deformity is recorded. Anterior, lateral, and oblique photographs should be obtained.

ANESTHESIA

Neck lifting can be performed under local anesthesia only, local anesthesia with sedation, or general anesthesia, depending on the extent of surgery to be performed. It is crucial that all preoperative markings be made before local anesthesia is infiltrated and with the patient in the upright position. The ideal cervicomental crease is identified using a paper tape measure. This line varies between patients, but is approximately at the level of the hyoid bone.

DETAILS OF PROCEDURE

A customized surgical approach is used to address the specific areas to be corrected with a neck lift. For patients who have fat deposits with excellent skin tone, lipectomy is a good option and suction or ultrasound-assisted liposuction can be performed through an incision placed behind the submental crease. If more aggressive lipectomy is required, two incisions anterior to the mastoid can be used for greater access.

Liposuction can be combined with procedures that alter the tone of the platysma. For example, the classic Giampapa procedure involves plicating the platysma muscle and placing 2 permanent suspension stitches that interlock in the muscle bellies and are anchored laterally to the mastoid bone. Another option for patients with submental fullness and minimal signs of facial aging is direct excision. This involves excision of some redundant skin and preplatysmal or subplatysmal fat. The redundant neck skin can then be excised as an ellipse. Several techniques have been described, all of which consist of a

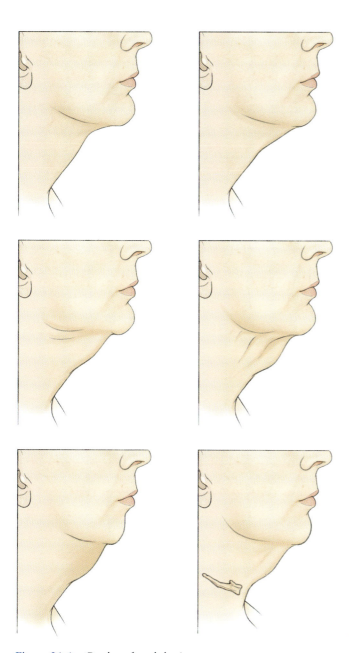

Figure 21-1   Grades of neck laxity.

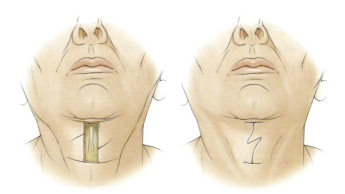

Figure 21-2   Design of Z-plasty for skin closure.

midline, nearly to the medial edge of the sternocleidomastoid (SCM). The platysma is folded in the midline using 4-0 polydioxanone suture to achieve a more tailored neck and give the skin flaps medial movement. The Z-plasty limbs are marked at 60 degrees and designed to be approximately 1.5 to 2 cm in length. The flaps are incised, carefully elevated, and transposed. Subcutaneous absorbable sutures are used to secure the limbs. A combination of running and interrupted polypropylene sutures is used to close the skin edges (Figs. 21-2 and 21-3). The superior border of the wound should be truncated before reaching the apex of the chin to hide the scar under the chin. The inferior edge of the wound should end superior to the suprasternal notch. Importantly, direct excision is indicated for a select group of patients who are willing to accept an obvious submental scar.

If a patient has lax skin and poor platysmal tone, the fibrous attachments of the superficial platysmal fascia must be freed from the dermis. A combination of preauricular and postauricular incisions are used for access. If the medial edges of the platysma muscles are free, a 3-cm incision placed 1 cm behind the submental crease is made. The inferomedial fibers of the platysma are incised over a distance of 1 to 2 cm, then the free medial edges are reapproximated with interrupted 4-0 Mersilene sutures. If the midline decussation is intact, the muscle is imbricated to tighten the muscular sling and sharpen the cervicomental angle. The lateral platysmal fibers are plicated to the SCM fascia.

For patients who have lax skin, poor platysmal tone, and lipodystrophy, direct supraplatysmal defatting is also performed. The subplatysmal fat is then exposed by elevation of the medial borders of the platysma from the mentum to the level of the cricoid cartilage. The excess fat is then removed under direct vision with the Bovie cautery and scissors. Careful hemostasis must be obtained. Overresection of fat in the submental region can lead to a hollowed out submental appearance that is difficult to correct. A greater amount of fat can be removed at the

longitudinal excision that incorporates a Z-plasty at the level of the cervicomental crease (Fig. 21-2).

To perform a direct excision, the proposed cervicomental crease is marked with a surgical marker. This will be the line on which the arms of the Z-plasty will transpose to create the cervicomental crease. Next, the proposed, vertically oriented, elliptical excision of redundant tissue is marked. The redundant skin and subcutaneous tissue are excised with a scalpel. Using a combination of blunt dissection with scissors and blended electrodissection and coagulation, undermining is accomplished bilaterally from the excision site approximately 3 cm from

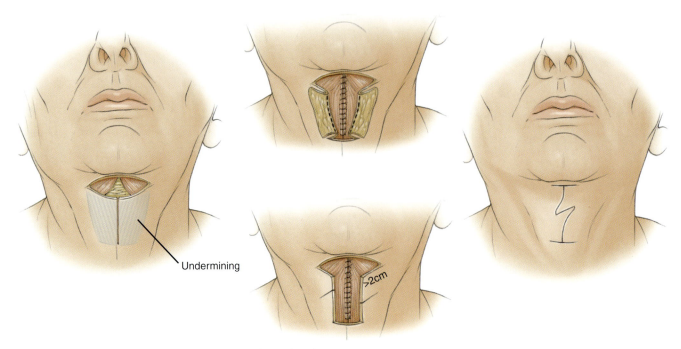

Figure 21-3   Platysmal plication followed by Z-plasty skin closure.

level of the hyoid, where it helps to deepen the cervicomental angle.

Once adequately exposed, the amount of platysmal laxity is evaluated, and, if necessary, excess muscle and fat are clamped and removed centrally in a conservative fashion to prevent undue tension on the suture plication.

In addition, releasing the muscle laterally by performing a myotomy either at the level of the hyoid or just caudal to the last muscle plication suture relieves some of the tension along the platysmal plication and allows the platysma to shift superiorly, creating a deeper cervicomental angle. This back cut or myotomy of the platysma is parallel to the inferior border of the mandible and away from the submandibular gland, facial artery, facial vein, and the facial nerve.

After adequate mobilization of the platysma, the edges of the muscle are grasped and overlapped in the midline. Platysmal plication is then performed with interrupted 3-0 Vicryl or 3-0 silk sutures from the mentum to at least the level of the hyoid bone. It is important to bury the knots and create a smooth contour (Figs. 21-4 and 21-5).

To give greater definition to the body and angle of the mandible, a suspension suture (Vicryl) can be placed from 1 cm below the mandibular border in the submental platysma to the mastoid fascia. This suture helps define the neck from the cheek, provides support for the often ptotic submandibular gland, and assists in reestablishing the contour. This suspension suture is not recommended in thin-skinned individuals, because it may result in palpability or surface irregularity.

PEARLS

An individualized approach must be used and the ideal combination of techniques requires careful analysis. Evaluation of the chin is essential to formulating the appropriate neck rejuvenation treatment plan; a neglected ptotic chin pad can lead to an accentuated submental crease.

Adjuncts to surgical neck lifts, such as laser and botulinum injections, exist. In men, the scar often lies in hair-bearing skin that tends to heal better and be less noticeable. For female patients opposed to a facelift, submental liposuction followed by carbon dioxide laser coagulation of the underside of the flap is an option. Male patients often present with a greater degree of skin redundancy and tend to have a greater amount of recurrence of the aged appearance. These patients benefit from the inferomedial and inferolateral platysmal incisions and advancement/plication.

PITFALLS

On occasion, patients presenting for secondary facelift or neck lift have bulging of their submandibular gland. This presentation can be secondary to overaggressive liposuction during the primary procedure or just ptosis of the gland with attenuation of the deep fascia and gland capsule.

There are several nerve structures that must be protected from injury during cervical rejuvenation. The marginal mandibular branch of the facial nerve passes along

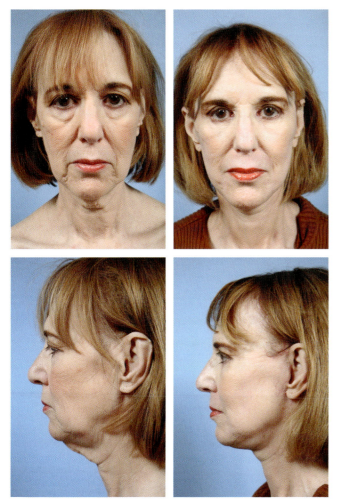

Figure 21-4   Patient 1. (Top and Bottom Left) Preoperative photographs. (Top and Bottom Right) Postoperative photographs taken following the described procedure.

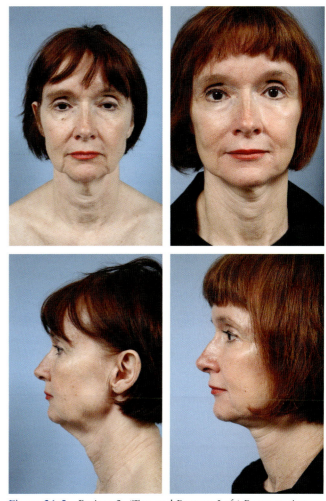

Figure 21-5   Patient 2. (Top and Bottom Left) Preoperative photographs. (Top and Bottom Right) Postoperative photographs taken following the described procedure.

the inferior border of the mandible and is covered along its course by platysmal fibers. Anterior to the facial artery, the marginal mandibular nerve is always superior to the mandibular border. The cervical branch of the facial nerve supplies the innervation entering the deep surface of the muscle superolaterally and is often injured without knowledge.

SUGGESTED READING

Bitner JB, Friedman O, Farrior RT, Cook TA. Direct submentoplasty for neck rejuvenation. *Arch Facial Plast Surg.* 2007; 9(3):194-200.

Ellenbogen R, Karlin JV. Visual criteria for success in restoring the youthful neck. *Plast Reconstr Surg.* 1980;66(6):826-837.

Feldman JJ. Corset platysmaplasty. *Plast Reconstr Surg.* 1990; 85(3):333-343.

Gradinger GP. Anterior cervicoplasty in the male patient. *Plast Reconstr Surg.* 2000;106(5):1146-1154; discussion 1155.

Haiavy J. Reoperative face and neck lifts. *Oral Maxillofac Surg Clin North Am.* 2011;23(1):109-118, vi-vii.

Hancox JG, Eaton JS. Anterior cervicoplasty: neck rejuvenation using local anesthesia. *J Am Acad Dermatol.* 2008;58(3): 430-433.

Prado AS, Parada F, Andrades P, Fuentes P. Platysma chemical denervation with botox before neck lift. *Plast Reconstr Surg.* 2010;126(2):79e-81e.

Rohrich RJ, Rios JL, Smith PD, Gutowski KA. Neck rejuvenation revisited. *Plast Reconstr Surg.* 2006;118(5):1251-1263.

Roy D. Neck rejuvenation. *Dermatol Clin.* 2005;23(3): 469-474, vi.

Chapter 22. Open Approach to the Overprojecting Tip

C. Spencer Cochran, MD; Jack P. Gunter, MD

INDICATIONS

An incremental approach to tip deprojection in open rhinoplasty is indicated for patients who have an overprojecting nasal tip. Factors that contribute to tip support, and thus tip projection, include: (a) the length and strength of the lateral crura; (b) the length and strength of the medial crura; (c) the fibroelastic attachments connecting the feet of the medial crura to the caudal septum; (d) the ligamentous attachments between the lateral crura and the upper lateral cartilages; (e) the suspensory ligament over the septal angle connecting the cephalic margins of the domes; (f) the septal angle; and (g) the nasal skin.

PREOPERATIVE PREPARATION

A thorough preoperative nasal examination and analysis of preoperative photographs should be performed. Using computer morphing software or tracing paper enables the surgeon to estimate the planned tip projection. If preoperative analysis indicates that one goal of rhinoplasty is to decrease tip projection, the surgeon needs to be able to control the decrease incrementally.

ANESTHESIA

General anesthesia with endotracheal intubation is preferred for this procedure. This allows the patient to be completely still for the duration of the procedure and allows for a protected airway.

POSITION AND MARKINGS

The patient is placed in the supine position. After adequate anesthesia is administered, the patient's nasal passages are packed with one-inch gauze strips saturated with a topical decongestant such as oxymetazoline or phenylephrine. The soft-tissue envelope is injected with approximately 5 mL of 1% lidocaine with 1:100,000 epinephrine, and the patient is prepped and draped in a sterile fashion.

The planned transcolumellar incision is marked as an inverted V or chevron shape across the narrowest portion of the columella and extends around the columellar roll to terminate on the midportion of the medial crura.

DETAILS OF PROCEDURE

Increased tip projection may be a result of any one of the aforementioned factors; usually it is the result of a combination of the factors, and therefore requires a stepwise or incremental approach. After each factor is addressed, the effect on tip projection should be assessed by redraping the soft-tissue envelope.

The transcolumellar incision is created with a no. 15 blade scalpel and connected with infracartilaginous incisions that follow the caudal border of the lateral crura. The nasal soft-tissue envelope is elevated from the tip and nasal dorsum to expose the osseocartilaginous framework. The soft-tissue envelope should be widely undermined from the lateral crura toward the piriform aperture because destabilization of the nasal tip occurs when the soft-tissue envelope is elevated in the open approach, allowing for a modest amount of deprojection.

Sever the ligamentous attachments between the lateral crura and the upper lateral cartilages (Fig. 22-1) and divide the suspensory ligament traversing the septal angle that connects the cephalic margins of the domes (removal of the cephalic margin of the lateral crura has the same effect). After the suspensory ligament has been divided, patients with a prominent septal angle may require judicious trimming of the lower portion of the cartilaginous dorsal septum. This can help prevent a "polly-beak" deformity resulting from excess dorsal septum in the supratip area.

If additional deprojection is required, the fibroelastic attachments between the feet of the medial crura and the caudal septum should be released (see Fig. 22-1). This is accomplished by dividing the lower lateral cartilages in the midline to allow elevation of mucoperichondrial flaps on either side of the caudal septum beginning at the septal angle and extending to the nasal spine area. Alternatively, a full transfixion incision will effectively free the medial crura from the septum.

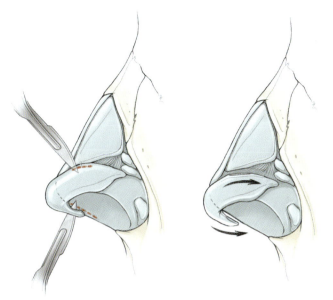

Figure 22-1   Decreasing tip projection by release of the ligamentous attachments between the lateral crura and upper lateral cartilages and release of the fibroelastic attachments between the medial crura and caudal septum.

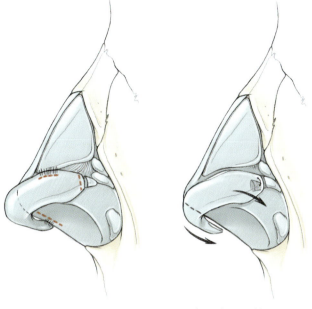

Figure 22-2   Decreasing tip projection by release of ligamentous and fibroelastic attachments with transection and overlap of lateral crura.

When all other factors have been addressed and the desired decrease in tip projection still has not been achieved, the length and strength of the medial and/or lateral crura must be altered. The lateral crura are usually altered first because they often play a more significant role in tip support than the medial crura. First, undermine the vestibular skin from the undersurface of the lateral crura just anterior to the lateral crus-accessory cartilage junction and vertically transect the lateral crus to allow them to overlap. Manually set the tip back to the desired position, overlap the cartilages to the desired amount, and suture the overlapping segments together (Fig. 22-2). This maneuver is then repeated on the opposite side. Supporting the area of overlap with lateral crural strut grafts may be required in patients with weak lateral crura to prevent external valve collapse. It is also important to note that when the lengths of the lateral crura are shortened but the medial crural lengths (or their attachments to the caudal septum) remain the same, there is a resulting upward rotation of the nasal tip.

When the medial crura are excessively long and the medial crural footplates impede retrodisplacement of the nasal tip, the medial crural footplates can be dissected from beneath the columellar skin and trimmed the appropriate amount. The medial crura may also be shortened by undermining the vestibular skin from the crura anteriorly where they meet the intermediate crura. The intermediate crura can then be transected vertically, which will allow them to be overlapped the desired amount.

The overlapped segments are then sutured together (Fig. 22-3). Shortening the intermediate crura can move the tip-defining points downwards, thereby decreasing the height of the infratip lobule (Figs. 22-4 to 22-10).

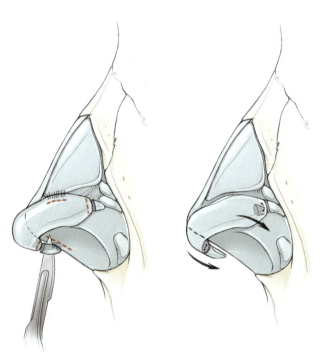

Figure 22-3   Decreasing tip projection by release of ligamentous and fibroelastic attachments with transection and overlap of lateral and intermediate crura.

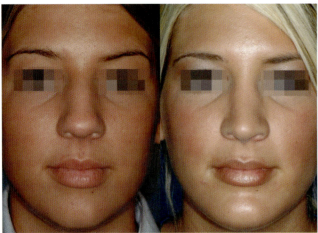

Figure 22-4   Preoperative (left) vs. postoperative (right) views of a primary rhinoplasty patient whose modest decrease in tip projection was achieved by ligamentous/fibroelastic release alone.

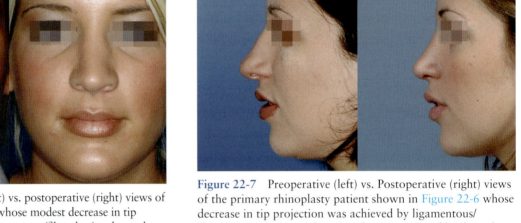

Figure 22-7   Preoperative (left) vs. Postoperative (right) views of the primary rhinoplasty patient shown in Figure 22-6 whose decrease in tip projection was achieved by ligamentous/fibroelastic release combined with transection of her lateral crura. Note the resulting upward rotation of her tip.

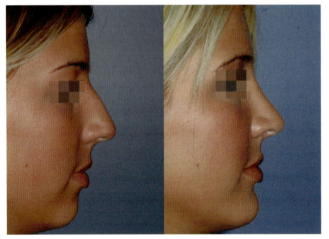

Figure 22-5   Preoperative (left) vs. Postoperative (right) views of a primary rhinoplasty patient shown in Figure 22-4 whose modest decrease in tip projection was achieved by ligamentous/fibroelastic release alone.

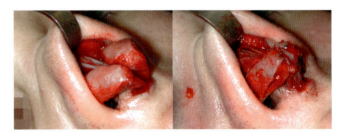

Figure 22-8   Intraoperative view of patient in Figure 22-6 showing shortening of lateral crura after transection and overlap with resulting upward rotation of the tip.

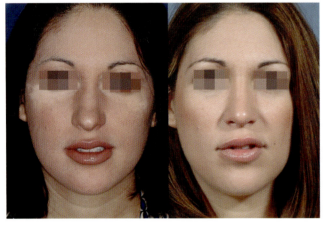

Figure 22-6   Preoperative (left) vs. Postoperative (right) views of a primary rhinoplasty patient whose decrease in tip projection was achieved by ligamentous/fibroelastic release combined with transection of her lateral crura. Note the resulting upward rotation of her tip.

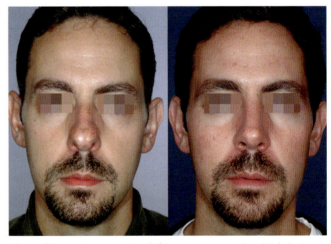

Figure 22-9   Preoperative (left) vs. postoperative (right) views of a primary rhinoplasty patient whose decrease in tip projection was achieved by ligamentous/fibroelastic release combined with transection of his lateral crura. Lateral crural strut grafts were used to correct his convex lateral crura and support his lateral crural-accessory cartilage junction.

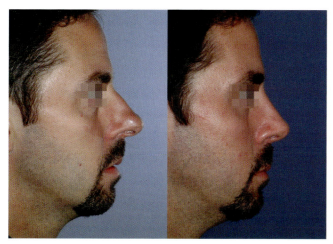

Figure 22-10 Preoperative (left) vs. Postoperative (right) views of same primary rhinoplasty patient shown in Figure 22-9 whose decrease in tip projection was achieved by ligamentous/fibroelastic release combined with transection of his lateral crura. Lateral crural strut grafts were used to correct his convex lateral crura and support the lateral crural-accessory cartilage junction.

PITFALLS

• Skin thickness is often the limiting factor in the amount of possible tip deprojection because the skin must be able to shrink around the osseocartilaginous framework for the nose to have sufficient tip definition.

• Changing the length of the lateral crura or medial crura can have the potential to affect rotation.

• The surgeon should be cognizant of the possibility of alar base flaring and be prepared to correct the flaring with an alar base resection.

PEARLS

• Multiple factors contribute to tip projection. Incrementally eliminating these factors will allow the surgeon to decrease tip projection in a controlled manner.

• When the ligamentous attachments and fibroelastic attachments are eliminated, the main support to the tip comes from the length and strength of the lower lateral crura, especially in an open rhinoplasty where the support from the skin has been eliminated.

• When transecting and overlapping the lateral crura, placement of lateral crural strut grafts can help prevent medial collapse of the lateral crus-accessory cartilage junction.

SUGGESTED READING

Johnson CM Jr, Godin, MS. The tension nose: open structure rhinoplasty approach. *Plast Reconstr Surg.* 1995;95:43.

PetroV MA, McCollough EG, Hom D, Anderson JR. Nasal tip projection: quantitative changes following rhinoplasty. *Arch Otolaryngol Head Neck Surg.* 1991;117:783.

Rich JS, Friedman WH, Pearlman SJ. The effects of lower lateral cartilage excision on nasal tip projection. *Arch Otolaryngol Head Neck Surg.* 1991;117:56.

Tardy ME Jr, Walter MA, Patt BS. The overprojecting nose: anatomic component analysis and repair. *Facial Plast Surg.* 1993;9:306.

Chapter 23. Open Approach to the Underprojecting Tip

Diana C. Ponsky, MD; Bahman Guyuron, MD, FACS

INDICATIONS

Rhinoplasty is performed to correct displeasing disharmonies of the nose and incongruences with the rest of the facial features. Functional compromise and aesthetic anatomic flaws of the underprojected nasal tip is one of the most important nasal imperfections to correct. The underprojected nasal tip can result from loss of tip support, as in acquired tip ptosis, or from inadequate tip projection relative to the aesthetic ideal. Because nasal tip anatomy and facial features vary widely between patients, there is no single surgical technique that can be routinely applied in all patients to correct the underprojected tip.

It is essential that adequate preoperative facial analysis be performed, and the surgical plan formulated in the surgeon's mind prior to surgery based on the nasal pathology and patient's desires. Goals and limitations must be understood and discussed prior to surgery. At the time of surgery, once the soft-tissue envelope is elevated, adequate exposure of the intended nasal structures may modify the surgical plan to some degree.

An external or open rhinoplasty approach is often preferred as it provides maximal exposure of the lower lateral cartilages, upper lateral cartilages, middle nasal vault, and bony nasal vault. These structures can be manipulated in a more precise fashion, and cartilage grafts can be accurately sutured into place, which is of particular importance in increasing nasal tip projection.

Contraindications to aesthetic rhinoplasty exist in patients who have medical problems such as uncontrolled diabetes, coagulopathies, or other chronic medical conditions that render elective surgery and anesthesia unsafe.

PREOPERATIVE PREPARATION

Careful analysis and study of the patient's facial features, with evaluation of standardized (frontal, base, lateral, oblique) photographs, or life-sized photographs, is crucial. Our preference is the use of life-sized photographs to perform frontal and profile view analysis. Complete nasal analysis, as well as its relationship to the chin, is also required. A thorough intranasal exam and digital palpation of the nose must be performed. The patient's goals and realistic expectations are discussed in detail. The external columellar scar is discussed with the patient. Any alar or nasal base modifications and the scar are also discussed.

Obtaining a detailed and complete medical and surgical history is necessary to understanding a possible iatrogenic or acquired cause of the underprojected nose. Medical history, such as inflammatory disease and infections, should be explored. A detailed account of past rhinoplasties should be elucidated. Additionally important is the need to assess for substance abuse, especially cocaine. All aspirin and nonsteroidal antiinflammatory agents should be discontinued at least 2 weeks before surgery. Smoking and steroid use may retard the healing process and should be stopped prior to surgery. The diagnosis of nasal tip underprojection requires a precise assessment of the nasal proportions and angles. Several reports and formulas have been developed to define the ones that constitute the aesthetic ideal. Analysis of facial proportions and landmarks, including the radix, nasal dorsum, nasal length, tip rotation, and tip projection, are essential.

In general, one should start with noting the different zones of the face and whether the facial thirds are in equilibrium. The nasofrontal angle (radix) is evaluated. The apex of the radix should lie between the upper lid eyelashes and the supratarsal fold with the eyes in neutral gaze. This is typically 4 mm deep in men and 6 mm deep in women. The aesthetic nasal dorsum should lie approximately 2 mm behind and parallel to a line from the radix to the tip-defining points in women and 1 mm behind in men.

Tip rotation and projection are addressed in profile view. Rotation is determined by the nasolabial angle, and is ideally between 103 and 108 degrees in women and between 95 and 100 degrees in men. In determining projection, a line is drawn from the alar-cheek junction to the tip of the nose. Projection is ideal if 50% to 60% of the nasal tip lies anterior to a vertical line adjacent to the most projected part of the upper lip. Alternatively, the Byrd method can be used where the tip projection is two-thirds or 0.67 of the planned postoperative (or the ideal) nasal length. Ideal nasal length in this approach is 0.67 of the midfacial height. Other methods can be used, including Crumley's 3-4-5 triangle.

The physical examination includes looking at both the external and internal nose. The external examination includes observation in the anterior, profile, oblique, and basal view, examining the nose for symmetry, proportionality, and flaws and deformity. The skin quality is noted: thin, medium, or thick. Thick skin can often drag down the nasal tip. Palpation of the nose can reveal the strength or weakness of the supporting skeletal framework as well as any irregularities of the firm radix or supple nasal tip. Understanding the patient history can help identify areas of scarring, contracture, resection, and previous grafting. The influence of the depressor septi muscle during animation on both frontal and profile views should be assessed.

The internal examination is important for evaluating the presence of any septal perforations and to assess the quality and quantity of the internal lining. Attention to the functional aspects of the nose should not be overlooked. Investigating for septal deviation, hypertrophic turbinates, and internal and external valve competence are part of a complete nasal examination. Any functional abnormalities should be addressed with the patient and included in the operative planning. If compromised nasal function is determined or suspected, or facial trauma has occurred, radiography and CT scans of the nose and paranasal sinuses should be obtained.

In addition to the nasal examination, consideration of possible donor sites for cartilage, soft tissues, and, in the case of trauma, bone grafts should be made. The most likely locations for cartilage are the septum, the auricle, and the costal cartilages.

The armamentarium for correction of nasal tip underprojection involves the use of onlay grafts, shield grafts, columella strut, septocolumella sutures, lateral crural steal, and footplate approximation. Nasal spine and maxillary augmentation can also give the illusion of increased projection. The Fred technique can be specifically used in patients with excess columella show and underprojected tip. The techniques of nasal correction of inadequate tip are quite complex and cannot be used interchangeably. It demands 3-dimensional consideration. A cephalic trim of the lower lateral cartilages requires reapproximation of the domes by suture, otherwise it results in unexpected widening of the tip. In general, a tip graft and transdomal suture will be suitable when the infratip lobule is deficient. The columella strut and septocolumellar suture suspension are a better choice when the columella is short.

ANESTHESIA

General anesthesia is employed, usually via an endotracheal tube or a laryngeal mask. Local anesthesia using 1% lidocaine with 1:200,000 epinephrine is injected into the soft-tissue plane. Once vasoconstriction is achieved from the initial injection, the nose is infiltrated with 0.5% Marcaine containing 1:100,000 epinephrine for further vasoconstriction.

POSITION AND MARKINGS

The patient is placed in supine position, with the entire face exposed and the eyes lubricated and taped closed with sterile Steri-Strips. The face is prepped in sterile fashion, nasal hairs are trimmed, and the nasal vestibule is cleaned with cotton tip swabs. The midpoint of the nose is marked for reference in the glabellar region, and the position of the midpoint of the incisors-philtral column is marked in cases where there is vertical facial asymmetry.

A stairstep transcolumellar incision is marked on the skin, above the flaring of the medial crura, extending into marginal incisions bilaterally.

Brilliant green or methylene blue is kept on hand for markings intraoperatively when working in multiple layers.

DETAILS OF PROCEDURE

The open approach to rhinoplasty using the transcolumellar stairstep incision is preferred. The incision is marked out on the midcolumella, and extended into bilateral marginal incisions, placed 1 to 2 mm caudal to the caudal margin of the lateral crura. The skin soft-tissue envelope is elevated off the cartilaginous lateral crura and extended cranially to expose the cartilaginous and bony dorsum. Dissection should extend just enough laterally to expose the upper lateral cartilage, but no more lateral than that. The bony vault can be exposed with a periosteal elevator up to the nasion. Any bony-cartilaginous hump reduction or maneuvers can be performed at this time. The septoplasty can be performed through the open or closed technique, depending on the severity of the deviation. The deviated portions of the cartilaginous septum, the vomer plate, and the perpendicular plates are removed. The flap is placed back in position and repaired using 5-0 chromic running quilting sutures. Any spreader grafts needed should be placed prior to osteotomies, which is next undertaken. A medial osteotomy is performed. A low-to-low lateral osteotomy is performed.

Maneuvers to improve nasal tip projection include columella strut, caudal extension grafts, septocolumellar sutures, transdomal sutures with or without lateral crural steal, tip grafts, plumping or shield grafts, and

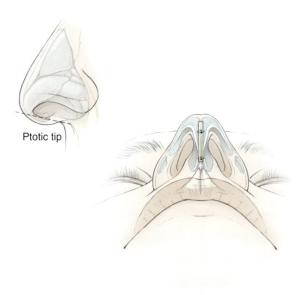

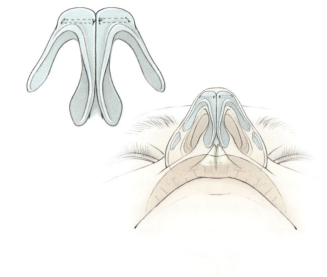

Figure 23-1   Schematic showing the use of the columella strut. It is secured in position between the medial crura. The columella strut is the most predictable and stable way to enhance tip projection.

Figure 23-2   Transdomal or interdomal sutures can be used to increase tip projection by 1 to 2 mm, and also to refine a broad or trapezoidal tip. If more projection is needed, a "steal" of the lateral crura can also be implemented.

premaxillary or nasal spine grafts to give the illusion of projection.

A columella strut provides the most predictable and stable means of increase in tip projection. It is the best means to strengthen the tip structure for the patient with a short columella, and effectively corrects the dependent tip deformity, especially on those patients for whom the condition is worsened on smiling. The strut is placed between the medial crura to augment tip projection, or to correct buckled medial or intermediate crura. The strut typically measures approximately 2 to 2.5 cm in length, 3 to 4 mm in width, and 1 to 2 mm in thickness. It is fashioned from the straightest portion of the septal cartilage if possible. Auricular or rib cartilage would be harvested when septal cartilage is not available. The strut is sutured in place using 5-0 clear nylon or PDS (polydioxanone suture) (Fig. 23-1).

Tip projection can be enhanced with transdomal sutures in cases where there is a broad or trapezoidal tip. Horizontal mattress transdomal sutures or interdomal sutures can be used. The transdomal suture increases lobule length by 1 to 2 mm. However, one needs to implement alar rim grafts because transdomal sutures tend to depress the lateral crura by pulling the domes together. In some cases, the transdomal sutures can be extended to "borrow" the lateral crus to lengthen the medial crura and effectively increase projection (and rotation). In cases where a larger bite of the lateral crura is taken, this is considered a "steal" of the lateral crura to lengthen the medial leg of the tip tripod (Fig. 23-2).

Approximation of the footplates will create more stability to the columella and also increase the tip projection, as will fixation of the medial crura to the caudal border of the septum in an anterior position, known as the Fred technique (Fig. 23-3). This is only applicable in certain patients, however, particularly those with long cephalo-caudal length and excess columella show. Patients must be forewarned of increased nasal rigidity since the tip and septum become a single unit.

Tip augmentation using an onlay tip graft is suitable for a patient with normal columella length and inadequate infratip lobule volume. It is fashioned from septal cartilage and sutured in position using clear 5-0 nylon or PDS to increase tip projection and improve tip contour. This can be carved from harvested septal cartilage or conchal or rib cartilage when necessary. We use the Tip Punch (Fig. 23-4) to create the tip graft, although the graft can also be custom crafted without this punch. An onlay graft is used when isolated projection deficiency exists.

If anterior and caudal lobule deficiencies coexist, a shield graft enhances projection and corrects the caudal lobule deficiency (Fig. 23-5).

Augmentation of the nasal spine and maxillary advancement also provide increased tip projection. These techniques are used only on those patients with deficiency of the premaxilla or anterior nasal spine. Application of a columella strut, augmentation of the nasal spine, and suspension of the footplate/medial crura will result in cephalic rotation of the tip.

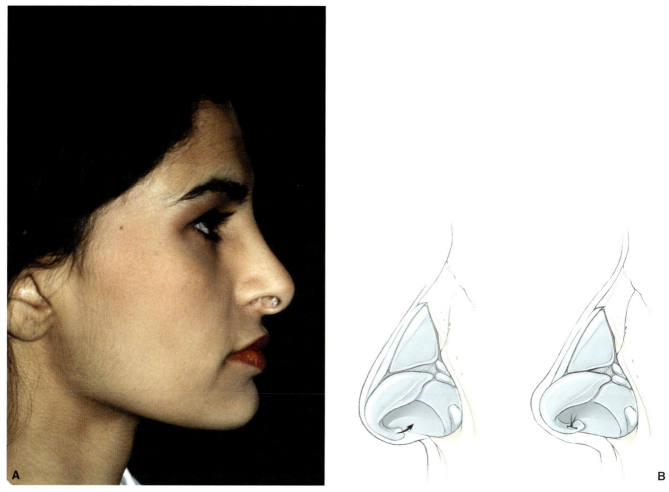

Figure 23-3   The Fred technique fixates the medial crura to the caudal border of the septum. This is helpful in patients with excess columella show.

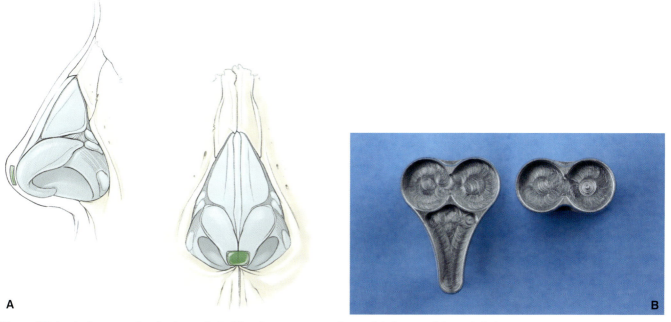

Figure 23-4   **A.** An example of a tip graft. **B.** The Guyuron tip graft punch helps simplify graft fashioning.

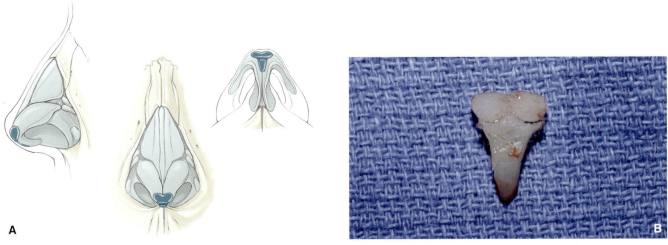

Figure 23-5 **A.** Schematic of a shield or shear graft. **B.** Actual graft obtained by using the Guyuron tip graft punch.

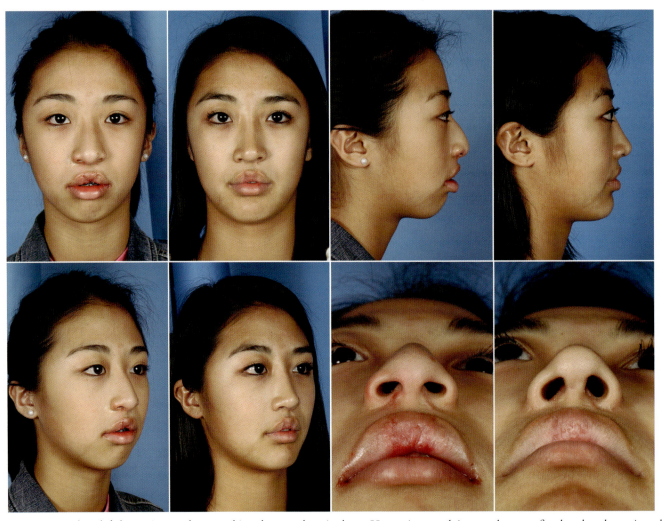

Figure 23-6 This cleft-lip patient underwent rhinoplasty and genioplasty. Her main complaint was her unrefined and underprojected nasal tip. Using a combination of a columellar strut, the Guyuron punch for a tip graft, and interdomal suturing techniques, she demonstrates an increase in tip projection by 3 to 4 mm, and improved tip refinement. She is shown 2-years post-operatively.

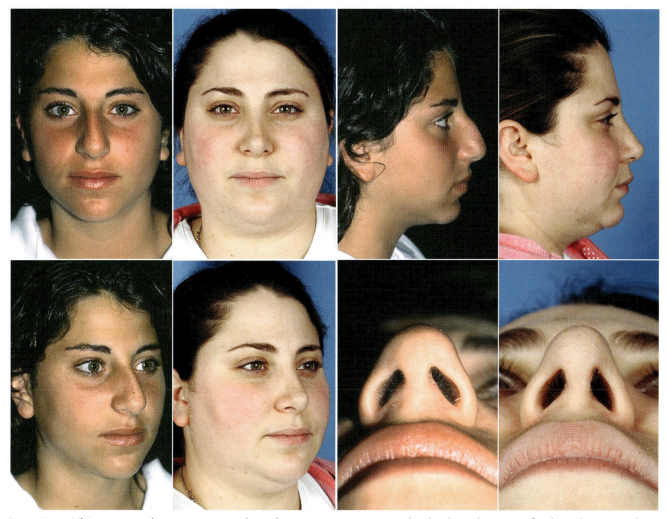

Figure 23-7   This patient is shown preoperatively, and at 10-years postoperatively. She shows her new refined nasal contour after removal of dorsal hump, and enhancement of her tip projection. The techniques used include interdomal sutures with a lateral crural steal. The projection is maintained a decade later.

PITFALLS

A successful aesthetic rhinoplasty operation is one in which both the surgeon and the patient are satisfied. This requires careful preoperative discussion and planning. Expectations of both parties should be realistic; in particular, the patient should be determined to be psychologically sound.

Blank the patient should be counseled that most of the tip augmentation techniques may result in stiffness of the tip. Addressing this possibility will reduce the patient's dissatisfaction. Be wary of the patient with thin skin and strong alar cartilages as these allow visible irregularities years after surgery.

Complications after rhinoplasty include the common postsurgical wound infection, hematomas, and dehiscence. Rhinoplasty is one of the most challenging operations, and revisions are common. By meticulous preoperative planning, careful patient selection and realistic expectations, one can decrease the revision rate.

PEARLS

There is no other operation as rewarding as that of a successful aesthetic rhinoplasty in balancing overall facial harmony (Figs. 23-6 and 23-7). This is only achieved through careful patient selection and meticulous preoperative planning. The surgeon should be familiar with all options for increasing tip projection and rotation. In the use of cartilage grafts, beveling the edges of grafts ensures that it blends easily into the surrounding tissue. If the patient has thin skin, the beveled edges will be less palpable and less visible. This will decrease potential postoperative complications, skin dimpling, and palpable irregularities.

SUGGESTED READING

Byrd HS, Hobar PC. Rhinoplasty: a practical guide for surgical planning. *Plast Reconstr Surg.* 1993;91:642-654.

Crumley, RL, Lanser M. Quantitative analysis of nasal tip projection. *Laryngoscope.* 1998;98:202-208.

Guyuron B, Behmand RA. Nasal tip sutures part II: the interplays. *Plast Reconstr Surg.* 2003;112(4):1130-1145.

Guyuron, B, Jackowe, D. Modified tip grafts and tip punch devices. *Plast Reconstr Surg.* 2007;120(7):2004-2010.

Guyuron B. Precision rhinoplasty. Part I: the role of life-size photographs and soft-tissue cephalometric analysis. *Plast Reconstr Surg.* 1988;81:489-499.

Sajjadian A, Guyuron B. An algorithm for treatment of the drooping nose. *Aesthet Surg J.* 2009;29:199-208.

Chapter 24. Closed Approach to Rhinoplasty

Rodger H. Brown, MD; Daniel A. Hatef, MD;
Jamal M. Bullocks, MD; Samuel Stal, MD

INDICATIONS

The debate about whether to use the open or endonasal approach to rhinoplasty has been ongoing on for many years. The majority of rhinoplasty procedures can be performed in an endonasal or closed approach, but some surgeons believe there are advantages to using the open approach in more difficult cases such as secondary or cleft rhinoplasties. The open approach involves an external incision across the columella that will lead to a scar. This incision usually heals well, but it can occasionally lead to an unsightly scar and/or notching (Fig. 24-1).

The patient's nasal deformity should be assessed preoperatively, and the surgeon needs to determine whether he or she is capable of correcting that deformity through an endonasal approach or whether wider exposure will be needed. Most experts would agree that simple dorsum, tip, and septal problems can easily be addressed with the closed approach. In more complex problems, the decision

between closed versus open depends on the extent of the deformity, the techniques planned, the patient's desires, and the surgeon's experience.

PREOPERATIVE PREPARATION

The preoperative consultation should consist of a complete examination of the external nasal features, the internal nasal anatomy, and the relationship of the nose to other facial features. In endonasal rhinoplasty, it is important to be able to look at the nose externally and understand what underlying structural abnormality is causing each deformity. Unlike in open rhinoplasty, there is limited ability to visualize the underlying framework during the operation. Correct evaluation and diagnosis of the underlying deformity allows the surgeon to plan what procedures and techniques will be used during the operation. If the preoperative evaluation is incorrect, the procedures performed will not correct the deformities and may make them worse. This is one of the biggest criticisms of the closed approach, but if one becomes skilled at the preoperative evaluation and diagnosis, the endonasal approach can allow for a shorter and less-traumatic approach to rhinoplasty, yielding equal or superior results.

The preoperative exam should be performed in the same organized manner with each patient to develop a routine. This will make the surgeon more efficient and accurate in assessment and diagnosis. One good way to approach it is in a top-down, external-to-internal fashion. Begin with evaluation of the radix, followed by the dorsum, tip, columella, ala, nostrils, and external nasal valve. Examine the internal structures, which include the septum, turbinates, and the internal nasal valve, with a nasal speculum and adequate lighting.

ANESTHESIA

Endonasal rhinoplasty may be performed under local anesthesia only, local anesthesia and sedation, or general anesthesia. Regardless of technique, the infiltration of

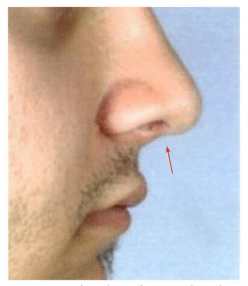

Figure 24-1 Picture of notching after open rhinoplasty incision across the columella.

local anesthetic with epinephrine is effective to limit bleeding, allow better visualization, and better define tissue planes.

The local anesthetic preparation is begun by packing the nose with cottonoids soaked in 4% cocaine or Afrin (oxymetazoline) to create a vasoconstricted state. Afrin causes vasoconstriction only, while cocaine will cause a more intense vasoconstriction and also act as a local anesthetic. Cocaine has the potential for causing cardiac complications, and should be used with caution in patients at risk for such complications; the dose should be strictly limited to 4 mg/kg. Next, the nasal structures are infiltrated with 1% lidocaine with 1:200,000 epinephrine. Usually only 5 to 10 mL are needed. Injection of too much local anesthetic can distort the soft tissues and make intraoperative evaluation of results difficult. The local anesthetic solution should be injected at the radix, along the dorsum, along the ascending processes of the maxilla at the proposed osteotomy sites, along the septum, the alar-facial grooves, and a small amount over the lower lateral cartilages and tip. Small amounts should also be injected at the sites of any other proposed incisions.

POSITION AND MARKINGS

The patient should be placed in the supine position with a shoulder roll to create slight extension of the neck. The entire face should be prepped in the usual sterile fashion. If the patient is under general anesthesia, the eyes should be protected with lubricant and an occlusive dressing or corneal protectors. A sterile adhesive drape can be used to further isolate the mouth and endotracheal tube from the operative field. Finally, sterile towels are used to create a head drape as in other facial surgery. Given that all incisions are endonasal in the closed approach, no markings are absolutely necessary, but some find it helpful to mark the borders of the lower lateral cartilage, the midline of the tip, and the caudal end of the nasal bones.

DETAILS OF PROCEDURE

Incisions

An infra-, intra-, and/or intercartilaginous incision is made using a no. 15 blade with a sharp double hook to help evert the alar rim for exposure. The infracartilaginous, or marginal, incision is placed at the caudal border of the lower lateral cartilage (Fig. 24-2). An intracartilaginous incision overlies the lateral crus of the lower lateral cartilage and is carried through the mucosa and the cartilage; therefore, it is also called a cartilage splitting or transcartilaginous incision (Fig. 24-3). This allows for direct cephalic trim, but can make dissection and further tip modifications more difficult. An intercartilaginous incision is carried out over the scroll area, or the

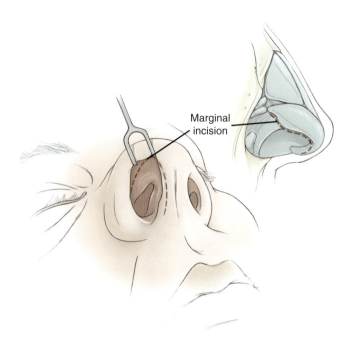

Figure 24-2 Illustration depicting infracartilaginous incision at the caudal edge of the lower lateral cartilage.

junction of the lower lateral and upper lateral cartilages (Fig. 24-4). A transfixion or hemitransfixion incision is made with the no. 15 blade through the membranous septum/columella at the caudal border of the cartilaginous septum to give access to the columella and septum (Fig. 24-5). A separate incision may be made at the alar

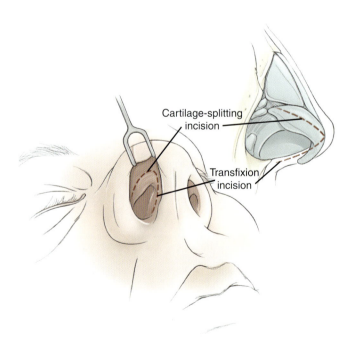

Figure 24-3 Illustration depicting intracartilaginous incision at the vestibular skin underlying the middle of the lower lateral cartilage.

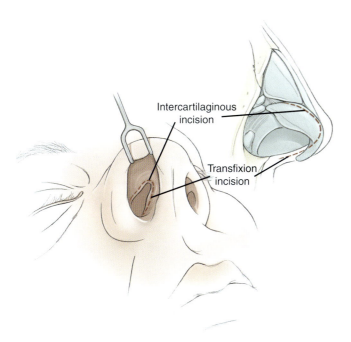

Figure 24-4 Illustration depicting intercartilaginous incision at the intranasal mucosa between the cephalic border of the lower lateral cartilage and caudal border of the upper lateral cartilage.

base later if an alar contour graft and/or alar base excision is planned.

Dissection

After making the above incisions, the cartilaginous and bony framework is dissected free from the overlying skin and soft tissue and mucoperichondrium/periosteum. This dissection is carried out in the subperichondrial and subperiosteal plane to preserve the integrity of the soft tissues and blood supply.

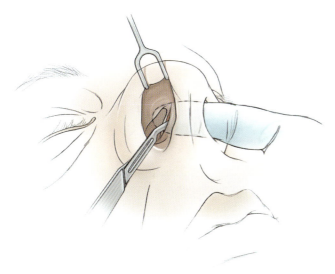

Figure 24-5 Illustration depicting transfixion incision to gain access to the septum with the endonasal approach.

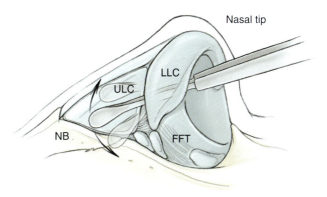

Figure 24-6 Illustration depicting subperichondrial dissection over the upper lateral cartilage. ULC, upper lateral cartilage; NB, nasal bone; LLC, lower lateral cartilage; FFT, fibro-fatty tissue.

The lower lateral cartilages are freed of their attachments using sharp tissue scissors, such as the Iris or Josephs. This allows for later modification of the cartilage and redraping of the soft-tissue envelope. Under direct observation with an Aufricht retractor, the soft tissue over the upper lateral cartilages is elevated up to the caudal edge of the nasal bones using sharp tissue scissors (Fig. 24-6). A periosteal elevator is then placed in the intra- or intercartilaginous incision and used to elevate the overlying soft tissues off of the medial nasal bones with care to prevent injury to the septal cartilage in the midline. A mucoperichondrial flap is dissected off the septum through the transfixion incision using a periosteal elevator. A mucoperiosteal tunnel is created, separating the septum from the upper lateral cartilages and the under surface of the nasal bones. These submucosal tunnels should be dissected prior to resection of the dorsum so as to maintain the integrity of the mucosa and prevent scarring and later stenosis.

Septum

The septum is accessed through the transfixion or hemitransfixion incision (Fig. 24-7). Dissection is performed as described above, elevating a mucoperichondrial flap and making mucoperiosteal tunnels. If caudal shortening is desired, as in the patient with a long nose or hanging columella, a strip of the caudal septum can be resected through the transfixion incision to shorten the nose and improve tip rotation. A swivel knife or septal scissors are then used to resect the septum for graft material or to excise deviated and abnormal segments. Care must be taken to leave at least a 1- to 1.5-cm L-strut dorsally and caudally for support (Fig. 24-8).

Dorsum

The bony portion of the hump can be reduced at this time by using a down-biting rasp placed through the

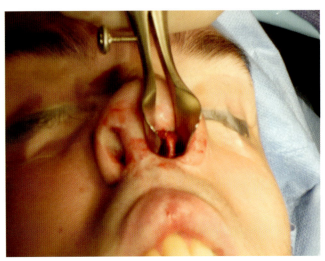

Figure 24-7   Intraoperative picture of septal exposure through transfixion incision.

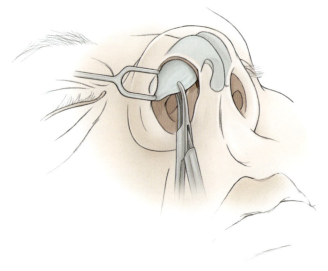

Figure 24-9   Illustration depicting delivery of the lower lateral cartilage.

intercartilaginous incision. Once this is complete, the cartilaginous portion is excised with a no. 15 or no. 11 blade. Reexamine the nasal profile externally multiple times during the hump reduction until the appropriate contour is achieved.

Tip

After a symmetrical dissection of the lower lateral cartilages has been performed as described above, the tip may be modified by a number of methods. Cephalic trim

can be performed directly using an intracartilaginous/transcartilaginous incision. If further tip work is necessary, an inter- and/or infracartilaginous incision would be beneficial to allow for delivery of the cartilages. By delivering the cartilages, the surgeon has improved visualization for more accurate trimming, and the domes can be accessed for suture modification (Fig. 24-9).

Osteotomy

The incision for performing the osteotomy is a stab incision through the vestibular mucosa above the inferior turbinate, near the base of the pyriform aperture. A periosteal elevator is then used to dissect in the subperiosteal plane at the pyriform aperture and the base of the ascending process of the maxilla where the osteotomy will be started. For a patient with pyramidal basilar lines, a low-to-high osteotomy pattern is used. In this case, a curved osteotome is inserted as low as possible on the pyriform aperture, and the osteotomy is carried out in a pyramidal fashion toward the proximal nasal bones. For a patient with parallel basilar lines, a low-to-low osteotomy pattern is used. In this case, a straight osteotome is used and the osteotomy is carried out more parallel to the dorsal nasal lines. If a medial osteotomy is needed, this can be performed through the intercartilaginous incision with a curved osteotome. In the severely deviated nose, double osteotomies may be indicated on one or both sides, in order to accurately relocate the dorsum.

Placement of Grafts

Once all other steps of the resection rhinoplasty are complete, many patients will benefit from the placing of grafts to maintain structure or camouflage abnormal underlying

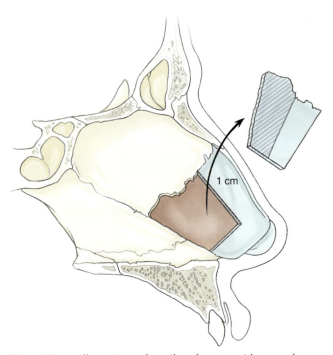

Figure 24-8   Illustration of cartilage harvest with septoplasty, leaving a 1-cm L-strut for support.

1 cm

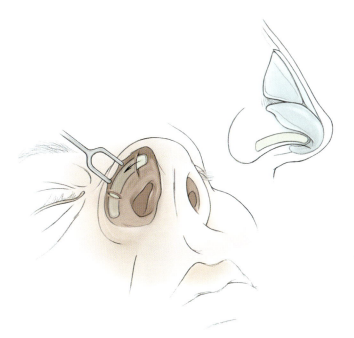

Figure 24-10   Illustration depicting technique for placement of alar batten graft through medial end of infracartilaginous incision.

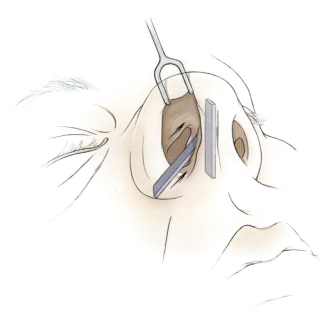

Figure 24-11   Illustration of columellar strut graft insertion into pocket through transfixion incision.

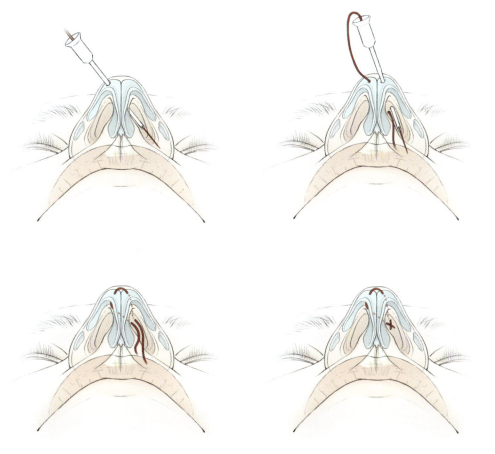

Figure 24-12   Illustration depicting suture securitization of tip grafts by passing suture back and forth percutaneously.

anatomy. These grafts include possible tip, columellar strut, spreader, or dorsal onlay grafts. The open approach allows for direct visualization of graft sites and allows easy access for fixation; however, the endonasal approach can also be used to successfully place and secure all these grafts through the previously discussed incisions. A tip or alar graft can be placed into a subcutaneous pocket through the medial end of the infracartilaginous incision (Fig. 24-10). The columellar strut graft is placed through the transfixion incision (Fig. 24-11). The spreader and dorsal onlay grafts can be placed through intercartilaginous incisions and sutured to the dorsal septum and/or upper lateral cartilages. It may be more difficult to secure the grafts in place using the closed approach, but it can be successfully done by passing suture back and forth through each side or by temporarily securing it with transcutaneous sutures (Fig. 24-12).

Closure

Since all incisions are endonasal, they are closed with 3-0 or 4-0 chromic gut suture.

PITFALLS

The biggest pitfall with the use of the closed approach is a limited ability to completely visualize the underlying osseocartilaginous framework. In inexperienced hands, this may lead to misdiagnosis of deformities and/or inadequate correction. To avoid this, it is important to become an expert at the preoperative evaluation and hone the ability to diagnose the underlying abnormality by external evaluation. Some patients have substantial asymmetry of their lower lateral cartilage not apparent on external appearance of the nose, which will not be recognized by the closed approach without cartilage delivery.

PEARLS

- Infracartilaginous incisions with delivery of the lower lateral cartilages allows for the best access in patients who need significant tip modification.
- In patients with a simple dorsum, tip, or septal problem, the closed approach avoids the increased operative time, increased dissection, and destruction of tip support associated with the open approach (Fig. 24-13).

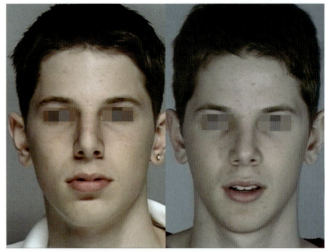
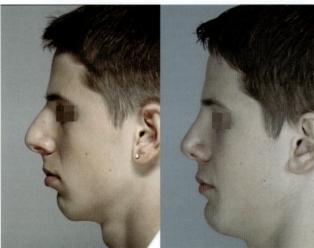

Figure 24-13   Preoperative and 6 months postoperative pictures of closed rhinoplasty to reduce dorsal hump in a 17-year-old male.

- The closed approach can be combined with alar base resection without concern for devascularizing the tip.
- The closed approach avoids the potential undesirable scars that can result from transcolumellar incisions.

SUGGESTED READING

Sheen JH. Closed versus open rhinoplasty—and the debate goes on. *Plast Reconstr Surg*. 1997:99(3):859-862.

Sheen JH, Sheen A. Basic technique. In: Sheen JH, Sheen A. *Aesthetic Rhinoplasty*. 2nd ed. St. Louis, MO: Mosby; 1987: 173-250.

Chapter 25. Principles of Approaches in Secondary Rhinoplasty

Ronald P. Gruber, MD; Meryl Singer, MD; Kenton Fong, MD

INDICATIONS

The indication for performing a secondary rhinoplasty depends upon whether the needs of the patient are reasonable and can be met by the surgeon. Photographic imaging analysis is extremely helpful in making this determination as it allows the surgeon to give the patient some idea of what can be done and allows the patient to give feedback as to what the patient does or does not like about the imaged result. It is often prudent not to attempt major revisions for at least one year after the most recent nasal surgery, although earlier surgery may be performed with the understanding that the desired final result may be more difficult to obtain. Evaluation of the nasal skin quality is one of the most important initial considerations. Very-thick-skin patients are less amendable to the open rhinoplasty approach because the transcolumellar incision aggravates postoperative edema and causes subsequent fibrosis that mars the final sculpted result. One common subset of secondary rhinoplasty patients that is useful for illustrative purposes is the overresected short-nose patient. These cases often require dorsal augmentation, septal extension grafts, tip grafts, spreader grafts, columellar strut, intercartilaginous grafts, rim grafts, and suture techniques, all of which illustrate secondary rhinoplasty techniques in general.

PREOPERATIVE PREPARATION

Most patients require at least 2 consultations prior to surgery. The most important aspect of the informed consent is warning the patient that a touch-up or revision might be necessary. This occurs in at least 20% of cases. On the morning of surgery, it is important that the surgeon has thought out a clear game plan prior to beginning the operation. It can be extremely helpful to perform mock surgery with the photo imager before going to the operating room.

ANESTHESIA

Most rhinoplasties can be performed under conscious sedation. Intramuscular Vistaril (hydroxyzine HCl) 100 mg (for its antiemetic effect) and an analgesic, for example, Demerol (meperidine HCl) or Nubain (nalbuphine HCl), are given in the preoperative holding area. Intraoperatively, the patient receives intravenous Versed (midazolam HCl) as needed to achieve adequate sedation as well as a onetime dose of intravenous ketamine 30 to 50 mg prior to local anesthetic injection. The dose of ketamine allows for 5 minutes of complete dissociation during the normally unpleasant injection process. Local anesthesia consists of a mixture of Xylocaine and Marcaine (bupivacaine HCl) with fresh 1:200,000 epinephrine concentration. If general anesthesia is used, the concentration of epinephrine may be increased to 1:100,000. To facilitate elevation of the nasal skin flap and minimize the risk of skin perforation, the nose is typically hyperinfiltrated with 20 to 30 mL of local anesthetic in the subcutaneous space, septal mucosa, and turbinates. Using this technique, no topical anesthetics are necessary and osteotomies may be performed.

POSITION AND MARKINGS

The patient is positioned in the supine position and the face is prepped with Castile soap or dilute Betadine (povidone-iodine). Working with loop magnification makes it difficult to appreciate the gestalt of the sculpted result. Therefore, it is ideal to have a video camera and monitor in the operating room that give the surgeon a true lateral view of the patient. Otherwise, it is helpful for the surgeon to occasionally walk to the other side of the patient to get a fresh perspective. For open rhinoplasties, an inverted V incision at the narrowest point in the columella is used unless the patient has a different scar from the primary surgery.

DETAILS OF PROCEDURES

Most secondary rhinoplasties need adequate exposure in order to perform detailed and accurate sculpting of the underlying framework; consequently, most major secondary rhinoplasties require an open approach. As mentioned above, to facilitate elevation of the flap with minimal risk of skin perforation the nose is hyperinfiltrated with 20 to 30 mL of local anesthetic into the subcutaneous space, septal mucosa, and turbinates.

Soft-tissue Release to Lengthen the Nose

The anterior septal angle is exposed first because it is easiest to locate when there is significant scar tissue. From there the mucoperichondrium is elevated off the caudal septum and the upper lateral cartilages are released from the dorsal septum (Figs. 25-1 to 25-3). A double hook is placed on the tip cartilages to retract the lower lateral cartilages (LLCs) from the upper lateral cartilages (ULCs). Using a pair of scissors, a gap is created between the ULCs and LLCs (Fig. 25-4).

Donor Cartilage

If septal cartilage is available, it should be harvested from the septum leaving an L-shaped strut that is at least

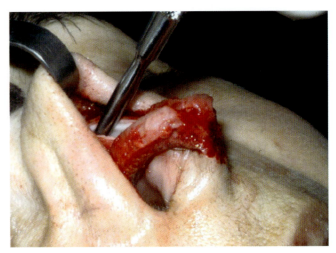

Figure 25-2 Intraoperative view showing beginning release of upper lateral cartilage and mucoperichondrium from septum.

1 cm in width. If not, ear cartilage works well. A retro-auricular incision is made to expose the concha cymba and concha cavum. When the cymba and cavum are properly exposed, they have a kidney shape. Removal can be accomplished without significant alteration to the shape of the ear. However, the patient may lose a few degrees of prominence. The graft is pinned to a silicone block, which facilitates carving. The cymba is separated from the cavum. Despite the fact that the cavum is slightly concave, it can be used in total as a septal extension graft. The cymba is pinned to the block and split down the middle. To remove its curvature and strengthen it, the cymba is pinned to the block concave side down and a 5-0 PDS (polydioxanone) mattress suture is placed on each side of the graft to shape the cartilage. The graft then becomes strong and straight enough for intercartilaginous or columellar strut grafts.

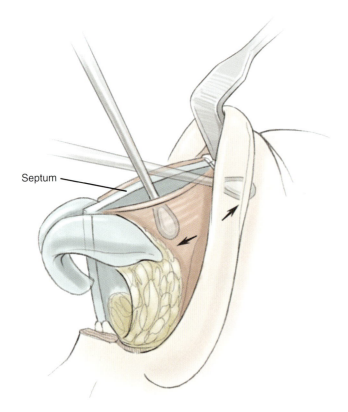

Septum

Figure 25-1 Schematic of releasing upper lateral cartilage and septal mucoperichondrium.

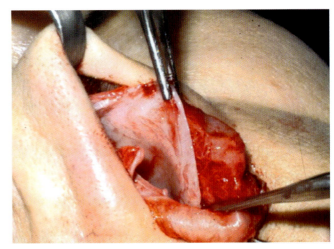

Figure 25-3 Intraoperative view showing completed release of upper lateral cartilage and mucoperichondrium from septum.

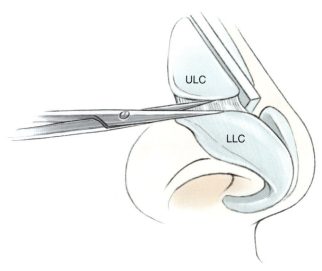

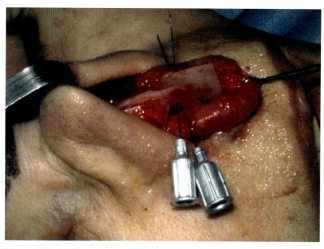

Figure 25-6   Intraoperative view showing attachment of septal extension graft to septum.

Figure 25-4   Schematic of separating upper from lower lateral cartilage after hyperinfiltrating underlying mucous membrane.

Septal Extension Graft

A cartilaginous graft is applied unilaterally to the dorsal aspect of the septum (Figs. 25-2 to 25-6). If septal cartilage is available, it makes an ideal septal extension graft because of its straight shape and thickness. However, enough septal cartilage must be saved for the intercarti-

laginous graft, which takes first priority because the intercartilaginous graft must be thin. If there is not enough septal graft, the concha cymba can be used after straightening with sutures as described above. The cavum is pinned to one side of the septum, allowed to protrude caudally for as many millimeters as desired for nasal lengthening, and then sutured to the septum with a few 5-0 PDS mattress sutures.

Intercartilaginous Graft

To prevent postoperative alar retraction that can occur after lengthening the nose with a septal extension graft, an intercartilaginous graft is placed between the ULCs and the LLCs (Figs. 25-7 and 25-8). Septal material is ideal but a cymba graft will work as well. It is sutured end to end to the ULC. However, the other side of the graft is placed deep to (under the lip of) the cephalic edge of the LLC.

Tip Graft

The tip graft is made from the concha cavum (of the other ear), which has a slight curvature that is ideal for a tip graft. The cavum is pinned to a silicone block. A silicone sizer (Miltex Co., York, PA)—usually a medium size works best—is pinned on top of the graft and the tip graft is created in cookie-cutter fashion.

Dorsal/Radix Augmentation

For large dorsal augmentation, a rib graft works best, and the fifth rib in the inframammary area is ideal. Either the anterior half of the rib or the entire rib, if necessary, can be harvested. Alternatively, diced cartilage wrapped in fascia is another excellent choice. For smaller augmentations, fascia alone may work well. Despite its ideal shape, septal cartilage grafts are seldom used for dorsal augmen-

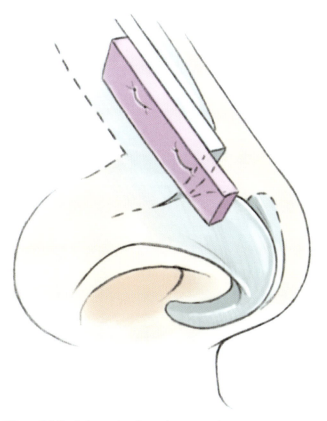

Figure 25-5   Schematic of attaching septal extension graft to septum.

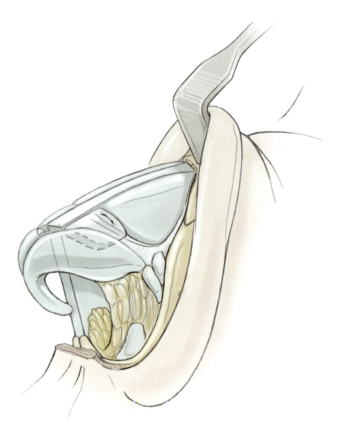

Figure 25-7 Suturing intercartilaginous graft to caudal edge of upper lateral cartilage and slipping caudal edge of graft under the edge of the lower lateral cartilage.

tation because they are usually needed for other purposes, as described above.

Columellar Strut

In the short/small nose, the tip is often deficient to the point that a tip graft alone is insufficient to accomplish

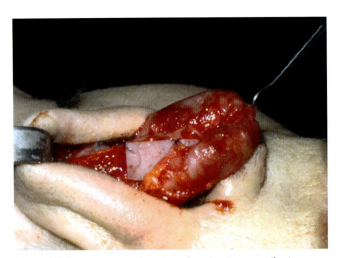

Figure 25-8 Intraoperative view showing intercartilaginous graft in place.

the task of tip projection without making the tip lobule too large and unaesthetic. Thus, a columellar strut may be required to provide support and project the tip. If septum is unavailable, concha cymba works well if first prepared and straightened as described above and in the accompanying video. It is passed into a tunnel made between the middle crura and sutured to the middle crura with 5-0 PDS sutures.

PITFALLS

- When a patient is lying down it is difficult to appreciate if the nasolabial angle is appropriate. Sitting the head of the bed up at the end of the case helps avoid underprojection.
- The patient with thick skin may develop severe postoperative edema and fibrous tissue deposition that mars the surgical result. The closed rhinoplasty approach should be considered for these patients to preserve columellar circulation and minimize scarring.
- Fibrous deposition may mar a surgical result, particularly in secondary cases. Therefore, keep dissection undermining to a minimum.
- If temporalis fascia is used for padding the tip or augmenting the dorsum or sides of the nose, it must be sutured down. Otherwise, it tends to shrink and thicken to 3 times its original thickness and severely distorts the intended result.

PEARLS

- The surgeon should stress to the patient the relatively high revision rate in rhinoplasty (unlike other aesthetic procedures).
- Analysis is half the case. Mock surgery helps with analysis.
- The transcolumellar scar is rarely a problem and is usually not a reason to avoid the open approach.
- Working with a model makes it easier to do biological sculpting (Fig. 25-9).
- Hydrodissect with local anesthesia to facilitate dissection and avoid perforations.
- Grafting generally gives better results than resection because it stretches the skin and mitigates fibrous tissue deposition.
- Thin-skin areas may need soft-tissue augmentation to avoid contour irregularities caused by cartilage grafts. Temporalis fascia is an ideal choice.
- Septum is the donor site of choice for cartilage grafts. If it is unavailable, ear cartilage is an excellent choice because its shape can be controlled with suture techniques.

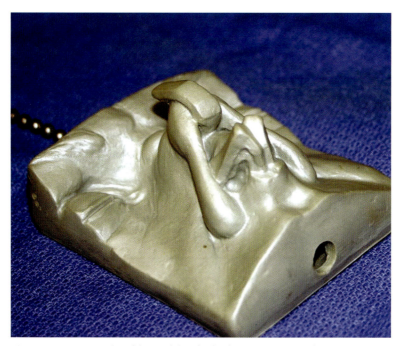

Figure 25-9 Autoclavable model (which also acts as a nasal retractor at surgery) used to help sculpt nasal tip cartilages (Miltex Co.).

PHOTOGRAPHY

The patient in Figures 25-10 to 25-14 had overresection during a primary rhinoplasty leaving the nose short, dorsally deficient, and tip deficient (front, side, and basal views). The Gunter diagrams (Figs. 25-10 and 25-11) demonstrate: (1) release of the ULCs and mucoperichondrium of the septum; (2) attachment of a septal extension graft; (3) release of the gap between the ULCs and LLCs;

(4) the insertion of an intercartilaginous graft (placed under the lip of the LLCs); and (5) removal of the silicone implant and replacement with rib graft.

The postoperative views (Figs. 25-12 to 25-14) at greater than 1-year in followup demonstrate that the nose is longer, the nostril show is improved, and alar retraction was prevented by lengthening the side wall with the intercartilaginous grafts.

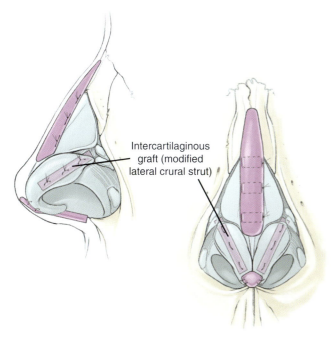

Intercartilaginous graft (modified lateral crural strut)

Figure 25-10 Gunter diagram of maneuvers performed.

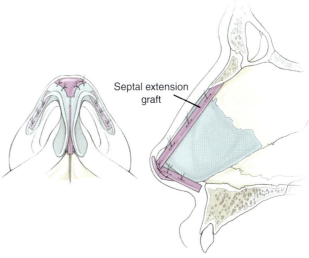

Septal extension graft

Figure 25-11 Gunter diagram (alternative views) of maneuvers performed.

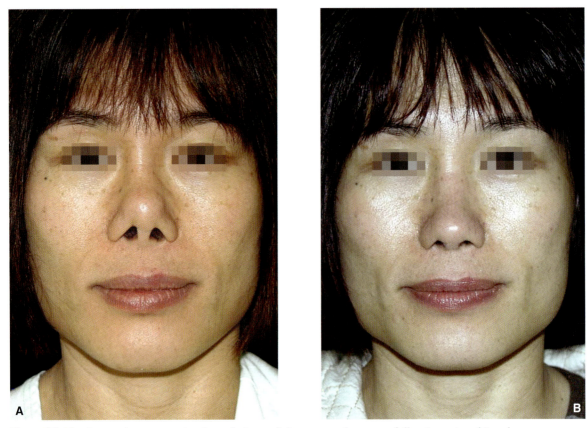

Figure 25-12   Pre- and postoperative frontal views of short, turned-up nose following prior rhinoplasty at greater than 1 year follow up.

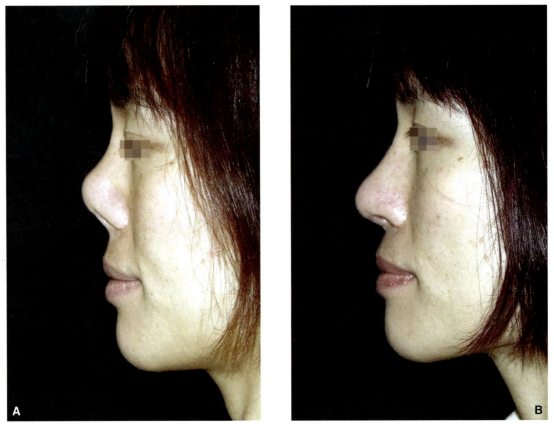

Figure 25-13   Pre- and postoperative side views of turned-up nose following prior rhinoplasty.

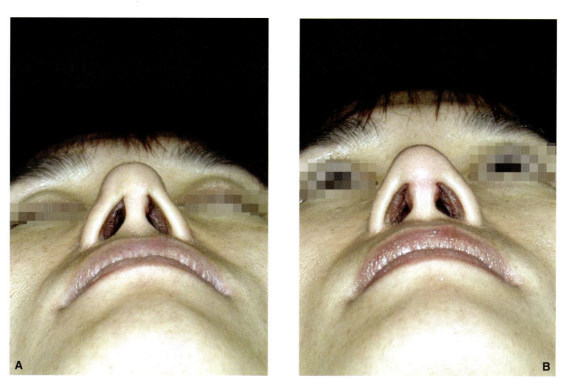

Figure 25-14   Pre- and postoperative basal views of short, turned-up nose following prior rhinoplasty at greater than 1 year follow up.

Chapter 26. Rib Grafting

C. Spencer Cochran, MD; Jack P. Gunter, MD

INDICATIONS

Although septal cartilage is generally considered the preferred grafting material in rhinoplasty, severe deformities or a paucity of available septal cartilage requires alternative sources of grafting material. This is particularly true in patients who require dorsal augmentation and in secondary rhinoplasty patients with structural deformities resulting from previous procedures.

PREOPERATIVE PREPARATION

The choice of which rib to harvest depends on the planned use and grafting requirements, because the amount of cartilage required dictates whether the cartilaginous segment from one rib, rib and a portion of another, or the entire cartilage segments of 2 ribs need to be harvested. The surgeon should choose the cartilaginous portion of the fifth, sixth, or seventh rib that provides a straight segment long enough to construct all required grafts. If additional grafts are needed, a part or the entire cartilaginous portion of an adjacent rib may be harvested.

In older patients, ossification of the cartilaginous ribs can make graft preparation difficult and preclude its use. A preoperative CT scan of the ribs and sternum can help delineate the extent of calcification in patients in whom there is a high index of suspicion. In this case, some surgeons recommend diced cartilage within a temporalis fascia wrap.

ANESTHESIA

General anesthesia with endotracheal intubation is preferred for this procedure. This allows the patient to be completely still for the duration of the procedure and allows for a protected airway.

POSITION AND MARKINGS

The patient is placed in the supine position. After adequate anesthesia is administered, the patient is prepped and draped in a sterile manner. In female patients, the incision is marked slightly above the inframammary fold and measures 5 cm in length (Fig. 26-1). In males, placement of the incision is not as important unless there is a hair-bearing area in which the incision can be camouflaged. If not, the incision is usually placed directly over

the chosen rib to facilitate the dissection. Although rib cartilage can be harvested from either the patient's right or left side, harvesting rib cartilage from the patient's left side allows for a 2-team approach.

DETAILS OF PROCEDURE

The skin is incised with a scalpel, and the subcutaneous tissue is divided with electrocautery. Once the muscle fascia has been reached, the surgeon palpates the underlying ribs and divides the muscle and fascia with electrocautery

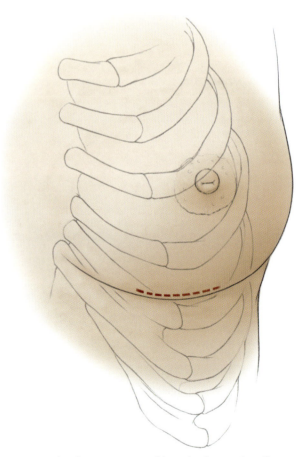

Figure 26-1 The skin incision (*red line*) for harvesting rib cartilage in female patients is placed parallel and slightly superior to the inframammary fold and measures approximately 5 cm.

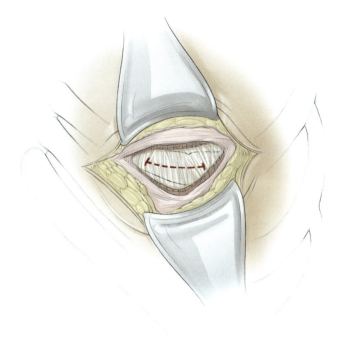

Figure 26-3 After the muscle has been divided, the perichondrium is incised (*red dashed lines*) along its long axis to expose the underlying rib cartilage. Perpendicular cuts at the medial and lateral aspects of the central incision facilitate reflection of the perichondrium.

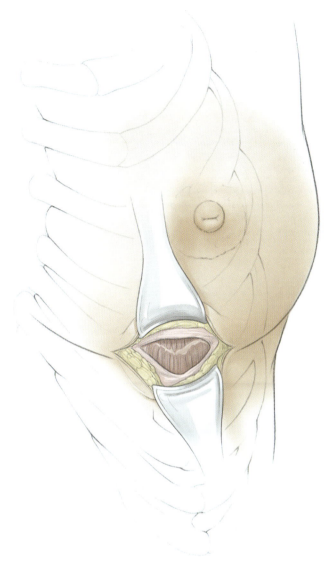

Figure 26-2 After incising the skin, dissection is carried out down through the subcutaneous tissue, and the surgeon divides the muscle and fascia with electrocautery directly over the cartilaginous portion of the chosen rib.

dissection is then continued circumferentially along the length of the cartilaginous portion of the rib until the posterior aspect of the rib is exposed. A curved rib stripper completes the posterior dissection (Fig. 26-5). The curved rib stripper is slid back-and-forth along the rib, taking care to stay between the cartilage and perichondrium until the undermining is complete. Perichondrial tears should be avoided so that a tight postoperative closure can later be accomplished to help "splint" the wound, which aids in relieving postoperative pain.

The final step involves separating the cartilaginous rib from its medial attachment near the sternum and laterally at the bony rib. This is performed by making a partial thickness incision perpendicular to the long axis of the rib using a no. 15 blade at the aforementioned junctions (Fig. 26-6). The cartilaginous incision can then be completed with the sharp end of a Freer elevator using gentle side-to-side movement. Once the cartilage segment is released both medially and laterally, the graft is easily removed from the wound and placed in sterile saline until the surgeon is ready for fabrication. If more grafting material is required, a portion of cartilage or the entire cartilaginous part of an adjacent rib should then be harvested in a similar fashion.

After hemostasis is achieved, the donor site is checked to ensure that no pneumothorax has occurred. The wound is filled with saline solution and the anesthesiologist applies positive pressure into the lungs. If no air

directly over the cartilaginous portion of the chosen rib (Fig. 26-2). The rib is exposed from its sternal attachment medially to the bony-cartilaginous junction laterally. Identification of this junction is facilitated by the subtle change in color at the interface: The cartilaginous portion is generally off-white, whereas the bony rib demonstrates a distinct reddish-gray hue.

After exposing the selected rib, an incision is made through the perichondrium along the long axis of the rib (Fig. 26-3). Perpendicular cuts are also made in the perichondrium at the most medial and lateral aspects of the cartilaginous rib to facilitate reflection of the perichondrium.

A Dingman elevator is then utilized to elevate the perichondrium superiorly and inferiorly from the cartilaginous rib (Fig. 26-4). The subperichondrial

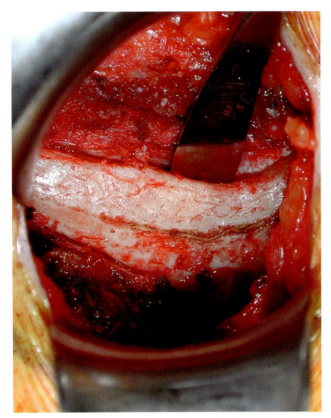

Figure 26-4   Intraoperative view of perichondrial elevation from the superior aspect of the cartilaginous rib using a periosteal elevator.

leak is detected, a pneumothorax can be excluded. A 16-gauge Angiocath catheter is inserted through the skin and placed in the bed of the wound to allow instillation of a long-acting local anesthetic at the conclusion of the procedure. The wound may then be closed in layers

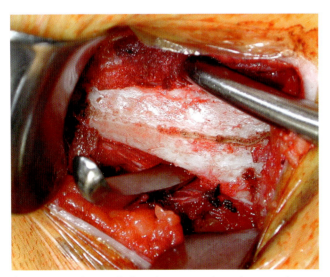

Figure 26-5   A curved rib stripper completes the posterior dissection. Care should be taken to stay between the rib and perichondrium to avoid a pneumothorax.

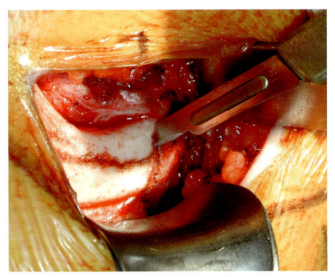

Figure 26-6   Intraoperative view of separating the cartilaginous rib laterally at junction of the bony rib.

using 2-0 Vicryl sutures. Particular attention should be directed at reapproximating the perichondrium and muscle fascia layers tightly to prevent a palpable or visible chest-wall deformity. A tight closure also helps "splint" the wound and reduce postoperative pain. Skin closure is carried out using deep dermal and subcuticular 4-0 Monocryl sutures.

After the rib cartilage has been harvested, it can then be fashioned into the desired grafts. Before carving of the grafts is begun, silicone sizers are used to estimate the shape and size of the needed grafts. The silicone sizers are prefabricated by the surgeon. Molds of anatomically shaped dorsal onlay grafts and columellar struts are carved in a paraffin wax block in an assortment of shapes and sizes. RTV (room temperature vulcanizing) silicone is mixed and poured into the molds and left for 24 hours to polymerize before trimming to their final form.

Graft warping can occur in autogenous rib cartilage and lead to long-term postoperative distortions of nasal shape. The utilization of stabilizing K-wires placed through the center of large grafts, such as dorsal onlay grafts and columellar strut grafts, has been a successful technique to counterbalance the tendency of the grafts to warp. A smooth 0.028-inch K-wire is drilled longitudinally through the center of the graft. The 0.028-inch K-wire is removed and replaced with a threaded 0.035-inch K-wire placed within 2 to 3 mm from the cephalic end of the graft and cut flush with the caudal end. The same routine is used for placing the internal K-wire in the columellar strut except that the K-wire within the columellar strut should extend three-fourths the length of the graft and 8 to 10 mm of the K-wire should be left exposed at the graft base, which will be seated into a drill hole created in the maxilla. The cartilage grafts with the internal K-wires are then carved into similar but slightly larger shapes of the

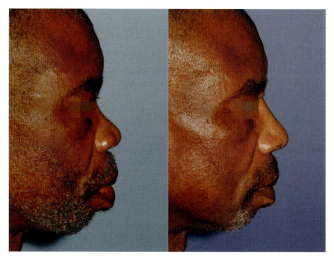

Figure 26-7 Preoperative (*left*) versus postoperative (*right*) views of a primary rhinoplasty patient in whom rib cartilage grafts with internal K-wires were used as a columellar strut to increase his tip projection and a dorsal onlay graft to augment his dorsum.

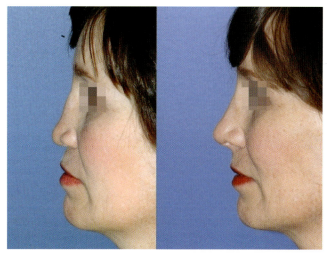

Figure 26-9 Preoperative (*left*) versus postoperative (*right*) views of a secondary rhinoplasty patient in whom rib cartilage grafts with internal K-wires were used as extended spreader grafts, dorsal onlay graft and a columellar strut to correct a saddle-nose deformity.

selected sizers. To avoid warping of smaller grafts, we follow the principle of carving balanced cross sections originally described by Gibson and later substantiated by Kim et al. (Figs. 26-7 to 26-9).

PITFALLS

- Ossification of the cartilaginous rib is a concern in patients older than age 50 years. A limited CT scan of the ribs and sternum can help delineate the extent of rib calcification.
- A pneumothorax is an uncommon complication of rib cartilage harvest. If an air leak is detected from the pari-

etal pleura and the lung parenchyma has not been injured, a red rubber catheter can be inserted through the pleural tear. The wound is closed in layers over the catheter. The anesthesiologist applies positive pressure into the lungs while the catheter is placed on suction and removed.

PEARLS

- The fifth, sixth, and seventh ribs often provide a cartilaginous segment long enough to construct all required grafts. If additional cartilage is needed, it can be harvested from an adjacent rib.
- A tight closure of the perichondrial and muscle fascia layers helps to prevent a palpable or visible chest wall deformity and also helps "splint" the wound to reduce postoperative pain.
- Balanced cross-sectional carving of rib cartilage can decrease its tendency to warp. For rib cartilage that exhibits significant degrees of warping, internal stabilization of large grafts such as dorsal onlay grafts and columellar strut grafts with centrally placed K-wires can decrease the likelihood of postoperative distortion.

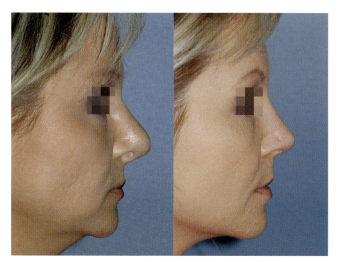

Figure 26-8 Preoperative (*left*) versus postoperative (*right*) views of a secondary rhinoplasty patient whose nasal tip deformity was corrected using rib cartilage grafts without K-wire stabilization as a columellar strut and lateral crural strut grafts.

SUGGESTED READING

Gibson T. Cartilage grafts. *Br Med Bull*. 1965;21:153.

Gunter JP, Rohrich RJ. External approach to secondary rhinoplasty. *Plast Reconstr Surg*. 1987;80:161.

Kim DW, Shah AR, Toriumi DM. Concentric and eccentric carved costal cartilage: a comparison of warping. *Arch Facial Plast Surg*. 2006;8(1):42-46.

Chapter 27

Spreader Grafting

Brian M. Parrett, MD; Samuel J. Lin, MD, FACS

INDICATIONS

There are multiple indications for spreader grafts including:

1. Improving airway obstruction at a narrowed internal nasal valve is a common indication. This indication can occur from trauma or, more commonly, from overresection of the dorsal septum and upper lateral cartilages during prior rhinoplasty. Patients may present with an inverted V deformity. The grafts act as volume expanders, moving the upper lateral cartilage away from the dorsal septum, thus increasing the valve angle.

2. The widening of an excessively narrowed middle vault or camouflage asymmetry of the middle vault. Asymmetry of the middle vault may be addressed with placement of a unilateral spreader graft or with placement of spreader grafts of unequal thickness. In a crooked nose, a unilateral spreader graft is placed on the concave side and will laterally displace the upper lateral cartilage to correct the concavity.

3. Correcting or stabilizing of dorsal septum deviations that occur after nasal trauma.

4. Using spreader grafts in primary rhinoplasty as a preventative measure. They are useful in patients prone to middle vault collapse, especially patients with "narrow nose syndrome" with short nasal bones, weak upper lateral cartilages, and thin skin. These grafts can correct avulsion or destabilization of the upper lateral cartilage from nasal bones that may occur during nasal bone rasping. In this situation, suturing the upper lateral cartilages to the septum can help prevent middle nasal vault collapse, and spreader grafts prevent excessive narrowing of the nose and preserve an adequate nasal valve.

PREOPERATIVE PREPARATION

Adequate time in patient consultation and preoperative planning is essential. A thorough history and physical should be performed to rule out other causes of nasal obstruction, including allergic rhinitis, chronic sinusitis, nasal polyps, deviated septum, and external nasal valve collapse. A detailed intranasal examination should be performed with special attention paid to the septum, internal and external nasal valves, and turbinates. A Cottle test may be performed. The typical angle between the dorsal septum and the upper lateral cartilage measures 10 to 15 degrees. A smaller angle increases airflow resistance. A history of prior septoplasty is important for technical planning in regards to cartilage harvest. The first choice for spreader grafts is the septal cartilage; other options include conchal and rib cartilage.

ANESTHESIA

Monitored conscious sedation with local anesthesia or general anesthesia is suitable for this procedure. Regardless of the anesthesia chosen, a local anesthetic with a vasoconstrictive agent should be infiltrated into the surgical field for anesthesia and bleeding control.

POSITION AND MARKINGS

The patient is placed in the supine position and prepped and draped in the usual sterile fashion for head and neck surgery. The patient's head and shoulders may be placed on a doughnut and a shoulder roll, respectively. Markings are made for an open or closed rhinoplasty approach. For more complex reconstructions, as well as for the more novice rhinoplasty surgeon, an open approach is preferable. Markings are also made for cartilage harvest and depend on harvest site.

DETAILS OF PROCEDURE

Spreader grafting begins with the harvesting of cartilage, most often septal cartilage via a septoplasty approach. Following the harvest of cartilage, spreader grafts are placed via a closed or open rhinoplasty approach.

Following injection of local vasoconstrictive/anesthetic agents, the appropriate rhinoplasty incisions are made with a no. 15 blade. Dissection proceeds to obtain exposure of the entire middle vault including the dorsal septum and upper lateral cartilages. If necessary, hump reduction and medial osteotomies should be performed prior to spreader graft placement; lateral osteotomies can be performed before or after graft

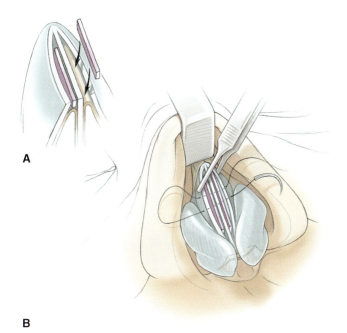

Figure 27-1 **A.** Vertically oriented spreader grafts are placed in submucoperichondrial pockets between the upper lateral cartilages and the septum. **B.** Spreader grafts are sutured into position with horizontal mattress sutures that go through the dorsal edge of the upper lateral cartilages, the spreader graft, and the dorsal edge of the septum. The graft's length extends from the osteochondral junction, or even under the bony arch, to the caudal border of the upper lateral cartilage. More recently the use of extended spreader grafts has come into existence; these grafts may extend to the anterior septal angle and further in certain cases.

placement. Using a no. 15 blade followed by a Cottle or Freer elevator, divide the upper lateral cartilages from their attachments to the dorsal septum in the submucoperichondrial plane. Special care must be taken to enter into the subperichondrial plane and avoid tearing the mucosa. Spreader grafts will be placed into pockets between the upper lateral cartilages and dorsal septum; this lateralizes the upper lateral cartilage(s), improves the airway, and widens, if indicated, the appearance of the middle vault (Fig. 27-1).

Fashion rectangular spreader grafts by incising the harvested cartilage to the proper dimensions. The grafts should be relatively straight and the length should extend from the osseocartilaginous junction to the anterior septal angle. The height is usually 3 mm and the appropriate thickness depends on the desired functional effect without causing excessive widening; this is usually 1 to 3 mm. If the cartilage is thin, 2 grafts can be stacked to reach the desired thickness. Insert the grafts into precise subperichondrial tunnels, taking care to preserve the mucosa. Spreader grafts can be temporarily held in place with a 25-gauge needle through the upper lateral

cartilages, spreader grafts, and septum. The spreader grafts are secured with several mattress sutures (5-0 polydioxanone, Monocryl, or Vicryl vs. 5-0 nylon) through the upper lateral cartilage, the spreader graft, and the septum. Alternatively, engage all structures (upper lateral cartilage to spreader graft to septum to spreader graft to upper lateral cartilage) with a single mattress suture. Do not cinch the mattress sutures too tightly.

The above description focuses on the more commonly used vertically oriented spreader grafts; horizontally oriented spreader grafts have also been described (Fig. 27-2). In practice, the senior author has found horizontal

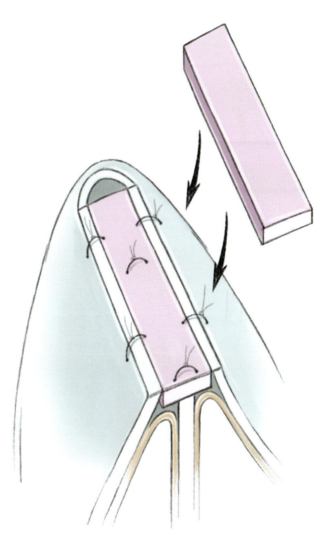

Figure 27-2 A horizontally oriented spreader graft is a dorsal graft that is inset between the dorsal upper lateral cartilages to form a T with the dorsal septum. The width of the spreader graft is adjusted depending on required displacement of the upper lateral cartilages. The dorsal septum must be lowered approximately 1 mm to account for the thickness of the graft. The graft is then sutured to the dorsal septum and to the dorsal upper lateral cartilages as shown.

spreader grafts infrequently indicated except for patients with the most severe inverted V deformities or traumatic midvault narrowing, and in specific cases where a preexisting saddle-nose finding is present preoperatively.

PITFALLS

Do not miss other causes of nasal obstruction; thus, a complete preoperative evaluation is critical. Pay close attention to the intranasal examination for septal perforations, turbinate hypertrophy, septal deviation, atrophic mucosa, and polyps. Additionally, a careful history is important to elicit ongoing nasal steroid spray usage, asthma, chronic sinusitis, prior surgery, prior trauma, and/or chronic Afrin usage.

Care should be taken to avoid overwidening of the middle vault, which should be no wider than the bony vault and narrower than the nasal tip. If excessive width or asymmetry is noted, the grafts should be repositioned or narrowed.

Spreader grafts may be placed through a closed or open rhinoplasty approach. The former relies upon accurate and consistent pocket development for graft placement. The latter approach utilizes accurate suture technique with the entire nasal cartilage framework exposed.

PEARLS

Double-check middle-vault width and symmetry after applying spreader grafts. Careful palpation will allow precise assessment of middle-vault width. Experience is required to develop reliable surgical judgment regarding the appropriate width and length of spreader grafts. In addition, careful palpation of the nasal skin envelope during the procedure will prevent postoperative patient queries about graft palpability.

SUGGESTED READING

Constantian MB, Clardy RB. The relative importance of septal and nasal valvular surgery in correcting airway obstruction in primary and secondary rhinoplasty. *Plast Reconstr Surg.* 1996; 98(1):38-54.

Sheen JH. Spreader graft: a method of reconstructing the roof of the middle nasal vault following rhinoplasty. *Plast Reconstr Surg.* 1984;73(2):230-239.

Toriumi DM. Management of the middle nasal vault in rhinoplasty. *Oper Tech Plast Reconstr Surg.* 1995;2(1):16-30.

Chapter 28. The Twisted Nose

Richard A. Bartlett, MD, FACS

INDICATIONS

The twisted nose is a distinct subclassification of the deviated nose. A deviated nose is uniformly deviated to the right or left like a tilted building. The twisted nose deviates to the right and left in a serpentine manner. Although the deviated nose may be noticeable, the twisted nose often has a bizarre appearance, which can affect self-confidence, social interaction, and even employment opportunities because of the perception of a history of trauma. These factors are the major driver for patients seeking correction.

Virtually all twisted noses have an associated deviated septum and obstructed nasal valves causing nasal airway obstruction. Correction of the twisted nose offers the opportunity to improve the patient's functional status. Even if the patient is not currently symptomatic, the potential for postoperative obstruction exists if these anatomical deformities are not accounted for.

Correction of the deviated nose should always be considered a combined aesthetic and functional procedure.

PREOPERATIVE PREPARATION

A thorough history should be obtained. The etiology of the twisted nose includes asymmetric growth and development, congenital deformities, such as cleft lip and palate, or facial clefts, trauma, or previous surgery. The underlying cause of the problem will have implications for surgical planning and preparation of the patient. If the patient has a nose that is twisted as a result of asymmetric growth but has had no previous procedures, the surgeon can be reasonably sure that the underlying cartilage framework and septum are intact and will be available for grafting. The unoperated nose will allow an easier dissection, fewer soft-tissue issues because of scar tissue, and a less-complicated postoperative course.

Congenital cleft deformities are often associated with underlying skeletal anomalies, which may require augmentation with grafts or alloplastic materials. The traumatized nose or secondary deformity after surgery is often associated with attenuated cartilages and a septum that may have been harvested, fractured, or affected adversely by hematoma. The most severe example is the

patient with a massive septal perforation. Obtaining old operative reports can be helpful, but one should always assume that the septum may be unusable and prepare the patient for the possible harvest of auricular or rib cartilage (Fig. 28-1). This is good practice even if a CT scan indicates that the septum is intact since the actual quality of the cartilage can only be assessed when the specimen is in hand. It is best to discuss all possible donor sites during the preoperative visit.

Examination of the nose follows the general principles for rhinoplasty, including an analysis of the patient's functional status. Standardized photographs are taken. The use of computer imaging must be carefully considered. Sharing images with the patient is controversial, even in straightforward aesthetic patients, because of the concern that the patient may regard the image as an ironclad guarantee. Most surgeons who utilize computer imaging make it clear to the patient that the images are for planning and discussion but that the actual results may differ. With more complex patients, the chance of the result differing from an idealized image is greater, thereby increasing the chance for unrealistic expectations. Whether computer

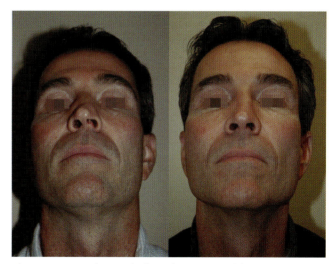

Figure 28-1 Before and after of a 47-year-old patient with twisted nose and septum. Open dorsal tip split approach with extended spreader grafts from auricular cartilage. Medial and lateral osteotomies.

images are used or not, it is best to emphatically and repeatedly tell the patient that their nose will be "better but not perfect." The surgeon can choose the best words to communicate this concept, but phrases such as "your nose will be better but still crooked" and "a perfect result is not possible" cannot be repeated too many times.

The standard risks of rhinoplasty are discussed but the patient should be informed that all risks are increased because of the complexity of correcting a twisted nose. It is not necessary to scare the patient, but full disclosure dictates that patients with a twisted nose should know that their situation is unusual and complicated. Families should be informed that the surgery will be longer. All patients should be told that there is an increased risk that a revision may be necessary. To have as much control and exposure as possible, an open technique is used. Patients should be informed that there will be an external scar and should also be prepared for alar base resections.

ANESTHESIA

Although rhinoplasty can be performed under IV sedation, it is often preferable for longer surgery to utilize general anesthesia. The fact that the remote operative site, including one or both ears and possibly a rib, may be accessed, makes general anesthesia the more conservative choice. Intubation with a RAE (Ring-Adair-Elwyn) endotracheal tube can lead to pressure on the lower lip, making it preferable to utilize a regular endotracheal tube taped with a narrow mesentery, similar to the technique used for tonsillectomy. A throat pack is always used.

POSITION AND MARKINGS

The patient is in a supine position with the head in a neutral position. The inside of the nose is cleansed of all particulate matter and prepped with povidone-iodine solution. Donor sites are prepped.

DETAILS OF OPERATION

An open technique is utilized. Various patterns for the columella incision have been described including a chevron, stairstep, and a modified W. Markings are made and the nose is infiltrated with 0.25% bupivacaine. If it is certain that a secondary donor site for cartilage grafts will be needed, then the grafts are obtained first. It is rare to harvest rib graft and the technique is described elsewhere in this text (see Chapter 26). For harvest of conchal cartilage, a postauricular incision is made in a location similar to an otoplasty incision. The floor of the conchal bowl is exposed using sharp dissection. It is important to harvest only the floor and not the vertical portion of the conchal bowl so as to avoid changing the prominence of the ear. To confirm the

dimensions of the harvest the posterior aspect of the bowl is marked by transferring the anatomical landmarks from anterior to posterior utilizing a 25-gauge needle and methylene blue. The posterior aspect of the bowl is then incised with a no. 15 scalpel. Sharp dissection utilizing an iris scissor on the anterior aspect of the bowl allows completion of the harvest with a curved scissor. Closure of the donor site is accomplished with a running 5-0 or 4-0 plain gut, running horizontal mattress suture. The suture is not tied after the last throw, but is left loose. A moistened sponge in placed in the conchal bowl and the head drape is rewrapped to apply compression. At the conclusion of the case the site is exposed, any accumulated blood is expressed and the suture is tied. This technique allows for a dry wound and avoids the use of a drain.

If the septum is to be harvested, it is accessed through a right or left side unilateral transfixion incision. The choice of right or left side incision is influenced by the presence of a right or left side septal and bony spur, which may require access to the crest of the maxilla. The transfixion incision is also used for access to the caudal septum and the anterior nasal spine. It is important to widely release mucosal attachments to deviated portions of the septum and at the junction of the upper lateral cartilages and the dorsal septum. The dissection is performed with a Cottle elevator beginning at the angle of the septum. In a twisted nose, the dissection can be difficult and the chance of perforating the septum or the mucosa is high. If the dissection is not going easily, it is better to complete the dissection from a dorsal approach rather than to persist.

After the intranasal chores are completed, the columella incision is made. The incision is carried lateral and anterior to the soft triangle. Before completion of the columella incision, undermining through the lateral incision is accomplished with an iris scissor. The columella incision is then completed sharply. The dissection is then carried in a cephalic direction by sharp dissection. In the case of secondary deformities, special care must be taken to avoid entering the wrong plane. It is not unusual to be dissecting above or below a previous cartilage graft or to puncture the underlying mucosa where portions of the caudal margin of the upper lateral cartilage have been overresected. With this knowledge in mind, care is taken and the dissection is often painstaking.

After exposure of the dorsum, the upper lateral cartilages are separated from the dorsum and any remaining mucosal attachments are teased away using a Cottle elevator. If necessary, the dissection is continued between the lower lateral cartilages for exposure of the caudal end of the septum from a "top-down" dorsal approach. Stay sutures can be placed at either dome to retract the lower lateral cartilages away from the septum. These maneuvers accomplish component separation in order to have as many degrees of freedom as possible, but also to expose the dorsal septum for inspection. The septum is usually an integral part of the "twist" and must be addressed; however, there may also be fractures or discontinuities of the dorsal/caudal strut from trauma or overaggressive surgery.

The reconstruction is then carried out in a cephalic to caudal direction (bones, septum/middle vault, then tip). The dorsum is reduced, if necessary. Lateral and medial osteotomies are carried out with in-out fracture as needed. Spreader grafts are then fashioned from the harvested graft material. The spreaders function not only to correct a narrow internal nasal valve, but also act as batten grafts to straighten and strengthen the septum. Scoring of the septum should not be done unless the scored area is then reinforced with a batten graft. It is often necessary to extend one of the spreader grafts into the area of the angle of the septum or the caudal septum to reinforce fracture sites or to correct caudal deflection. If the septum is displaced off the anterior nasal spine, it is now mobilized, shortened slightly, and sutured, to the spine with a 4-0 nylon or PDS suture. It is much easier to perform this maneuver through the transfixion incision because of its proximity to the anterior spine. Although it is possible to drill a hole in the anterior spine, in most patients a small hole can be created with an 18-gauge needle. This is a simple maneuver that minimizes equipment needs and avoids the risk of running a power instrument in a confined space with the risk of trauma to the surrounding soft tissue. Occasionally, an extended spreader graft which mimics the L-strut must be fashioned. If there is insufficient straight cartilage for this task a composite extended spreader graft can be fabricated by using PDS sheeting (Figs. 28-2 and 28-3).

The final component is the tip. A midline strut graft is placed between the medial crura and secured using two 6-0 nylon sutures. It is common for the lateral crura to be of unequal length and for the domes to have unequal projection. Often in twisted tips, the domes interdigitate and after they are dissected free, the discrepancy in the length of the medial or lateral crura is enhanced. Lateral crural

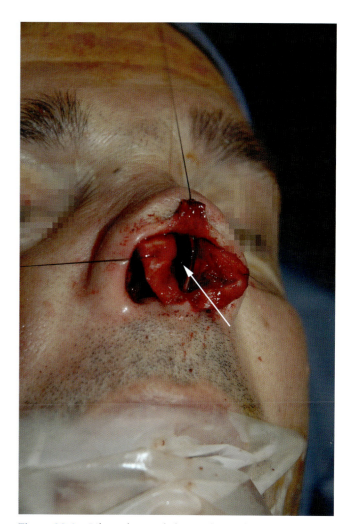

Figure 28-3 Bilateral extended spreader grafts on PDS (polydioxanone) sheet in place on both sides on septum (right arrow). Tip split approach.

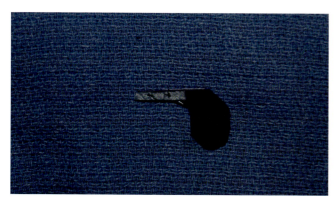

Figure 28-2 Prefabricated extended spreader graft on PDS (polydioxanone) sheet.

length can be equalized by differential resection of the domes or division of the lateral crura in a more lateral location. If the intrinsic tip shape is good, it may be preferable to resect laterally. If the discrepancy is addressed by resection of the domes, reconstitution of the domes with 5-0 nylon is followed by construction and placement of a shield graft. The final component of tip reconstruction is placement of a tip projection control suture (PCS) of 5-0 nylon between the medial crura and the caudal septum. The PCS can be placed with an anterior, neutral, or posterior position on the caudal septum to accomplish an increase, a maintenance, or a decrease in tip projection. With the skin redraped, the dorsal contour can be assessed and selective camouflage grafts can be applied using crushed cartilage.

The columella is closed with 6-0 nylon. All intranasal incisions are closed with 5-0 and 6-0 chromic. The dorsum is painted with benzoin or Mastisol and

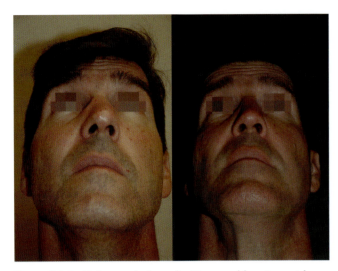

Figure 28-4   Before and after of a 51-year-old patient with a twisted septum and complete obstruction on the left. Open dorsal tip split with bilateral extended spreader grafts and PDS (polydioxanone) sheet.

Steri-Strips are applied, followed by application of an Aquaplast splint (Fig. 28-4).

PITFALLS

The primary pitfall is for the surgeon or the patient to underestimate the problem. By definition, the twisted nose is a complex case. Expectations must be managed carefully. The most effective exposure must be utilized (open approach), and multiple grafts employed. The patient must be prepared for multiple graft-donor sites. Because of the aggressive dissection and separation of mucosa from cartilage, prolonged swelling must be expected and the final result delayed, compared to a routine rhinoplasty. The chance of revision is higher than in simpler cases and should be made known to the patient in unequivocal terms.

PEARLS

- Prepare for the harvest of multiple grafts. The axiom so prevalent in reconstructive surgery—"figure out what you need and then get more"—applies.
- Take everything apart. Use an open approach. Expose all deviated cartilage and key junctions by release of mucosal attachments. Obtain the maximum degree of freedom through component separation. Utilize medial and lateral osteotomies. Separate the upper lateral cartilages from the dorsal septum. Fully mobilize the caudal septum off of the anterior nasal spine, if necessary.
- Utilize spreader grafts, strut grafts, tip grafts, dorsal, and caudal batten grafts.
- Tell patients that you can guarantee only one thing, "that your nose will not be straight."

SUGGESTED READING

Byrd HS, Salomon J, Flood J. Correction of the crooked nose. *Plast Reconstr Surg.* 1998;102(6):2148-2157.

Daniel Rollin. In: *Rhinoplasty: An Atlas of Surgical Techniques.* New York, NY: Springer; 2002:180-182 [chapter 5].

Guyuron B, Uzzo CD, Scull H. A practical classification of septonasal deviation and an effective guide to septal surgery. *Plast Reconstr Surg.* 1999;104(7):2202-2209.

Rohrich RJ, Gunter JP, Deuber MA, Adams WP. The deviated nose: optimizing results using a simplified classification and algorithmic approach. *Plast Reconstr Surg.* 2002;110(6):1509-1523.

Stuart JE, Kelly MH. Cartilage recycling in rtuno plasty: polydioxanone foil as an absorbable biomechanical scaffold. *Plast Reconstr Surg.* 2008;122(1):254-260.

Tebbetts JB. In: *Primary Rhinoplasty. A New Approach to the Logic and Techniques.* St Loics, MO: Mosby; 1998:340-350 [chapter 10].

Chapter 29. Septoplasty and Turbinate Reduction

Douglas M. Sidle, MD, FACS

INDICATIONS

The indications for septoplasty and turbinate reduction include situations where a patient complains of chronic nasal obstruction that is anatomical in nature and is refractory to medical therapy. Furthermore, turbinate reduction can be an effective means of reducing congestion and rhinorrhea.

PREOPERATIVE PREPARATION

A thorough history of the patient's nasal complaints should be obtained. A history or prior nasal surgery or trauma will tip the surgeon off to potential pitfalls. A history of sinusitis or allergies can complicate what would otherwise be a successful septoplasty and turbinate reduction. Cocaine and over-the-counter nasal decongestant abuse should be discontinued long before undertaking surgery. Nasal steroid spray use is safe in the perioperative period, but should be discontinued for 2 weeks preoperatively. Preoperative examination should confirm a deviation of either the quadrangular cartilage and/or the perpendicular plate of the ethmoid bone and vomer. Special attention should be paid to examination of the internal nasal valve whose primary contributors are the nasal septum, the caudal end of the upper lateral cartilages, the soft tissue of the pyriform aperture, and the head of the inferior turbinate.

ANESTHESIA

Most septoplasties are performed under general anesthesia to achieve both anesthesia and airway protection. However, septoplasty can be performed under conscious sedation or local anesthesia, even when performed with concomitant rhinoplasty. Regardless of the level of sedation chosen, the injection of 1% lidocaine with 1:100,000 epinephrine into the submucoperichondrial plane of the nasal septum helps reduce bleeding. Local anesthetic is also injected into the stroma of the inferior turbinates at the time of turbinate reduction. Additionally, cotton pledgets soaked with 4 mL of 4% cocaine can be placed into the nose preoperatively to provide further astringency and anesthesia. When there is concern for a patient's cardiac status, Neo-Synephrine (phenylephrine HCl) or oxymetazoline can be used on cotton pledges instead of cocaine. While allowing time for vasoconstrictive effects, the surgeon should reevaluate the septum and plan where the incision will be made based on each patient's anatomy (Fig. 29-1).

POSITION AND MARKINGS

The patient is placed in a supine position and prepped and draped in the standard sterile fashion for head and neck surgery. The patient's head may be placed on a doughnut for support and stability. The head of the bed may be raised slightly to aid in hemostasis. If the septoplasty is to be performed by an open approach, either with or without concomitant rhinoplasty, a midcolumellar incision is marked out prior to injection of local anesthetic. Generally, no marking is necessary when performing endonasal septoplasty, turbinate reduction, or rhinoplasty.

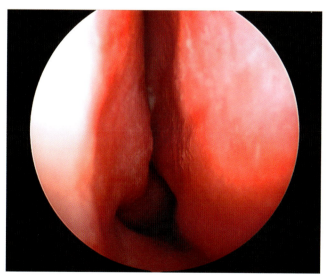

Figure 29-1 Anterior rhinoscopy view of the right nasal airway. The deviated nasal septum is impinging on the right inferior turbinate.

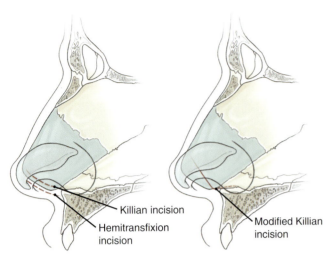

Killian incision
Hemitransfixion incision
Modified Killian incision

Figure 29-2   Types of endonasal septal incisions.

DETAILS OF PROCEDURE

A headlight is worn for both injection of local anesthesia and for the procedure itself. Following injection of local vasoconstrictive/anesthetic agent, incision is typically made in one of 3 ways: in the columellar skin for an open approach, in the membranous columella for a hemitransfixion incision, and on the septum itself for a Killian incision (Fig. 29-2). When a caudal deviation of the nasal septum is present, it may be necessary to approach the septum either through an open rhinoplasty approach or using a hemitransfixion incision. The hemitransfixion incision is placed on one side only of the membranous columella at the caudal border of the nasal septum. Retracting the columella aids in creation of the hemitransfixion incision and in dissection (Fig. 29-3). The

entire nasal septum can be exposed with either of these 2 approaches. If the deviated portion of the septum is more posterior (inside the nose), then a modified Killian incision can be used. The modified Killian incision is made inside the nose between 5 mm and 1 cm from the caudal border of the nasal septum and is directed from a high position 1 cm back on the septum downward to a position anterior to the nasal spine inferiorly. Angling the incision in this manner will help prevent tearing of the mucoperichondrial flap. Intranasal incisions are generally made with a no. 15 blade. Most right-handed surgeons find it easiest to start on the left side of the patient's nose, but the location and severity of the deviation will also determine incision location.

At first, it may be difficult to find the proper plane in which the flap will be elevated. Diligent slow dissection using a no. 15 blade at first, followed by a Freer or Cottle elevator, helps to delineate the bloodless submucoperichondrial plane. The proper plane has a distinct "gritty" feel with elevation of the flap and should be relatively bloodless. Wide undermining is performed on one side only, at first exposing the deviated portions of the cartilage and bone (Fig. 29-4). When the crooked portion of cartilage and bone are identified and exposed, the location of the transcartilaginous incision is chosen. This is usually just caudal or anterior to the area of the septum that needs to be removed and straightened. A no. 15 blade, a Freer elevator, or a Freer "D" knife is used to create the transcartilaginous incision, paying careful attention not to violate the contralateral mucoperichondrium (Fig. 29-5). Through the transcartilaginous incision, the contralateral mucoperichondrial flap is elevated only in the areas of the septum that need to be addressed and removed. To prevent destabilization of the nose, at least a 1-cm caudal and 1-cm dorsal strut of intact L-strut cartilage must remain

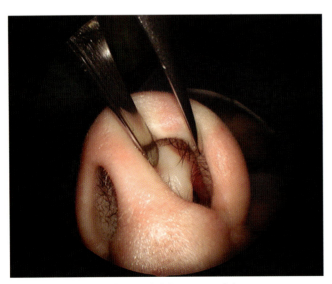

Figure 29-3   View of a caudal deviation of the septum to the left.

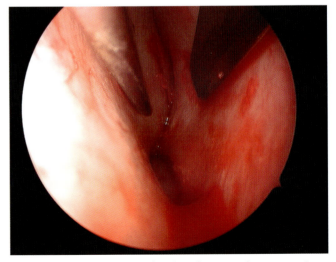

Figure 29-4   Dissection in the plane between the mucoperichondrium and the septal cartilage should he relatively easy and bloodless.

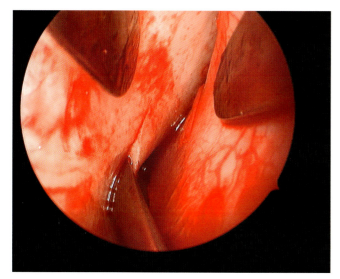

Figure 29-5   A trans cartilagenous incision is created with the Freer elevator.

(Fig. 29-6). Using septal scissors, elevators, and double-action instruments, the deviated portions of the quadrangular cartilage, vomer, and ethmoid plate are removed. Occasionally, it is necessary to remove a strong bony spur from the maxillary crest if it is contributing to the nasal obstruction. This is accomplished with mucosal elevation, gentle fracturing, or possibly an osteotome. Using a nasal speculum, the nose is examined internally to see if the obstructing septal elements have been removed. No cautery is generally necessary as bleeding is typically minimal. When the septum is straight, it is a good idea to replace some of the removed quadrangular cartilage for septal support. This is accomplished by removing any bony

elements and morselizing the twisted cartilage. Only straight cartilage is placed back between the septal flaps and into the cartilaginous defect. Replaced cartilage is not allowed to telescope over the caudal or dorsal segments of the L-strut.

The modified Killian or hemitransfixion incision is closed with interrupted 4-0 chromic stitches. Septal splints fashioned from silastic sheeting (Micromedics, St. Paul, MN) or plastic Bivalve Nasal Splints (Micromedics, St. Paul, MN) will aid in hematoma prevention and help to keep the septum straight. Splints can be removed anytime between postoperative days 4 and 7. Nasal packing is not typically necessary but can be achieved using simple Telfa (Covidien, Mansfield, MA) or an inflatable Merocel sponge (Medtronic Xomed Inc., Mystic, CT) in cases of excess bleeding. Patients are asked to begin saline irrigation of the nasal passages on postoperative day 3. This will aid in nasal hygiene and help with removal of the septal splints.

A turbinate reduction, or turbinoplasty, can also be accomplished by numerous techniques. The simplest is out-fracture of the inferior turbinates using any straight, blunt instrument (Fig. 29-7). Another simple method of achieving turbinate reduction is by submucosal unipolar cauterization. Here the surgeon inserts a 25-gauge spinal needle into each inferior turbinate and uses the Bovie cautery to pass current into the turbinate. Careful attention must be paid to not burn the sill of the nose during this procedure. Because the current disperses quickly upon contact with tissue, it is likely that only the head of the inferior turbinate is significantly affected with unipolar cautery. Likewise, bipolar cautery of the inferior turbinates can be performed using special turbinate bipolar needles, but is probably limited by the same drawbacks.

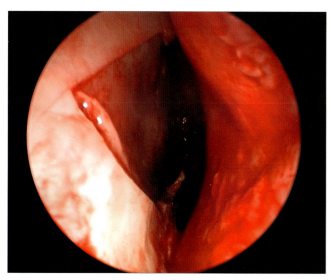

Figure 29-6   Maintenance of at least a 1 cm infact dorsal and caudal strut is vital to postoperative nasal support.

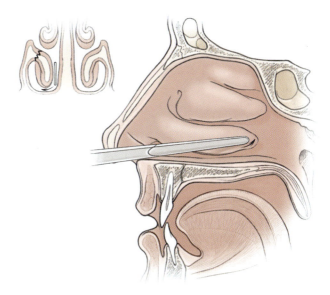

Figure 29-7   Outfracture of the inferior turbinate using a blunt instrument.

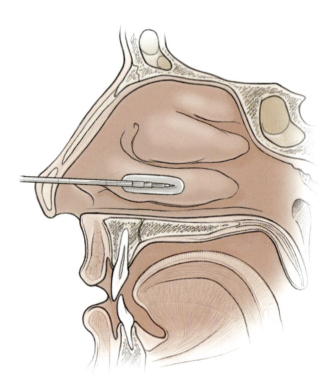

Figure 29-8 The radiofrequency turbinate reduction probe is buried in the stroma of the inferior turbinate. It is withdrawn slowly when activated.

Newer techniques used to reduce the inferior turbinates have been shown to be more effective; microdebrider-assisted turbinoplasty (MAT) and radiofrequency volumetric tissue reduction (RFVTR) turbinoplasty are safe and effective. MAT seems to have the best immediate and long-term results, but requires expensive specialized equipment, special training, and can be associated with significant bleeding. RFVTR, however, can be performed under local anesthesia, requires no nasal packing, and is associated with quick patient recovery. In RFVTR, the turbinate is first injected with local anesthetic and the RFVTR probe is inserted deep into the stroma of the turbinate and works along the entire length of the turbinate as the probe is withdrawn slowly (Fig. 29-8). In cases of severe turbinate hypertrophy, the probe may be inserted into 2 separate locations on each of the inferior turbinates. Of course, an inferior turbinate out-fracture procedure can be combined with any of the other methods.

PITFALLS

Although submucous resection of the septal cartilage is the classic septal surgery, it increases the risk of an iatrogenic septal perforation. Furthermore, it creates a situation where there may not be enough cartilage remaining for grafting during future rhinoplasty. Therefore, a history of prior nasal surgery should raise doubt that there is significant septal cartilage available for grafting when planning concomitant rhinoplasty. Morselizing, straightening, and replacing at least some part of the quadrangular cartilage aids in prevention of these potential problems. If a tear or rent occurs in one of the mucoperichondrial flaps, extra diligence should be exercised to keep the opposing flap intact to prevent a postoperative septal perforation. Undiagnosed sinusitis, choanal atresia, and nasal allergies can lead to a dissatisfied patient postoperatively, despite a nice, straight septum. To fully evaluate for these conditions, a nasal endoscopy may be necessary preoperatively. Finally, overresection of the septal cartilage can lead to destabilization of the nasal tip and nasal dorsum. This can lead to the dreaded saddle-nose deformity, creating an unsatisfactory functional and aesthetic outcome.

Resection of the inferior turbinates was a popular procedure for reducing nasal airway resistance that has fallen out of favor. The primary function of the turbinates is to humidify and warm air before it reaches the lungs. Resecting the inferior turbinates is associated with atrophic rhinitis, a debilitating nasal condition for some patients.

PEARLS

As described, there are numerous ways to approach the nasal septum. If an endonasal approach is chosen, the surgeon should opt for the hemitransfixion incision when the caudal septum is significantly deviated. Simply resecting the deviated portion of the caudal septum will result in significant change in nasal aesthetics and possibly nasal tip support. Replacing the straightened quadrilateral cartilage after removing the deviated and crooked portions of cartilage and bone will help prevent nasal septal perforations and further support the nasal framework. At least a 1-cm dorsal and 1-cm caudal strut should remain intact to prevent a saddle-nose deformity (see Fig. 29-6). Any method of turbinate reduction can be performed in conjunction with a turbinate out-fracture to optimize the results. Septoplasty and turbinate reduction are synergistic procedures when employed in the properly selected patient.

SUGGESTED READING

Joniau S, Wong I, Rajapaksa S, Carney SA, Wormwald PJ. Long-term comparison between submucosal cauterization and powered reduction of the inferior turbinates. *Laryngoscope.* 2006;116(9):1612-1616.

Liu CM, Tan CK, Lee FP, Lin KN, Huang HM. Microdebrider-assisted versus radiofrequency-assisted turbinoplasty. *Laryngoscope.* 2009;119(2):414-418.

Chapter 30. Chin Augmentation

Ryan Michael Garcia, MD; Bahman Guyuron, MD, FACS

INDICATIONS

Genioplasty is performed to correct horizontal and vertical discrepancies in the lower third of the face. The chin serves a pivotal role in balancing the overall aesthetic appeal and has a direct effect on the perception of other facial features. In particular, the inverse relationship of the chin and nose must be respected, as enhancement of the chin has the greatest effect on the appearance of the nose. A classification of chin deformities has been devised to help guide the surgical approach and various treatment options available.

The goals and limitations of each genioplasty procedure must be appreciated and the surgical plan individualized to the patient. Generally, osseous surgical options include simple burr reduction ostectomy, osteotomy with repositioning of the caudal segment (vertical and horizontal), osteotomy and grafting, or osteotomy and segmental sectioning. Other less technically demanding augmentation options include autologous grafting or the use of alloplastic implants. The benefits of shorter operative and recovery times associated with alloplastic implantation must be weighed against their limitations. For example, alloplastic implantation cannot significantly alter an undesirable cervicomental angle, and these procedures have guarded success in the correction of vertical and asymmetric chin deformities.

Genioplasty is contraindicated in a number of clinical situations. Genioplasty alone should not be performed in patients with severe facial disharmony where orthognathic surgery may be of better benefit. Furthermore, patients with advanced medical comorbidities, such as uncontrolled diabetes or uncorrectable coagulopathies, making surgical interventions and anesthesia unsafe, should not undergo elective genioplasty. Surgeons should caution the use of alloplastic implants in patients with immunocompromised conditions because of the increased risks of periprosthetic infections. On the other hand, patients in their sixth decade of life or older with minimal chin deformities may be better suited for an alloplastic implant as osseous corrections may be too extensive.

PREOPERATIVE PREPARATION

Careful preoperative soft-tissue cephalometric analysis using life-size photographs is critical to a successful aesthetic outcome. Vertical assessment of the chin is performed with frontal and profile view analysis. The ideal vertical face is divided into 3 equal sections (upper, middle, and lower face) by arbitrary lines drawn through the hairline, lower glabella, subnasale, and menton. The lower third of the face and lips are further analyzed by subdividing the lower face with a line through the stomion. The distance from the stomion to the menton should be twice the distance from the stomion to the subnasion. The female chin should have a single light reflection, whereas the wider and more rectangular male chin has a double light reflection.

Horizontal assessment of the chin is performed with profile analysis and aids the surgeon in balancing the inverse relationship of the nose and chin. Analysis starts with a tangent line drawn through the most projected portion of the upper lip, lower lip, and pogonion (anterior projection of the chin pad), thus creating Riedel's plane. Generally, if the chin lies posterior to the Riedel plane, then microgenia exists, whereas a chin that lies anterior represents a macrogenic chin. Next, a line drawn from the subnasion to the pogonion should make an 11 ± 4-degree angle to a line drawn from the glabella to the subnasion. The lips in profile are also analyzed in relation to any perceived chin deformity. Ideally, the upper lip is at the same level as the lower lip or slightly anterior to it. Upper lip deficiency is most often skeletal in nature and related to either relative (secondary to a deficient maxilla) or absolute mandibular prognathia.

Identifying chin asymmetry and then distinguishing the underlying cause are performed in both the vertical and horizontal plane. Vertical symmetry is confirmed when the chin lies within a line that is drawn through the midglabella, the tip of the nose, and the philtral dimple. Horizontal symmetry is confirmed by parallel lines drawn through the oral commissures and medial canthi. Nonparallel lines through the oral commissures can represent asymmetry secondary to distortion of the maxilla or

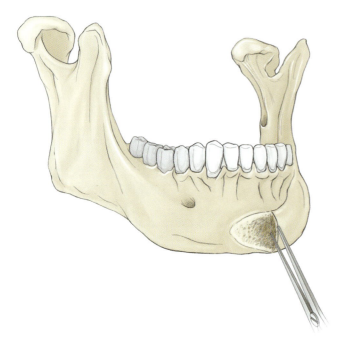

Figure 30-1   Macrogenic chin deformity can be managed with ostectomy using a large oval-tipped burr. The burr reduction is first completed on one half of the chin and measured precisely with a caliper prior to completing the opposite side. (Reproduced, with permission, from Guyuron B. Genioplasty. In: *Plastic Surgery: Indications and Practice*, Vol 2. St. Louis, MO: Elsevier; 2008:1536.)

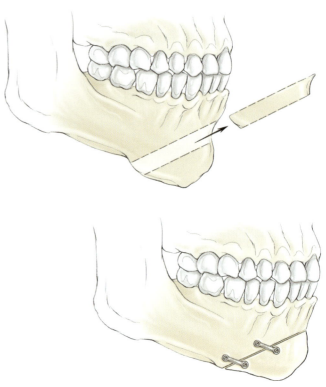

Figure 30-2   Microgenic chin deformity can be managed with osteotomy and repositioning of the caudal segment. Depicted is a chin with a combined vertical and horizontal deficiency which is corrected by positioning the caudal segment anterior and caudal with bone grafting.

mandible and orthognathic surgery may be necessary for proper correction. On the other hand, an asymmetric chin with a parallel intercommissural line is likely intrinsic to the chin and osseous genioplasty alone can be planned.

Vertical, horizontal, and combined chin deformities have been previously classified (Groups I to VII) based on the extent of bone or soft-tissue abnormality. Macrogenic chins (vertical, horizontal, or combined) are classified as Group I deformities and can be managed in a number of ways, depending on the extent of deformity. This includes simple burr ostectomy (Fig. 30-1); horizontal segment block or wedge resection (vertical); an osteotomy and caudal segment setback correction (horizontal); or a combined procedure, depending on the extent and plane of deformity present. Microgenic chins (vertical, horizontal, or combined) are classified as Group II deformities and can be managed by horizontal osteotomy and caudal segment repositioning (vertical), augmentation genioplasty, or horizontal osteotomy and caudal segment advancement (horizontal) (Figs. 30-2 and 30-3). Combined chin deformities (Group III) are defined as having an osseous excess in one plane and deficiency in the other plane. Horizontal excess and vertical deficiency can be corrected by an osteotomy with vertical advancement and posterior

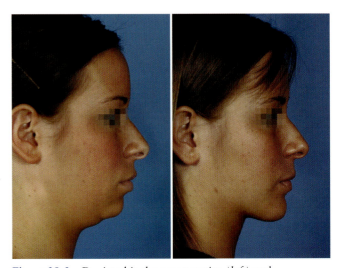

Figure 30-3   Depicted is the preoperative (*left*) and postoperative (*right*) profile view of a patient with a combined vertical and horizontal microgenic chin deformity that was corrected by osseous genioplasty. Submental lipectomy was also performed. (Reproduced, with permission, from Guyuron B. Genioplasty. In: *Plastic Surgery: Indications and Practice*. Vol 2. 2008:1536; Copyright Elsevier.)

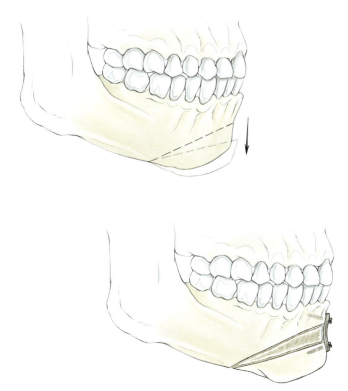

Figure 30-4 Combined chin deformities (defined as having an osseous excess in one plane and deficiency in the other plane) can be managed with ostectomy and repositioning of the caudal segment. Depicted is a chin with vertical excess and horizontal deficiency, which is corrected by completing 2 parallel osteotomies and removal of the cortical segment followed by cephalic and anterior repositioning of the caudal segment.

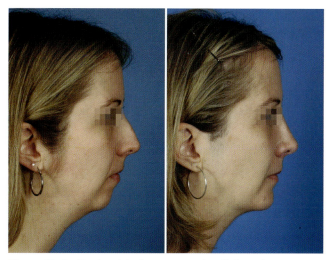

Figure 30-5 Depicted is the preoperative (*left*) and postoperative (*right*) profile view of a patient with a vertical excess and horizontal deficiency chin deformity. The patient underwent an osseous genioplasty with removal of a cortical segment and repositioning of the caudal segment. (Reproduced, with permission, from Guyuron B. Genioplasty. In: *Plastic Surgery: Indications and Practice*. Vol 2. 2008:1534; Copyright Elsevier.)

positioning of the caudal segment, whereas vertical excess and horizontal deficiency necessitates removal of an anterior cortical wedge along with cephalic and anterior repositioning of the caudal segment (Figs. 30-4 and 30-5). Asymmetric chin deformities (Group IV) are not well suited for alloplastic genioplasty secondary to the limited ability of a symmetric implant to correct an asymmetric deformity. Patients with an asymmetric chin but normal lower facial height are best treated by wedge osteotomy, osseous removal of the excessive side, and equal osseous grafting of the deficient side. Asymmetric chins with an excessive facial height require a closing wedge osteotomy with greater removal on the side of excess, whereas asymmetric chins with a deficient facial height require a single osteotomy with caudal repositioning and grafting of the deficient side. Pseudomacrogenic chins (Group V) are defined as having an excess of soft tissue demonstrated on radiographic studies and are best treated with resection through a submental incision. Pseudomicrogenic chins (Group VI) result from vertical maxillary excess along with a clockwise rotational deformity of the mandible. These deformities require orthognathic correction. Finally, witch's chin

deformities (Group VII) are characterized by soft-tissue ptosis and are corrected by an elliptical excision of soft tissue in the submental area.

ANESTHESIA

Osseous and alloplastic genioplasty procedures can be performed under general anesthesia with local anesthetic. The local anesthetic injection technique differs depending on the type and degree of genioplasty procedure. Simple burr ostectomy for reduction genioplasty requires an intraoral diffuse local infiltration of Xylocaine and 1:100,000 epinephrine, whereas more extensive procedures (osteotomy) require local anesthetic blocks at the mental foramen, within the soft tissues of the labial mucosa, and posterior to the mandibular symphysis (Fig. 30-6). Augmentation of the chin with autogenous or alloplastic implants performed through a submental incision require direct infiltration of the soft tissues with local anesthetic consisting of Xylocaine and 1:200,000 epinephrine.

POSITION AND MARKINGS

Genioplasty procedures are performed with the patient in a supine position. The head can be elevated slightly to aid the surgeon with complete visualization of the upper and lower face. Preoperative photographic analysis should be accessible throughout the operative procedure.

The intraoral incision is marked 1 cm distal from the sulcus of the labial mucosa with an anticipated length of

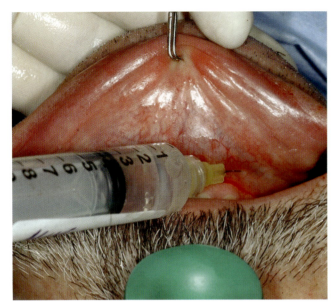

Figure 30-6 Intraoral infiltration of local anesthetic (Xylocaine) and a constricting agent (1:100,000 epinephrine) are used at the mental foramen, within the soft tissues of the labial mucosa, and posterior to the mandibular symphysis prior to incision.

approximately 4 cm. The submental incision site is marked a few millimeters anterior to the natural submental crease and measures approximately 3 to 3.5 cm in length. An additional vertical line is drawn perpendicular to the anticipated surgical incision at the middle of the chin (in reference with the glabella and nose) to serve as a reference point for the chin midline.

DETAILS OF PROCEDURE

Ostectomy

Burr ostectomy is indicated for mild horizontal and rarely for vertical macrogenia. After local anesthetic administration, an intraoral or submental incision is made. The incision should be planned such that a 1-cm cuff of mucosal surface and mentalis muscle remain on the gingival side to facilitate final tissue closure. The periosteum of the anterior surface of the mandibular symphysis is incised sharply with a scalpel and Bovie cautery, and then dissected bluntly in the cephalic and caudal direction using a periosteal elevator. Both mental foramina are exposed and the mental nerves are protected with gentle traction using a malleable retractor. The burr ostectomy is first completed on one half of the chin and measured with a caliper in order to precisely judge the extent of osseous removal (see Fig. 30-1). Once measured, the ostectomy is then repeated on the opposite side. The burr is used to taper the cortical surface superiorly and laterally to remove any irregularities. Thermal damage of the cortex is avoided throughout the procedure by copious

irrigation with normal saline and antibiotic solution. The surgical incision is closed with 4-0 chromic in a meticulous fashion by incorporating the mentalis muscle and the mucosal surface in each suture bite at the level it was divided. If a submental incision is utilized, the wound is repaired using 5-0 Monocryl for the periosteum, 6-0 Monocryl for the subcutaneous tissue, and 6-0 fast absorbable chromic for the skin.

Osteotomy and Caudal Segment Repositioning

The intraoral approach is performed as previously described with minimal caudal dissection of the periosteum posteriorly so as to preserve the periosteal perforating branches of the terminal lingual artery. Once the anterior cortical surface is visualized, a vertical score is made with an oscillating saw to mark the midline of the mandibular symphysis. Once the planned osteotomy site is confirmed, a wide oscillating saw blade is used to complete the central osteotomy. The osteotomy is then completed laterally with a narrow oscillating saw blade (Fig. 30-7). Thermal osseous necrosis is avoided by copious irrigation. The free caudal segment is then advanced or retracted to its desired position and secured by standard osteosynthesis techniques. A precontoured plate or standard plate that is contoured intraoperatively is used to fit the anterior symphyseal surface. Two unicortical screws are used on each side of the osteotomy to adequately secure the caudal segment (Fig. 30-8). When the lower facial height is in excess, 2 parallel osteotomies must be performed and the intervening cortical segment removed. In this situation, both central osteotomies are

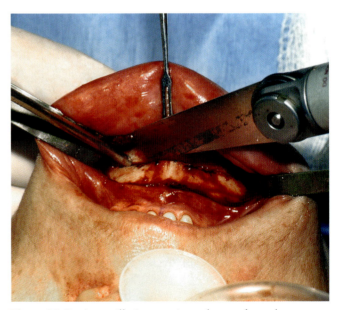

Figure 30-7 An oscillating saw is used to perform the genioplasty osteotomy. Once the central osteotomy is complete, a narrow saw blade is used to complete the lateral aspects of the osteotomy.

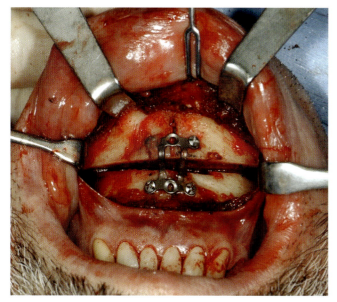

Figure 30-8 Following osteotomy, the free caudal segment can be advanced and secured with either a precontoured plate or a standard plate that is contoured intraoperatively to match the level of advancement. Depicted is a precontoured plate used to advance the caudal segment and secured with 2 unicortical screws on either side of the osteotomy. (Permission to reproduce this image was granted from Guyuron B. Genioplasty. In: *Plastic Surgery: Indications and Practice*. Vol 2. 2008:1522; Copyright Elsevier.)

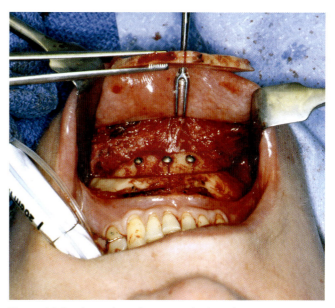

Figure 30-9 A number of osteosynthesis techniques are available to secure the caudal segment. When the caudal segment is positioned in a retracted or posterior position, 2 to 3 cortical screws can be used to adequately secure the 2 osseous surfaces. A cortical segment of approximately 3 mm was removed prior to internal fixation in this patient.

completed prior to performing the lateral osteotomies in order to keep the caudal segment secure. When the goal is to retract the caudal segment, 2 to 3 simple screws are adequate to fix the caudal and proximal segment (Fig. 30-9). The surgical wound is closed with interrupted 4-0 chromic sutures to incorporate the mentalis muscle and mucosal surface as described.

Genioplasty Augmentation

Advancements in technology and surgical techniques have changed the paradigm of genioplasty procedures toward an osseous approach. Despite this, augmentation procedures may still be indicated in patients with limited and extensive chin deficiencies. Potential autogenous grafts include bone (cranial, iliac crest, or nasal dorsum), cartilage (conchal or rib), or soft tissue (fat or dermis), whereas the most common alloplastic implants are silicone or porous polyethylene. When the choice is made to perform implanted augmentations, it is our preferred method to place these grafts or implants subperiosteal so as to minimize migration, chin dimpling, soft-tissue injury, and distortion if contracture occurs. Specific details are described regarding alloplastic implants for augmentation.

The submental incision is preferred over the intraoral incision so as to reduce the risks of periprosthetic infection, cephalic migration, and surgical wound dehiscence.

Additionally, the submental incision allows access to the anterior submental area along with the superficial and deep cervical elements, thus, facilitating additional interventions such as lipectomy or manipulation of the platysma and/or anterior belly of the digastric muscles. The submental incision is placed a few millimeters anterior to the natural submental crease. After the skin is incised, the subcutaneous tissue is dissected with electrocautery to the periosteum. The periosteum is incised sharply and elevated as previously described using an Obwegeser elevator to create a pocket that is large enough to accommodate the desired implant. The implant is inserted one side at a time and the midline of the implant is aligned with the vertical mark drawn on the skin. Bone erosion can be limited by placing the alloplastic implant caudally in the area of dense cortical bone. Meticulous surgical closure is performed in a serial fashion. The periosteum is closed followed by the dermis with 5-0 Monocryl. The skin is closed with interrupted 6-0 catgut sutures.

PITFALLS

Achieving mutual satisfaction between the surgeon and patient is always the goal with aesthetic procedures. Careful patient selection and adequate education are paramount during the preoperative visit. Surgeons should be cautioned when encountering patients with unrealistic expectations, underlying psychologic disorders, or dissatisfaction with prior surgical procedures despite a physically good aesthetic outcome.

Patients with long-face deformities who present for genioplasty should be counseled regarding their overall facial structure and the limitations of genioplasty. The long-face deformity can be exacerbated with genioplasty and maxillary intrusion should be considered in conjunction. Patients with excessive soft tissue of the chin preoperatively may also have an undesired result following reduction genioplasty if the soft tissue component is not addressed at the time of surgery.

Complications following genioplasty procedures are uncommon and can be reduced with adequate preoperative planning and meticulous surgical technique. Postoperative chin asymmetry, overcorrection, and undercorrection are most commonly the result of failing to detect a preexisting deformity or poor surgical planning. Minor postoperative imperfections should be observed as bone and soft-tissue remodeling may improve the aesthetic result. Larger, more significant postoperative deformities require revision surgery and may be best suited prior to osseous union. Soft-tissue ptosis or iatrogenic witch's chin deformity can occur after chin ostectomy or implant removal. These deformities are treated similar to native Group VII chins, with an elliptical excision of the soft-tissue excess through a submental incision.

Tooth devitalization is a rare but serious complication associated with osseous genioplasty. The average length of the lower canine is 25.5 mm; placement of the osteotomy an additional 5 mm caudal (30.5 mm caudal to the occlusive edge of the mandibular canines) will avoid iatrogenic injury to the dental nerve roots. Additionally, the mental nerve is protected by placing the osteotomy 5 mm caudal to the mental foramen. Dental root exposure and sensitization of the teeth can occur with an incision placed too close to the gingiva.

Surgical site wound dehiscence and infections are uncommon complications after osseous genioplasty secondary to the abundant vascular supply of the lower face. Should these complications occur, they are resolved by early debridement of the surgical site and antibiotic therapy. Metallic implants can be retained in most circumstances unless they are exposed or become loose.

Genioplasty with alloplastic implants has a limited capacity to change the cervicomental angle when compared to osseous genioplasty. Malpositioning and dislodgement occurs more frequently with implants placed over the periosteum and requires revision surgery with either repositioning of the implant or conversion to an osseous genioplasty. Some level of osseous bone resorption should be anticipated after alloplastic augmentation, particularly with silicone and acrylic implants. Resorption is minimized by positioning the implant caudally in an area of increased bone density. Soft-tissue distortion and dimpling secondary to capsular retraction requires implant removal and conversion to an osseous genioplasty. Lip retraction requires surgical revision with additional subperiosteal dissection with cephalic elevation and boney suspension of the soft tissues. Surgical site dehiscence, infection, and implant exposure require implant removal and can be minimized by proper incision placement and meticulous closure.

PEARLS

The outcome following genioplasty is generally pleasing as correction of any chin deformity benefits and balances overall facial harmony. A thorough preoperative evaluation is an essential component to obtaining a satisfactory result. The preoperative visit should include a complete history, physical examination, cephalometric analysis with life-sized photographs, and proper classification of each patient's chin deformity to help guide the surgical approach. Surgeons should be familiar with all the genioplasty options available and should understand the goals and limitations of each. The senior author recommends the utilization of osseous techniques, whenever possible, because of the versatility in correcting the majority of chin deformities. Surgical complications and unsatisfactory outcomes can be minimized with proper surgical planning and meticulous surgical technique. Proper placement of the surgical incision is paramount in facilitating the procedure, adequate closure without lip ptosis or contracture, and avoidance of undesired postoperative complications. The neurovascular structures are protected throughout the procedure and osteotomies are placed distal to their expected anatomic course. Augmentation procedures (autograft or alloplastic) are placed subperiosteal to diminish the potential complications of migration, dislodgement, and skin dimpling.

SUGGESTED READING

Cohen SR, Mardach OL, Kawamoto HK Jr. Chin disfigurement following removal of alloplastic chin implants. *Plast Reconstr Surg.* 1991;88:62-66; discussion 67-70.

Guyuron B, Kadi JS. Problems following genioplasty. Diagnosis and treatment. *Clin Plast Surg.* 1997;24:507-514.

Guyuron B, Michelow BJ, Willis L. Practical classification of chin deformities. *Aesthetic Plast Surg.* 1995;19:257-264.

Guyuron B. Precision rhinoplasty. Part I: the role of life-size photographs and soft-tissue cephalometric analysis. *Plast Reconstr Surg.* 1988;81:489-499.

Guyuron B, Raszewski RL. A critical comparison of osteoplastic and alloplastic augmentation genioplasty. *Aesthetic Plast Surg.* 1990;14:199-206.

Riedel R. An analysis of dentofacial relationships. *Am J Orthod.* 1957;43:103-119.

Chapter 31. Perioral Rejuvenation: Lip Lift, Corner Mouth Lift, and Direct Excision of Nasolabial/Marionette Looseness

George Weston, MD; Robert Sigal, MD; Byron Poindexter, MD

INDICATIONS

These procedures use a direct approach to the aging mouth/perioral area and are indicated when other procedures are thought to be inadequate for delivering a desired result (Fig. 31-1). They are designed to create a more youthful mouth where procedures with remote incisions (ie facelift/midface lift) are insufficient. They are most commonly performed simultaneously with a facial rejuvenation but may be performed independently when the patient's concerns are focused exclusively on the perioral area. Indications require the patient to have reasonable expectations and be willing to have the resulting scar as the trade-off for a better contour. These procedures are not indicated for perioral wrinkling or thinning, but can be combined with resurfacing or fat/filler injections when appropriate.

PREOPERATIVE PREPARATION

Patient selection is the most important factor in determining postoperative satisfaction with these procedures. The consultation is critical for exploring the patient's expectations for a result and the patient's willingness to have a potentially visible scar as the tradeoff for a more youthful mouth. It is explained that although the scars heal well and are barely noticeable from inches away, they are ultimately unpredictable and no guarantees can be given about scars or results. The plastic surgeon must be able to show and describe what result can be reasonably expected, both with and without these procedures, so that the patient can choose and be 100% responsible for his or her choice. This process is actually no different for any other cosmetic surgery except that the plastic surgeon must trust that the patient *really* is willing to have a scar as the tradeoff. We routinely prescribe oral antiviral therapy to begin one day prior to direct perioral procedures.

ANESTHESIA

Either local, monitored conscious sedation or general anesthesia is appropriate for these procedures.

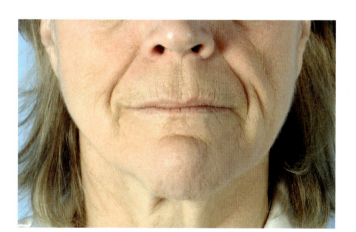

Figure 31-1 Typical patient for perioral rejuvenation with direct excisions.

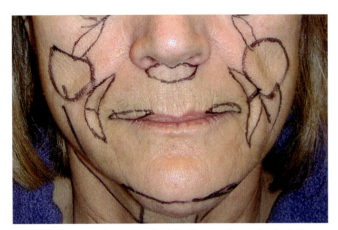

Figure 31-2 Markings for facial rejuvenation to include lip lift, corner mouth lift and direct excision nasolabial/marionette looseness.

POSITION AND MARKING

The list of procedures and surgical plan is confirmed with the patient the morning of surgery prior to marking (Fig. 31-2). Markings are then performed in the sitting position. Upon completion of the markings, a mirror is given to the patient and the details of the surgical plan are again confirmed and any final questions are answered.

Lip Lift

The lip lift is performed to shorten the elongation of the upper lip that occurs with aging. Ideally, this will allow 1 to 2 mm visibility of the upper teeth when the lips are slightly parted in repose. This procedure will also slightly evert more of the upper lip vermilion, making a thin upper lip appear fuller.

A wavy ellipse is marked in the crease beneath the nostril sill (Fig. 31-2). The nostril sill should not be violated and the scar should be *in* the crease, not in the nostril. The width of the ellipse is determined by the surgeon's aesthetic judgment as the amount necessary to mimic the shorter lip of youth. Although there are no rigid rules or mathematical formulas as to how short the upper lip should be, a length shorter than 10 to 12 mm from the nostril sill to upper lip vermilion will make the upper lip appear too short. Allowance should be made for 1 to 2 mm of redroop postoperatively.

Corner Mouth Lift

The corner mouth lift procedure is designed to correct the downturned lateral upper lip that can convey an appearance of aging or unhappiness. Although we (and other authors) have described variations of the technique that leave a scar outside the corner of the mouth, we now almost never use these techniques because the resulting scar outside the commissure runs perpendicular to natural perioral wrinkles and can be noticeable. The technique described here is a simple skin ellipse excision for vermilion exposure that accounts for 90% to 95% of our procedures.

A line is marked along the lateral lip vermilion extending from the commissure medially toward the cupids bow precisely at the junction of the skin with the vermilion (Fig. 31-2) An asymmetrical ellipse (or rounded triangle) is then drawn above this line, and tapered to the medial vermilion end point. The initial vector of this ellipse is directed toward the ipsilateral lateral canthus. The lateral portion of the ellipse is greater than the medial portion, allowing for more elevation toward the commissure than medially. The skin excision can be extended up to the peak of the cupids bow if necessary but should not, in our opinion, violate the area between the philtral columns. Scars here tend to contract, flatten the contour of the cupids bow, and become noticeable or obviously "operated."

Direct Excision of Nasolabial/ Marionette Looseness

Direct excision of the looseness at the lower nasolabial/ marionette area should be considered when a facelift/ midface lift is inadequate to tighten this area. This is determined during consultation by simulating the facelift by lifting the cheeks with the fingers. The patient is shown this technique with a mirror. If the simulation shows an inadequate result, the facelift will also be inadequate and a direct excision should be considered.

The length of looseness to be excised is marked with a line just medial to it, beginning superior to the looseness in the nasolabial crease and extending inferiorly far enough to excise any marionette laxity (Fig. 31-2). The "stretch" technique is used to determine the amount of skin to be excised). The cheek is stretched up while the marking pen is held in place at the medially marked line. Holding the pen stable, the skin is stretched down and a dot is marked. The process is repeated along the line and the dots are connected to form an ellipse to be excised.

DETAILS OF PROCEDURES

These procedures are simple full-thickness skin excisions. Occasionally, a small amount of subcutaneous fat needs to be excised in the lower nasolabial excision to reduce any bulge. The skin edges are backcut for 1 to 2 mm to allow for skin eversion and closure is with 6-0 Vicryl and 6-0 Prolene sutures. Resurfacing can be performed simultaneously if desired (Figs. 31-3 and 31-4).

PITFALLS

For any cosmetic surgery, patient dissatisfaction is usually because of either (a) a poor result (from design, execution, or healing); (b) an unexpected complication (from

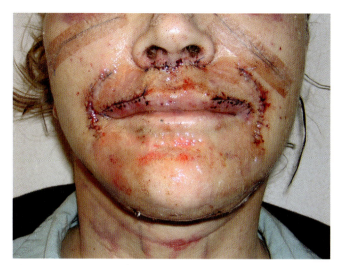

Figure 31-3   Post-op day 1. Note perioral dermabrasion with direct skin excisions.

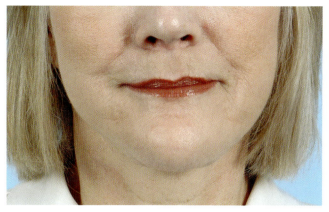

Figure 31-4   Close-up view shows scars barely visible at 4 months post-op.

infection, hematoma, or scaring); or (c) the patient's inappropriate expectations (of no visible scar, perfect symmetry, 100% correction of the flaw, etc). Our most common design flaw has been undercorrection from being too timid with our estimates for skin excision. Skin relaxes back slightly and with more experience we have learned to allow for it. Indented scars are the most common scar flaw, but are rare. This is avoided with good subcuticular suture technique. As with any procedure, patient's expectations should be aligned so that they expect a visible scar from inches away, no perfect symmetry, and less than 100% correction of any flaw. Improvement is stressed as the goal, not perfection.

PEARLS

The lip lift is designed to lift the central upper lip. It should most commonly be combined with the corner mouth lift to prevent an exaggerated "Kewpie Doll" effect. We do not believe that extending the lip lift around the nasal alae will adequately lift the corner of the mouth and may widen the nasal base.

We caution against performing a lip lift in a patient who has incisal show even if they have a long upper lip. Shortening the lip of this patient may result in excessive tooth show or even produce a "gummy" smile.

When excising the lower nasolabial looseness in combination with a facelift, we perform this excision first as this area looks, at first, adequately corrected at the end of the facelift. When the swelling and tightness relax, we have discovered that it was not adequately corrected.

The mouth and perioral area should be looked upon as a whole unit of the face. Many procedures are now available and are chosen based upon the patient's anatomy, desires, and willingness to weigh risks and benefits. Partial corrections, such as fat injections to a long lip, look odd, and should be avoided.

SUGGESTED READING

Poindexter BD, Sigal RK, Austin HW, Weston GW. Surgical treatment of the aging mouth. Seminars in Plastic Surgery 2003;17:199-208.

Chapter 32. Alloplastic Volumizing Augmentation of Midface and Mandible Sections

Edward O. Terino, MD, FACS

ALLOPLASTIC AUGMENTATION

Six Basic "Principles" Applied to All Alloplastic Volume Alterations of Any Aspect of Facial Anatomy

1. *Purpose.* The purpose of volume alterations aligns completely with the optimum goal of aesthetic facial surgery, that is, the 3-dimensional restructuring of facial form and balance.

2. *Principles of aesthetics.* Alloplastic volume alterations are highly effective in establishing the facial balance, which results from the symbiotic interrelationship of volume differentials and deficiencies within the zones of anatomy and interrelate the aesthetic regional segments of the face (Fig. 32-1). Correction of volume deficiencies in specific regions and zones constitute aesthetic balance.

3. *Predictability.* Alloplastic implants do not change over time. The materials from which they are made remain stable. Moreover, implants are fixed in location by encapsulating fibrosis, which constitutes the normal physiologic response.

4. *Precision.* Because alloplastic implants are volume devices with a noncompressible shape and form, their size and location are extremely critical. Small changes in the measurement, shape, and anatomic location of the facial implant create a much greater difference than 2-dimensional tightening of autogenous elastic facial tissues. This fact becomes more valid as aging and attenuation of the elastic subcutaneum occurs.

5. *Permanence.* The shape, size, and configuration of facial contours produced by alloplastic implants remain permanent. But depending on the material used, regional contours can be altered readily by an easy implant exchange. This is particularly true when using silicone rubber implants. Moreover, if the changes are considered undesirable, removal of the implants in most instances produces complete reversibility to the previous natural state without deformity or disfiguration.

6. *Practice.* Practice is absolutely necessary to understand fully the remarkable aesthetic changes that can be realized from alloplastic augmentation. The artistic expertise to use facial implants with predictability and precision can only be gained from experience. The technical aspects of the surgery are relatively simple and very easy for a novice to learn.

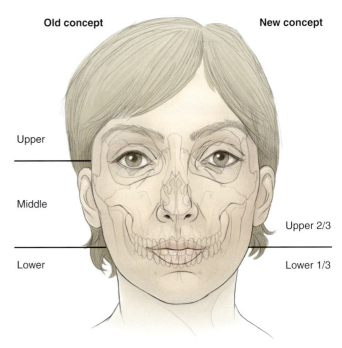

Figure 32-1 New aesthetic perception of a face: upper two-thirds and lower one-third.

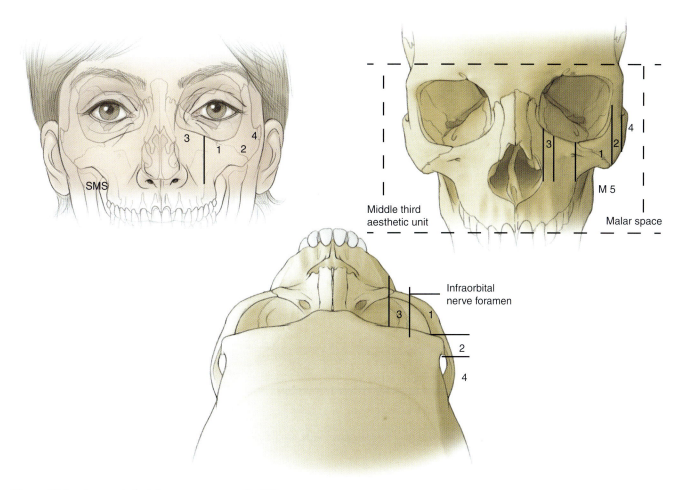

Figure 32-2   Anatomic facial contour zones of midface.

Indications

Alterations of facial volume and contour are easily predictable by using the practical model for anatomic analysis by skeletal facial zones (Fig. 32-2).

Zone 1

The implant is placed on the major body of the malar bone, producing a high strong malar bone contour. This is most frequently useful for young men who desire a well-defined sculpture appearance. It is also useful in young women who desire a more exotic look.

Zones 1, 2, and 3

Volumization of the lateral and suborbital region in patients who have a hereditary or posttraumatic deficient maxilla with suborbital and malar flattening. This can extend from the medial canthus to include the major body of the malar bone.

Zone 2 Procedures

Widening in the middle third of the zygomatic arch, which produces greater width to the upper third midface aesthetic segment. This can be desirable in someone with a narrow upper face.

Zone 3

Increased volume and shape in the paranasal tear trough and the suborbital areas. Volume deficiencies in these areas appear as a tired, hollow appearance. Isolated tear trough suborbital deficiencies may also be corrected.

Zone 4

The posterior third of zygomatic arch, according to the perception of the authors, never needs augmentation for aesthetic purposes. Surgical dissections in this zone could produce temporomandibular joint symptoms or permanent damage.

Malar Zone

The lower half of the midface can be called the submalar (SM) region, which exists beneath the lower border of the malar bone and lies on the surface of the masseter muscle. It is often deficient because of aging atrophy or heredity factors. Accentuation or contour improvements in this area are the most frequent reason for implants to be used. Submalar aging changes of the face as a result of facial atrophy causes a dissipated, emaciated appearance and the loss of youthful midfacial fullness.

Preoperative Preparation

The overriding most important principle with all allo-plastic facial implant surgery is to spend sufficient "communication time" with a patient to achieve a complete understanding of their contour goals and expectations. These must be understood with certainty and precision.

A computer imaging program is indispensable along with the "homework assignment" of having patients bring photographs of friends, family, earlier periods in their life, as well as pictures of models, actresses, and the like, who have contours in the malar midface region they would like to emulate ("ideal scene").

The limitations, as well as possible complications from the surgery, must be thoroughly discussed, as well as alternative methods of treatment such as injectable fillers, autologous fat transplants, and upper midface suspension techniques.

Anesthesia

Malar midface implant augmentation techniques require general anesthesia. Local anesthesia and monitored sedation are usually avoided because of the possibility of aspiration of blood or saliva. Copious injection of local anesthesia into the anatomic dissection areas to be implanted facilitates optimum hemostasis and easy anatomic planar dissection. Injected into each implantation site is 20 to 30 mL of lidocaine 0.25% with adrenaline 1:600,000.

Position and Markings

After using computer imaging and photos to decipher the patient's beauty ideal, both the patient and surgeon agree on a malar or submalar midface contour shape. The specific implant size is chosen on the morning of surgery. The patient is seen first in an examining room where the computer images and "game plan" are reviewed with the patient. A marking pen is used to outline the lateral orbital rim and the malar zygomatic bone in its entirety. The patient is asked to smile, which facilitates the marking of the submalar space below the lower border of the malar bone. The regional zones 1 through 4 and SM (submalar space) are also labeled on the face.

A variety of implant sizes and shapes are then demonstrated and discussed with the patient (Fig. 32-3). Together, a mutual agreement is reached about the exact implant location, size, and shape, which is determined by the computer image that was created, as well as from the photographs that the patient has brought in. Most commonly (99%), 4-mm thick implants in small, medium, large, and extralarge sizes are selected. The exact one is chosen by the implant surface area, which can be observed by placing an implant on the face within the confines of the malar-submalar-zone markings.

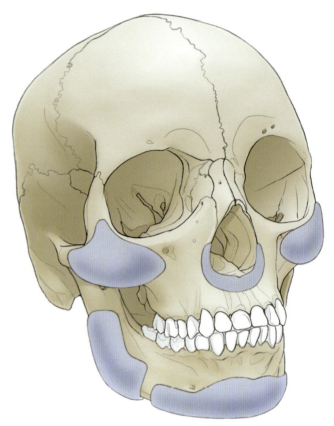

Figure 32-3   Anatomic-style implants used to imitate natural bony and soft-tissue contours in malar-midface and permeable regions.

Details of Procedure

After 30 years of experience and several thousand midface augmentations, the senior author has found that 2 approaches work best: (a) intraoral and (b) lower-eyelid subciliary and occasionally transconjunctival. It is also possible to put them through the superficial musculoaponeurotic system (SMAS) fascia in the zygomatic region underneath a facelift flap through a small 1-cm aperture directly down onto the bone in the lateral zone 1 area where it is certain that there are no branches to any important motor nerves.

Intraoral Approach

This approach has the least morbidity and is the easiest to perform. A 1-cm oblique incision is made through only the mucosa over the canine tooth with a 1-cm lateral extension. This creates an L-shaped incision. A 3-mm elevator is thrust directly through the incision beneath the orbicularis oris musculature and onto the inferior maxillary buttress, approximately 2 cm above the gumline over the third canine tooth. A 10- to 13-mm spatula elevator is used to dissect on the subperiosteal plane up the maxillary buttress to the major point of prominence where the masseter muscle and tendon arise from the anterior malar bone. The dissection is extended posteriorly on the bone

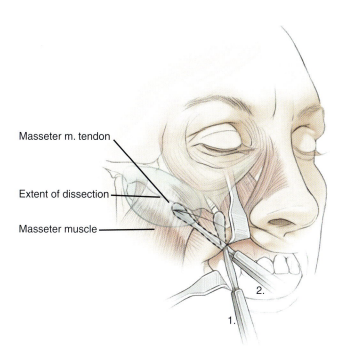

Masseter m. tendon

Extent of dissection

Masseter muscle

2.

1.

Figure 32-4   Minimally invasive intraoral dissection for placing midface implants.

to dissect the soft tissues from the major body of the malar bone (zone 1) and lateral over the midzygomatic arch (zone 2) (Fig. 32-4).

The dissection is oblique and extends laterally as it is carried superiorly on the maxillary buttress, making it a safe distance from the medial infraorbital foramen and nerve. When a tear trough or suborbital tear trough malar implant is inserted, the dissection must extend medially to carefully visualize and isolate the infraorbital nerve trunk and the foramen. In such cases, the dissection is carried above the infraorbital nerve foramen and along the infraorbital rim to the junction of the nasal bone and the maxilla.

By dissecting only on the subperiosteal bony surface, injuries are avoided to the zygomaticus major and minor, as well as the frontalis musculature. Also, significant muscle damage may stimulate capsular contracture or pain during the healing process.

The submalar space (zone SM) inferior to the lower border of the malar bone is augmented either to position a malar implant partially into a submalar position or to place a midface implant exclusively into the submalar region. The elevator is used to sweep in a downward direction from the malar bone to establish an adequate submalar space. The sweeping motion will lift the overlying tissues from the glistening, easy-to-identify tendinous covering of the masseter muscle.

This inferior space dissection must be done gently and not too far posterior in front of the ear where the

major trunks of the facial nerve to the zygomatic muscle group and the buccinators are located.

There are several limits to the dissection downward into the submalar area, depending on the decision of how much submalar volumization must be done for the "ideal scene" of the patient. The various sizes of malar implants range from 3- to 4-cm vertically in dimension. For an exclusive submalar augmentation, dissection with the elevator is begun along the inferior border of the malar bone and extended downward only. This prevents the natural tendency of implants to move upward during the encapsulation process, which occurs around all smooth-surface silicone rubber implants.

In many instances, to obtain the best contour, the implant should be placed 5 to 10 mm above the inferior malar bone margin so that it bridges the bone down into the submalar space on top of the tendinous masseter muscle surface. This essentially creates a new and vertically larger malar bone, making the submalar midface contour fuller, rounder and lower, that is, an "apple cheek" appearance. The decision to do this is made by the patient and the surgeon preoperatively.

Subcilial or Transconjunctival Approach

A 2.5-cm incision is made 3 mm below the lash line, extending only to the orbital rim laterally. A skin muscle flap is elevated above the orbital septum using a Freer elevator. The dissection is continued 4 to 5 mm down over the inferolateral margin of the orbital rim. At this point, the periosteum is penetrated with a sharp elevator. The subperiosteal dissection of the malar space is made with a larger elevator to expand it posterolaterally and inferiorly as necessary to accommodate the chosen implant.

For tear trough or suborbital extended malar implant placement, the subperiosteal dissection beneath the lower lid is extended medially along the orbital rim beneath the orbicularis oculi muscle to create the tear trough space (zone 3) and isolate the infraorbital neurovascular bundle. In more difficult cases, a combination approach (intraoral, plus lower lid) can be used to facilitate accuracy and minimize trauma.

Gentle dissection around the infraorbital nerve trunk under direct vision is essential in avoiding nerve damage. A keyhole aperture is made in the medial portion of the suborbital tear trough malar implant after measuring the distance of the infraorbital nerve from the nasal bone to the infraorbital rim. The implant is then placed to surround the infraorbital nerve.

The implant is securely sutured to the arcus marginalis, medial and lateral to the infraorbital nerve along the orbital rim with 4-0 Vicryl.

Proptotic fat may be attached to the anterior surface of the implant with 1 or 2 sutures to ensure a smooth lid-cheek junction. A transconjunctival approach may be used but is somewhat more difficult unless a lateral canthotomy is performed. The authors avoids canthotomies because of potential canthal angle irregularities or deformities following repair.

By staying above the orbital septum, the infraorbital fat will be contained so that it cannot protrude significantly and obscure clear visualization, not only of the anterior orbital rim, but also down into the malar and submalar region. It is necessary to look carefully and directly to create the space required to place a tear trough or suborbital tear trough malar implant. A malar implant can easily be placed through the lateral aspect of either a transconjunctival incision or a subcilial incision onto the major body of the malar bone and over into the midzygomatic arch (zones 1 and 2).

When a subcilial incision is utilized, a "canthal sling" canthopexy with 4-0 black nylon should be done to support the position of the lower eyelid, or even to alter its shape and configuration during the healing process. The sling is done with 4-0 black nylon and is placed two-thirds of the distance from the anterior orbital rim to the canthus when the tendon is retracted upward by using a small 2-Prong hook under the lateral raphe. The suture can be placed into the lateral rim periosteum from 2 to 5 mm above the natural lateral canthal location to tighten the lower lid and avoid lower lid scleral show or to create an almond-shaped, more attractive eyelid. This distance is precisely marked using a caliper and methylene blue ink.

A secondary support suture is placed into the skin muscle flap through the orbicularis muscle with 4-0 Vicryl secured to the periosteum at the new canthopexy location. More than 95% of the author's lower lid procedures remove very little skin and muscle, if any.

Pitfalls

The major pitfalls to successful malar midface alloplastic contour operations are as follows:

- It is critical to precisely determine the patient's "ideal scene," that is, the exact shape the patient wishes to attain for the region of his or her facial anatomy that the patient desires to change. This communication with the patient may take considerable time and must be as precise as possible.
- Knowledge of the regional zonal anatomy and of the various types of implants sizes and shapes that are available are definitely essential for the surgeon's choosing which implant to use and for determining the exact position to place it into.
- In malar-zygomatic augmentation by an intraoral approach, the path of dissection should be superior and lateral to avoid trauma to the infraorbital nerve.
- Tear trough and combined suborbital tear trough malar implants involve a visual dissection of the infraorbital foramen and nerve to specifically avoid trauma, which may result in nerve symptoms or deficits.

- The subperiosteal plane is the location for placing implants, because solid immobilization occurs and they feel like a natural part of the patient's normal bony anatomy. If implants are not subperiosteal, they can encapsulate in a deformed fashion and also can be mobile to palpation.
- Not creating an adequate pocket can trap an implant into a space and position that will not result in the proper shape the patient desires.
- The percutaneous needle fixation technique must be done by thrusting the needles posteriorly through the zygomatic tunnel to externalize them behind the temporal hairline to pull and hold the implant into proper position. Otherwise, a postoperative problem may occur that will need secondary correction.

Pearls

- Malar midface augmentation has minimal to no pain in the postoperative period. Edema, however, persists and final contour definition is not present until 1 year following surgery. This prolonged healing phase should be well communicated to the patient preoperatively and emphasized postoperatively.
- The authors have found that there is a long learning curve to understand how to determine the precise anatomic site necessary to achieve a patient's desired contour.
- Use of percutaneous needle fixation allows for adjustment if the implant is pulled too far posteriorly or is too anterior. Without removing the needles, the implant can be withdrawn and the posterior margin trimmed by 2 to 3 mm to allow it to be pulled more posterior in the zygomatic tunnel. Likewise, if it is positioned too far back, it can be pulled forward a bit even when the percutaneous suture is secured over a tonsil sponge by wetting the tonsil sponge and compressing it into a smaller volume. This allows the implant to be pulled more anteriorly.
- To achieve perfect symmetrical placement, the anterior margin of the malar implant can be secured to the masseter muscle and tendon with a 4-0 Vicryl suture.
- Both intraoral incisions should remain open until the position of both midface implants are visualized and adjusted to be precisely symmetrical prior to closure.
- Lateral canthopexy is an essential operation for the surgeon to master for all lower-eyelid procedures, and especially when an implant is placed or a midface dissection is performed with suspension techniques. The canthopexy is used to aesthetically adjust and shape the palpebral aperture in its horizontal dimension and to prevent downward healing forces from producing ectropion.
- The authors feel that imaging the patient's face contours with the computer is indispensable for the purposes of

clarifying both the patient's specific desire and to provide the surgeon with the maximum data for precise size, shape, and position placement.

- Repeated antibiotic solution irrigations (1 g Ancef [cefazolin sodium] in 1 L Ringer lactate) should be done along with maximum "no touch" technique for the implant. The implant should be introduced on a clamp with sufficient retraction of the incisional margins so that there is the least contact with the intraoral mucosa and external skin.

- Implants should not be left lying on the instrument table or on the paper drapes. Implants should be soaking in antibiotic solution and sterilization prep solution (Techni-Care [chloroxylenol]) at all times until ready to be used.

- Occasionally an implant can be palpated and observed by the surgeon to be slightly out of position within the first 10 days following surgery. If and when this is the case, the surgeon can perform gentle but firm pressure manipulation to "mold" (position) the implant properly. Then the patient can be taught a similar routine to be done 2 to 3 times a day until the periimplant capsular formation stabilizes it 2 to 3 weeks following surgery.

- Inadequate postoperative sequelae, such as malposition of the lower-eyelid position after canthoplasty, or discrepancy of the size, shape, or position of the implant can be easily corrected within the first 18 days following surgery before the maximum biochemical healing phase occurs (18 to 28 days). After this time, postoperative surgical intervention may aggravate scar tissue formation and produce further symptoms and patient problems.

CHIN–MANDIBLE AUGMENTATION

Indications

Volume and contour deficiencies of the lower third facial aesthetic segment in one or more regional anatomic zones:

1. *Central mentum* for anterior-posterior projection.
2. *Midlateral* to widen the lower mandibular facial segment on frontal view.
3. *Posterolateral* to widen and give definition to the posterior mandibular angle and ascending ramus.
4. *Submandibular* to vertically lengthen a "short" lower facial third mandibular aesthetic segment (to add volume improvement to the hereditary or acquired prejowl sulcus, etc).

Preoperative Preparation

It is critical in alloplastic facial contouring surgery that the surgeon completely understand the patient's contour goals and expectations with precision. To this end, the authors find it invaluable to have the patient bring magazine photos of faces illustrating their "ideal scene" chin-jawline shape and/or photos of themselves at a different time in their life when they may have had an appearance more preferable to them.

A computer imaging program has been found to be indispensable for clarifying the exact shape the patient desires ("ideal scene").

Finally, the limitation of the techniques must be stressed, along with the possible complications and their resolution.

Anesthesia

For chin implants only, monitored sedation, general anesthesia, or local anesthesia are equally suitable. However, insertion of mandibular angle implants is best performed with general anesthesia to avoid possible aspiration problems.

Copious dilute (lidocaine 0.25% with adrenalin 1:600,000) local anesthetic solution (20 to 30 mL injected into each site) is critical to facilitate optimum hemostasis and easy anatomic planar dissection.

Position and Markings

In an examination room, the mandibular outline is drawn on the patient's face in a sitting position with a black marking pen. The regional zonal anatomy is also labeled. The precise location of the underlying mental nerves and foramina are marked in red to serve as an external guide for the surgeon's internal dissection, which is designed to avoid inflicting damage to them.

A 2- to 3-cm submental incision is designed centrally in either a natural submental crease, or just anterior to it.

For large implants (7- to 9-mm projection) or a vertical extension implant (4-mm vertical and 4-mm projection), the incision *must* be placed a minimum of 10 mm posterior to the submental crease to allow for the significant anterior displacement of the soft-tissue mound of the chin, which occurs and which can possibly prevent the scar from being obscured by the overhanging central mentum chin prominence.

The intraoral approach is performed through a 2 mm central incision horizontally through the mucosa only. The mentalis muscles are then separated centrally in a vertical fashion to gain access to the central mentum subperiosteal bone surface. Then the space is expanded laterally beneath the mental nerve and along the inferior border of the mandible. The mental nerve must be clearly visualized to not traumatize it.

Mandibular angle implants are placed using intraoral incisions 2.5 cm in length, which are created anterior to the last 2 molar teeth and extend posterior and over the transition of the angle into the ascending ramus.

A 1.5-cm cuff of mucosa and muscle should be left adjacent to the bone and away from the gingival buccal sulcus to facilitate an excellent watertight closure with 4-0 Vicryl suturing, either by interrupted or continuous techniques.

All procedures are preceded by copious 20 to 30 mL of 0.2% lidocaine with 1:600,000 adrenalin injected into each operative site using a 25-gauge needle and trying to get under the periosteum.

All procedures entail dissection only on the subperiosteal plane to ensure firm adherence and complete immobilization to the bone of silicone rubber implants by encapsulation.

Whenever dissections are off the bone, the elevator must be used gently to prevent unnecessary traumatization of muscle tissue resulting in excessive bleeding and hematoma formation, or even dreaded nerve transection, avulsion, or stretching resulting in numbness, paresthesia, or hypoesthesia.

Details of Procedure for Chin Implantations

Subperiosteal tunnels are dissected laterally on each side of the midline by degloving the muscle attachments along the anterior inferior border of the mandible. The tunnels are made 1 cm longer than the proposed implants to facilitate insertions and avoid buckling or folding of the end of the implant tail if the space is too short.

In the great majority of cases, the mental nerve exists 5 to 10 mm above the inferior border and directly below the first premolar tooth. It should always be visualized with a lighted retractor so that the implant is placed under and *not* over it. The ability to move the implant easily side-to-side as well as passing a Freer elevator gently over and under it gives reassurance of the correct position of the implant wings.

The center of the mentum and the center of the implant must be accurately identified and marked by some means.

The implant is secured to the inferior muscles and periosteum with three 4-0 Monocryl sutures— one placed centrally and the other 2 placed 1 cm laterally, thereby securing the implant and preventing horizontal and rotational movement.

On layered muscle, subcutaneous and subcuticular closure is carefully performed with 4-0 Monocryl and a Steri-Strip glued onto the incision with benzoin for 2 weeks. No other compression or stabilizing dressing is necessary.

Mandibular angle implants are inserted similarly on a subperiosteal level by degloving the inferior and posterior border at the angle. Special attention must be taken to clearly avulse or transect (by careful electrocautery) the dense, tendinous origin of the masseter, which may be present right at the angle.

Tendinous disinsertions also must be performed all the way up the ascending ramus to create an adequate space for the proper positioning of a Taylor silicone rubber angle implant. A preselected Taylor mandibular angle silastic implant (8, 10, or 12 mm of lateral projection) is inserted by placing a curved Kocher clamp along the anterior, thin, L-shaped margin and introducing it through the incision, into the prepared space with a posterior then superior upward thrust, quickly removing the clamp. A 10-mm wide Obwegeser spatula elevator is then judiciously used to adjust the space wherever necessary to accurately position the implant over the angle properly.

The elevator lifts the positioned implant up from the bone to allow clear visualization to give the surgeon certainty that the location of the implant is in correct position over the mandibular angle.

All implant surgeries are accompanied by copious frequent antibiotic solution (1 g Ancef [cefazolin sodium] in 1 L Ringer lactate) irrigations.

Once again, a secure, one layer, muscle and mucosa closure is done with 4-0 Vicryl continuous or interrupted sutures. No dressing is applied.

Pitfalls

The most crucial pitfalls to successful chin-jaw implant operations are the following:

- Incomplete communication with the patient. It is critical to precisely determine the patient's exact shape and contour desires.

- Not understanding the regional zonal anatomy and the variety of implants that are available. This compromises the surgeon's ability to choose which implant should go into which regional zone to accomplish the patient's ultimate goals.

- Not visualizing the mental nerve to avoid traumatizing it, which can cause disturbing transient or permanent nerve symptoms or deficits.

- Not releasing the muscles along the anterior-inferior mandibular border to prevent an implant from riding too high on one side or both.

- Creating too big a pocket superiorly or inferiorly, as well as by releasing the inferior muscle attachments too much. This can allow an implant to be too low or an implant wing to slip below the mandibular border and cause a visible or palpable deformity.

- When placing mandibular implants, not properly degloving the inferior border, the ascending posterior border, and, specifically, the tendon at the angle of the mandible sufficiently to allow an implant to remain in an adequate posterior position.

- Not putting an elevator beneath the mandibular angle implant to visualize its position precisely over the mandibular angle.

- Not placing a small elevator over and under a chin implant after placement to ensure that the posterior end of the implant wing is not buckled or folded upon itself.

- Not listening sufficiently to the patient's complaints after surgery to enable you to exchange an implant or change its shape if the original procedure was not to the patient's satisfaction.
- Not having precise and clearly understandable signed written agreements to explain the type of postoperative situations for which the doctor will or will not take a certain amount of financial responsibility if the patient has "issues" with the results.

Pearls

- Inject local anesthesia liberally into all of the tissues you will be dissecting into, especially beneath the periosteum.
- Always make certain that you are subperiosteal with your dissection.
- Develop an adequate space—not too big and not too small—to allow a comfortable fit for the implant.
- Be gentle and do not traumatize anterior soft tissues or tissues around the mental nerve.
- Know the various sizes and shapes of implants and their optimum uses for both chin and mandible contouring. Select one according to the patient's desire and your accurate communication and perception of their "ideal scene."
- Learn to use a computer imager for facial contouring and facial surgery; it is indispensable.

- Under direct vision, make certain that chin and mandibular angle implants are in proper position.
- Use antibiotic irrigation solution (1 g Ancef [cefazolin sodium] in 1 L Ringer lactate) repeatedly.
- As much as possible, do not touch the implants to the external skin or the internal oral mucosa.
- Thoroughly soak implants in antibiotic solution and sterilizing solution (Techni-Care [chloroxylenol]) before insertion.
- Make certain that closure of the mucosa and muscle is secure whether using intermittent sutures or continuous suture techniques.
- Do not manipulate or pull on the cheek or lip tissues to examine the incisions following surgery unless absolutely indicated and necessary.
- Photographically document postoperative changes frequently following surgery to demonstrate continuous healing changes with contour improvements to the patient.
- Know the healing curve of the human body, that is, maximum strength scar tissue formation at 3 to 4 weeks, lasting for 3 months, then slowly diminishing swelling and edema resulting in a return of flexibility and softness of the tissues by 6 months with final healing at 1 year.

Chapter 33. Midface Rejuvenation

Michael J. Yaremchuk, MD, FACS

INDICATIONS

The attributes of an attractive, youthful midface and periorbita include a narrow palpebral fissure, a short lower lid, and a convex midface with full cheeks. Aging causes descent of these structures with rounding of the palpebral fissure, lengthening of the lower lid, and loss of cheek prominence. Resuspension of the midface soft tissues (subperiosteal midface lift) can rejuvenate the midface and lower lid by restoring the youthful contours. Augmentation of the infraorbital rim with alloplastic implants can be a useful adjunct to midface soft tissue resuspension for patients who lack adequate skeletal projection in this area. It not only supplies attractive midface convexity, but also a platform on which to reposition the midface tissues (Fig. 33-1).

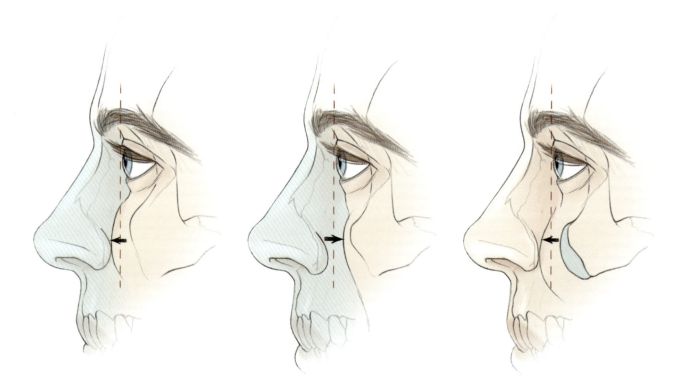

Figure 33-1 Globe-orbital rim relationships have been categorized by placing a line or "vector" between the most anterior projection of the globe and the malar eminence and lid margin. (*Left*) Positive vector relationship: In the youthful face with normal globe-to-skeletal rim relations, the cheek mass supported by the infraorbital rim lies anterior to the surface of the cornea. The position of the cheek prominence beyond the anterior surface of the cornea is termed a positive vector. (*Center*) Negative vector relationship: In patients with maxillary hypoplasia, the cheek mass lies posterior to the surface of the cornea. The position of the cheek prominence posterior to the anterior surface of the cornea is termed a negative vector. (*Right*) "Reversed" negative vector relationship: Alloplastic augmentation of the infraorbital rim can reverse the negative vector.

PREOPERATIVE PREPARATION

During the preoperative consultation, digital images of the patient are reviewed. Midface descent with loss of the cheek-lid interface is most obvious on lateral views. Smiling elevates the cheeks and provides a simulation of the proposed surgery.

Patients with "dry eyes" symptoms are informed that their symptoms may be aggravated immediately after surgery. Most often eye dryness is improved and even eliminated by the midface surgery, which elevates the lower lid margin, thereby providing more corneal coverage.

ANESTHESIA

General anesthesia is preferred because it allows optimal intraoral preparation and intraoperative airway protection.

POSITION AND MARKINGS

The patient is placed in the supine position, prepped, and draped in the usual sterile manner for head and neck surgery. A throat pack is placed.

DETAILS OF PROCEDURE

Overview

The midface lift described here involves the subperiosteal degloving of the midface soft tissues, their vertical elevation, and suture fixation to drill holes in the infraorbital rim or an infraorbital rim implant. This procedure is performed through access afforded by periorbital, intraoral, and temporal approaches (Fig. 33-2).

Hemostasis

Midface lifting procedures have a reputation for prolonged periods of postoperative edema. Convalescence need not be greater than other facial rejuvenative procedures if attention is paid to dissection in the subperiosteal plane.

Steps are taken to minimize soft tissue trauma and to assure hemostasis. The operative site is infiltrated with a long-acting anaesthetic solution containing epinephrine for hemostasis. Because the majority of the dissection is done in the subperiosteal plane, infusion is done directly on bone with only enough injectate to affect the plane of dissection. Use of a 27-gauge needle for injection minimizes trauma. All mucosal incisions and the majority of the subperiosteal dissection is done with the needle-tip electrocautery using the coagulation mode. Epinephrine-solution-soaked neurosurgical patties are placed after dissection of an area and are not removed until that area is repositioned or closed. The subperiosteal midface plane is always drained using a suction drain. A drain with a trocar tip exits from the temporal scalp.

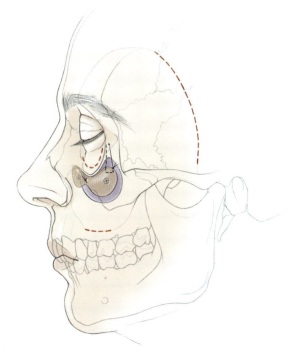

Figure 33-2 Overview of subperiosteal midface lift utilizing alloplastic augmentation of the infraorbital rim. I prefer a transconjunctival retroseptal incision (*broken line*), often with the lateral extent of a lower lid blepharoplasty incision (*solid line*) to expose the infraorbital rim. This approach preserves the integrity of the lateral canthus and hence, the palpebral fissure. Transcutaneous blepharoplasty or transconjunctival with lateral canthotomy incisions are alternative approaches that provide greater exposure but are accompanied by a greater risk of palpebral fissure distortion. An intraoral incision (*illustrated*) is used to access the lower midface skeleton and to identify and protect the infraorbital nerve. The temporal area is accessed through a temporal incision (*solid line*) or a bicoronal incision. The lower lid and midface soft tissues are freed by subperiosteal dissection. The implant is immobilized with titanium screws. Sutures secure the elevated midface soft tissues to the infraorbital rim implant (or to drill holes made in the boney rim if implants are not used).

Periorbital Access

Various combinations of incisions may be used to expose the infraorbital rim while mobilizing adjacent lid and midface soft tissues. My preference is to combine a transconjunctival retroseptal incision with an upper gingival buccal sulcus incision (see Fig. 33-2). For additional exposure, the lateral extent of the lower lid blepharoplasty incision can be added to the transconjunctival approach. The transconjunctival incision can be connected with the lateral blepharoplasty transcutaneous incision with a lateral canthotomy. These additional incisions prolong palpebral edema and risk canthal distortion. The lower lid skin or lower lid skin-muscle flaps are other alternative approaches.

Midface and Lower-Lid Mobilization

Through a temporal (or bicoronal) incision, the lateral orbital soft tissues are mobilized. The superficial layer of the deep temporal fascia is incised at the level of the zygomatic frontal suture to expose the superficial temporal fat pad. This dissection is carried inferiorly until it reaches the zygomatic arch and lateral orbital rim previously exposed through the lateral blepharoplasty incision. Using the intraoral incision, the midface soft tissues are separated from the underlying skeleton and masseter muscle. This allows "en bloc" elevation of the malar midface soft tissues and lower lid.

Implant Placement

In patients in whom the infraorbital rim is retrusive relative to the projection of the globe (flat or concave midface skeletons), the anterior projection of the infraorbital rim can be augmented with an implant specifically designed for this purpose. These infraorbital rim implants (Porex Surgical, Newnan, GA) are custom carved to meet the specific needs of the patient. Approximately 3 to 5 mm of augmentation at the infraorbital rim are employed. All implants are fixed to the skeleton with titanium screws (Synthes Corporation, Paoli, PA) as seen in Figures 33-3 and 33-4. Screw fixation is employed to eliminate the potential for any movement of the implant. Tightening the screw also eliminates any gaps between the posterior surface of the implant to the anterior surface of the facial skeleton. Gaps result in unanticipated increases in augmentation.

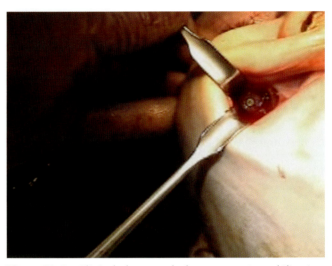

Figure 33-4   Clinical photograph shows screw immobilization of the inferior lateral aspect of the implant through intraoral access. Retractors are retracting the right upper lip and cheek. Illustration shows position of the infraorbital rim implant relative to the underlying skeleton and overlying the lip elevators.

Midface Elevation and Fixation

Sutures are used to elevate and secure the malar midface and lid soft tissues. Through the intraoral incision, 2 figure-of-eight sutures of 3-0 polyglycolic acid are used to purchase the midface soft tissues. These sutures incorporate the incised periosteum, origins of the released lip elevators and cheek subcutaneous tissue (Fig. 33-5). A suture placed at the midpupil level is passed through the lower-lid incision and secured to a drill hole placed in the infraorbital rim or to the infraorbital rim implant (Fig. 33-6). Another suture is placed in the lateral aspect

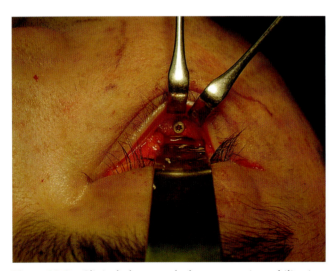

Figure 33-3   Clinical photograph shows screw immobilization of the infraorbital rim implant. Two Senn retractors are retracting the lower lid. A malleable retractor is retracting the orbital contents.

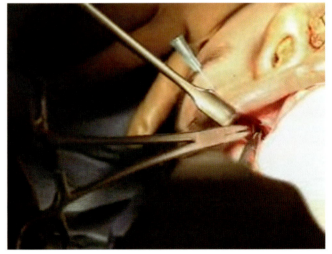

Figure 33-5   Clinical photograph shows suture elevation of the cheek mass during subperiosteal midface lift. Through an intraoral approach the cheek soft-tissue mass is being purchased with a figure-of-eight suture. A needle has been placed percutaneously at a point 3 cm beneath the lateral canthus.

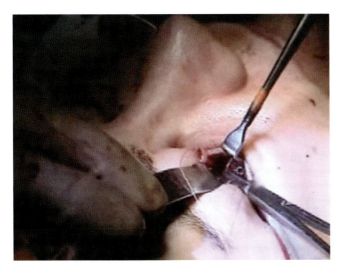

Figure 33-6 The suture elevating the midface is being tied to the rim implant.

of the malar fat pad (placed approximately 3 cm beneath the lateral canthus) and is tied to a drill hole placed in the lateral aspect of the infraorbital rim (or to the rim implant). The elevated suborbicularis oculi fat (SOOF) and adjacent musculature now rest on the infraorbital rim or augmented skeleton and help to support the freed and elevated lid margin.

Temporal Soft-Tissue Elevation

The temporal soft tissues are elevated and redistributed to avoid the "Madam Butterfly" look. A suction drain is placed beneath the composite lid-midface flap and exits the temporal scalp. A temporary stitch is placed to limit postoperative chemosis. Tape dressings are used to support the position of the lower lid and minimize bruising. Compressive dressings are not used because they direct fluid toward the more distensible lid soft tissues (Figs. 33-7 and 33-8).

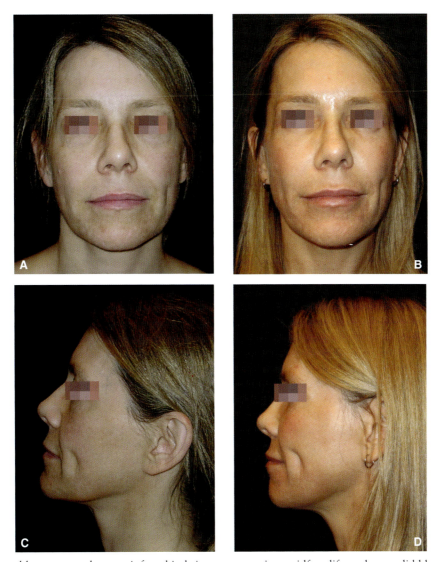

Figure 33-7 A 50-year-old woman underwent infraorbital rim augmentation, midface lift, and upper-lid blepharoplasty. A small amount of fat was also removed from her lower lids. **A.** Preoperative frontal view. **B.** One-year postoperative frontal view. **C.** Preoperative lateral view. **D.** One-year postoperative lateral view.

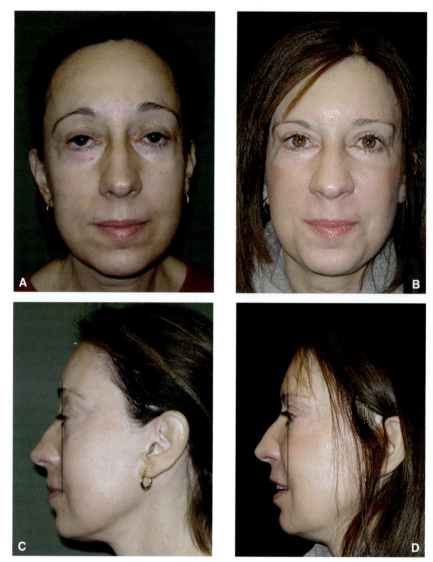

Figure 33-8   A 52-year-old woman had undergone previous browlift, rhytidectomy, and upper- and lower-lid blepharoplasty. Lower-lid retraction was treated by multiple canthopexies, spacer grafts, and full-thickness skin grafts. Dry-eye symptoms persisted. Infraorbital rim augmentation, midface lift, and lateral canthopexy resolved her symptoms. Her brows and hairline were repositioned. **A.** Preoperative frontal view. **B.** Three year postoperative frontal view. **C.** Preoperative lateral view. **D.** Three year postoperative lateral view. Note that the negative vector relationship on the frontal view has been transformed into a positive vector relationship on the postoperative view.

PITFALLS

Elevation of the midface musculature may cause temporary paresis with asymmetries during facial expression. This usually resolves within the first few weeks. It may persist considerably longer in certain patients. Likewise, trauma to the infraorbital nerve during retraction may result in numbness to the lip and paranasal tissues in the nerve's distribution. This is also a temporary finding.

PEARLS

- A temporary tarsorrhaphy stitch will help control postoperative chemosis.

- The use of cautery, epinephrine, and suction drains optimizes hemostasis and decreases postoperative morbidity.

SUGGESTED READING

Yaremchuk MJ. Improving periorbital appearance in the "morphologically prone." *Plast Reconstr Surg.* 2005;114(4): 980-987.

Yaremchuk MJ. Infraorbital rim augmentation. *Plast Reconstr. Surg.* 2001;107(6):1585-1592.

Yaremchuk MJ. Subperiosteal and full-thickness skin rhytidectomy. *Plast Reconstr Surg.* 2001;107(4):1045-1058.

Chapter 34. Otoplasty

Emily B. Ridgway, MD; Charles H. Thorne, MD

INDICATIONS

The indications for otoplasty include the patient with the prominent ear, constricted ear, Stahl's ear, or cryptotia. The prominent ear is most common, affecting 5% of the Caucasian population and is typically a result of 3 anatomical variants: underdevelopment of the antihelical fold, overdevelopment of the conchal bowl and wall, and a conchoscaphal angle greater than 90 degrees. The human ear obtains 85% of its final size by age 3 years. The ear width reaches its adult size by age 7 years for boys and 6 years for girls. The length matures to its adult size at age 13 years in boys and age 12 years in girls. Ear surgery is best addressed at younger ages as the ear becomes firmer, less malleable, and calcified with age. At infancy, the prominent ear can be addressed with nonsurgical molding. A myriad of techniques exist for otoplasty, indicating that there is not one definitive approach, and each surgery must be tailored to the individual patient. Advantages of the technique described here are its simplicity and reproducibility.

PREOPERATIVE PREPARATION

Adequate time in consultation and preoperative planning is essential. Patient and parent expectations and understanding of complications must be verified. The surgical technique varies with each patient; each of the components of the ear resulting in a prominent ear must be defined.

ANESTHESIA

Local anesthesia with monitored conscious sedation or general anesthesia is suitable for this procedure. In younger patients, general anesthesia is recommended.

POSITION AND MARKINGS

The patient is placed in the supine position, prepped and draped in the usual sterile fashion with both ears, and the retroauricular skin exposed. The patient's head may be placed on a doughnut.

The incision is marked along the retroauricular sulcus and less frequently on the posterior surface of the concha if a conchal excision is planned. If a lobular setback is planned, a triangular area of skin is marked for incision at the most medial area of retrolobular skin. The intended region of antihelical fold creation is marked.

Incision and Exposure

The procedure begins with the incisional injection of local vasoconstrictive/anesthetic agents. This aids in anesthesia and hemostasis but also in dissection of all soft tissue from the cartilage. The incision is then made with a no. 15 blade and the triangular retrolobular skin is excised. Using sharp dissection, the incision is then deepened through the subcutaneous tissues to expose the posterior surface of the concha, scapha, and medial portion of the helix. The ponticulus and any soft-tissue redundancy in the region posterior to the concha and/or lobule is excised if a conchal or lobular setback is planned. A region of the mastoid fascia suitable for conchal setback sutures is cleared of intervening soft tissue.

DETAILS OF THE PROCEDURE

The Antihelical Fold

When posterior exposure of the cartilage and hemostasis are complete, the antihelical markings are then pierced with a 27-gauge needle exposing the region of the intended antihelical fold on the posterior cartilage surface. These markings are then used to direct the placement of the Mustarde conchoscaphal sutures. These sutures are placed at multiple levels and are placed full thickness through the cartilage and anterior perichondrium but not skin at each site. In our opinion, permanent sutures provide the most reliable and durable results. The goal of the suture placement is to create a smooth fold along the full length of the antihelix that parallels the helical crus—beginning at the scaphal and triangular fossa region and extending down the length of the antihelix to the tail. These sutures redefine a conchoscaphal angle of less than 90 degrees (Fig. 34-1). We have found that both the Chongchet technique of sharply scoring the lateral scaphal cartilage and the Stenstrom technique of rasping the scapha in order to weaken the cartilage and form an antihelix are unnecessary and can be complicated by sharp anterior contour irregularities.

Conchal Reduction and Setback

The decision to proceed with a conchal reduction and/or setback is based on the individual characteristics that have led to the prominent ear deformity. The helix-to-mastoid distance should be 10 to 12 mm in the upper

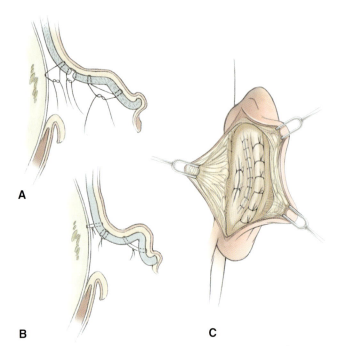

Figure 34-1 Otoplasty technique. The combination of Mustarde scaphoconchal sutures, conchal resection with conchal reapproximation, and a Furnas conchal-mastoid suture. **A.** Sutures placed. **B.** Sutures tightened to create the desired contour. **C.** Same sutures as seen through the retroauricular incision.

third, 16 to 18 mm in the middle third, and 20 to 22 mm in the lower third. Conchal hypertrophy is identified on examination by placing medial pressure on the helix, allowing visualization of a hypertrophied concha. This is addressed by a small crescent-shaped conchal excision. This crescent is removed at the junction of the conchal floor and posterior wall to avoid any visible contour irregularity. The conchal edges are reapproximated with multiple absorbable sutures. If indicated, the concho-mastoidal angle is further reduced by placing conchal-mastoid sutures as described by Furnas. Ideally, the conchal-cephalic angle is less than 90 degrees.

Lobular Setback

The lobular setback begins with triangular or fish-tailed skin excision from the posteromedial surface of the ear-lobe. The amount of skin excision is directed to leave enough for a retrolobular crease and surface for ear piercing. The second portion of the lobular setback is directed by 3-point suturing that brings both edges of the skin excision to the point of the concha at the retroauricular sulcus similar to the deep-dermis-to-scalp periosteum sutures described by Spira et al. When these sutures are tightened, the earlobe is setback without skin redundancy

or an irregular lobular contour. It is our experience that suturing the helical tail does not adequately address lobular prominence.

PITFALLS

- Skin excision is rarely indicated and can be complicated by widened hypertrophic scarring.
- All modalities or versions of abrading or weakening the cartilage on the anterior surface of the antihelix carry the risk of visible sharp irregularities.
- A straight antihelical contour is a surgical giveaway.
- Conchal mastoid sutures placed too far forward on the mastoid or too posterior on the concha will cause forward rotation of the conchal bowl and narrowing of the external auditory canal diameter.
- Avoid unilateral surgery, but also consider each ear individually, as different components of a prominent ear may exist on opposite ears.
- Severe pain postoperatively warrants dressing removal for evaluation of hematoma.
- Chondritis must be addressed with proper antibiotic regimen (usually IV) and prompt debridement of devitalized tissue because if untreated can lead to a permanent deformity.

PEARLS

- Know your normal anatomy and have an image in your mind of the intended ideal contour. The helix of both ears should be visible beyond the anithelix from the front view. The helix should have a smooth contour and should be symmetric in its distance from the head to the opposite ear at any point within 3 mm.
- Keep it simple.
- The techniques of otoplasty for prominent ear can be applied to a multitude of ear deformities requiring reconstruction.

SUGGESTED READING

Converse JM, Wood-Smith D. Technical details in the surgical correction of the lop ear deformity. *Plast Reconstr Surg.* 1963;31:118.

Hoehn J, Ashruf S. Otoplasty: sequencing the operation for improved results. *Plast Reconstr Surg.* 2005;115:5e.

Janis JE, Rohrich RJ, Gutowski KA. Otoplasty. *Plast Reconstr Surg.* 2005;115:60e.

Spira M, McCrea R, Gerow FJ, Hardy SB. Correction of the principal deformities causing protruding ears. *Plast Reconstr Surg.* 1969;44:150.

Thorne CH. Otoplasty. *Plast Reconstr Surg.* 2008;122:291.

Chapter 35. Upper Lid Blepharoplasty

Jerry W. Chang, MD; Sumner A. Slavin, MD

INDICATIONS

Upper lid blepharoplasty can be performed for patients who seek upper eyelid rejuvenation because of skin excess secondary to dermatochalasis of the upper eyelids. Steatoblepharon or fat protrusion in the upper eyelids caused by weakening of the orbital septum is also another indication. This chapter does not address correction of ptosis.

Blepharochalasis, which is a condition of the eyelids characterized by edema, erythema, and thin/excess skin, is a recurrent, inflammatory condition caused by increased immunoglobulin (Ig) E and subsequent histamine release. This condition is unlikely to be corrected surgically and must be distinguished from the other indications.

PREOPERATIVE PREPARATION

All patients undergoing upper lid blepharoplasty should have a complete history and physical evaluation. Special attention to ophthalmologic conditions should be given; these conditions include prior surgery, trauma, allergic reactions, excess tearing, thyroid disease, and dry eyes, as these may alter the surgical plan. Medications, including aspirin/anticoagulants, should be reviewed carefully; any medications that may affect clotting, including dietary supplements, should be discontinued at least 2 weeks preoperatively.

ANESTHESIA

Upper-lid blepharoplasty can be performed under local, monitored anesthesia care (MAC), or general anesthesia. It is our preference to perform this procedure under MAC or general anesthesia, in conjunction with local infiltration of 1% lidocaine with epinephrine.

POSITION AND MARKINGS

Preoperative markings should be made with the patient sitting upright in neutral gaze. It is important to slightly elevate the eyebrows manually while marking to avoid possible overresection. The eyelid crease (supratarsal fold) incision is marked first, usually just caudal (1 mm) to the existing crease. The supratarsal fold is approximately 8 to 9 mm superior to the ciliary margin in females and 7 to 8 mm in males. Next, the upper incision line is marked based on the amount of excess skin to be resected, which can be confirmed with a pinch test. The upper incision line should be at least 10 mm from the lower edge of the eyebrow as to not include any thick brow skin, which will lead to prominent scarring. The shape of the skin resection is lenticular with slightly fuller dimensions laterally. Ensure markings do not extend past the lateral orbital rim to prevent noticeable scarring laterally. Likewise, the medial markings should not extend past the medial canthus to avoid webbing in the nasal sidewall area (Fig. 35-1).

The excess fat pads (if present) are then marked with the patient in up and down gaze. The patient is placed supine on the operating room table in the standard fashion for head and neck procedures, with the neck in slight extension.

DETAILS OF THE PROCEDURE

Local anesthetic is carefully infiltrated just beneath the thin upper lid skin while taking care to avoid injection hematomas. After adequate time has passed for maximal vasoconstrictive effects of epinephrine to take place, the skin incisions are made with a fresh no. 10 blade just through skin and into the subcutaneous layer (Fig. 35-2).

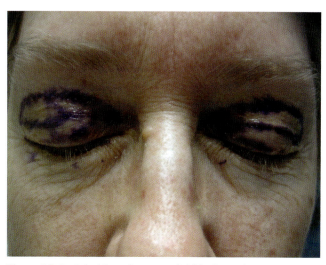

Figure 35-1 Markings for upper lid blepharoplasty.

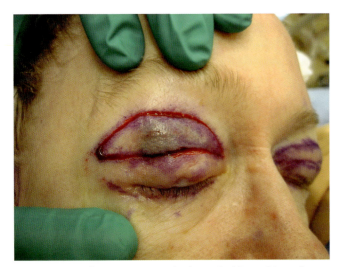

Figure 35-2   Skin incisions made through skin and into the subcutaneous layer.

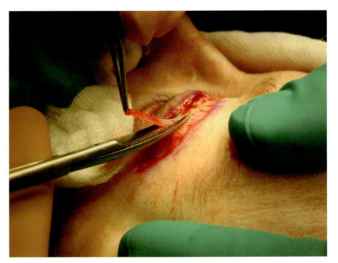

Figure 35-4   Resection of a strip of orbicularis muscle from lateral to medial and not violating the orbital septum.

Skin incision is facilitated by retraction provided by the surgical assistant to keep the upper lid skin taut. Care is taken to ensure that the scalpel blade is perpendicular to the skin surface at all times. Next, the skin is resected, starting laterally to medially with the no. 10 blade, staying in the subcutaneous plane and not violating the orbicularis muscle (Fig. 35-3). Careful hemostasis is achieved with a pinpoint cautery. Using Adson forceps to pinch the orbicularis at the very lateral edge of the skin resection to provide upward and lateral traction, a strip of orbicularis muscle is resected with curved Iris scissors, going from lateral to medial while taking care not to violate the orbital septum (Fig. 35-4). Once again, meticulous hemostasis must be established, especially along the cut orbicularis muscle edges.

Using preoperative markings as reference, small incisions are then made in the septum in the medial/nasal and central orbital fat compartments with tips of Iris scissors. Redundant fat will reveal itself with gentle global pressure. The medial/nasal fat is white, while the central fat is yellow. It is important to resect only the fat that protrudes through the orbital septum with gentle global pressure. The fat to be resected is the redundant fat that can easily be teased out and resected (Fig. 35-5). The protruding fat is clamped at the base, the fat is sharply resected, and the clamp and base are carefully cauterized. Any visible vessels are also cauterized to ensure perfect hemostasis. Tugging/pulling the fat aggressively will result in overresection and volume depletion, leading to a hollowed-out appearance of the eyes, giving

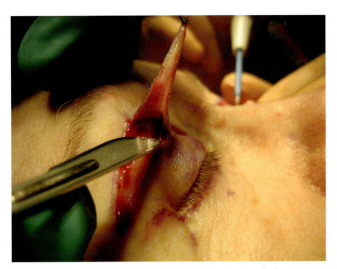

Figure 35-3   Resection of skin from lateral to medial staying in the subcutaneous plane and not violating the orbicularis muscle.

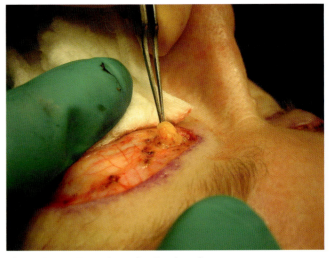

Figure 35-5   Resection of redundant fat.

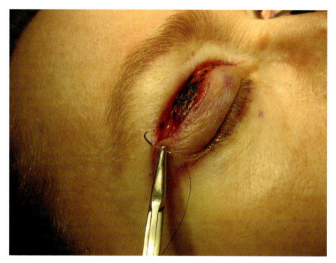

Figure 35-6 Closure of the incision with careful attention to everting skin edges.

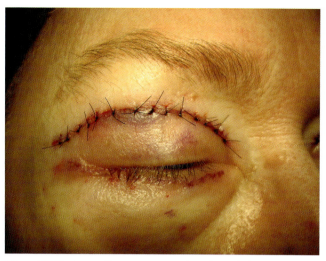

Figure 35-7 Immediate post operative view of the upper eyelid.

the patient an older look. Additionally, aggressive resection places neurovascular structures and extraocular muscles at risk for injury. Therefore, conservative resection of fat is always the rule.

After a final thorough inspection for hemostasis, the incision is closed with interrupted simple 5-0 nylon sutures, with careful attention to everting the skin edges (Figs. 35-6 and 35-7).

PITFALLS

- Avoid overresecting periorbital fat, as this leads to a hollowed-out and older appearance.
- Aggressive tugging on orbital fat when resecting places neurovascular structures and extraocular muscles at risk for injury.
- Without carefully everted skin edges upon closure, chance of dehiscence after suture removal increases.

PEARLS

- Skin incision is facilitated by retraction provided by the surgical assistant to keep the upper lid skin taut.
- Ensure skin incision is made with scalpel blade perpendicular to the skin surface at all times. Being conservative is the rule in fat resection.
- Sutures are removed 5 days postoperatively to minimize scarring.

SUGGESTED READING

Guyuron B, Hudak D. Periorbital rejuvenation. *Plastic Surgery: Indications and Practice*. Amsterdam, Netherlands, Saunders Elsevier; 2009:1427-1444.

Rohrich RJ, Coberly DM, Fagien S, Stuzin JM. Current concepts in aesthetic upper blepharoplasty. *Plast Reconstr Surg*. 2004;113:32e.

Trussler AP, Rohrich RJ. CME article: blepharoplasty. *Plast Reconstr Surg*. 2008;121:1.

Chapter 36. Senescent Ptosis

Kimberly A. Swartz, BA; Henry M. Spinelli, MD, FACS

INDICATIONS

Although there are many causes of ptosis, this chapter is limited to senescent, or involutional, causes of ptosis. It is important to confirm the ptosis is an isolated condition related to impairment of the upper eyelid retractor system, and not pseudoptosis secondary to conditions such as severe dermatochalasis, brow ptosis, hypertropia, blepharospasm, and enophthalmos. In cases of pseudoptosis, correction of the "ptosis" can often be achieved by addressing the primary cause.

PREOPERATIVE PREPARATION

To choose the correct ptosis-correcting procedure, degree of ptosis and levator function need to be assessed. Degree of ptosis is measured by assessing the distance from where the upper lid rests in primary gaze to the line bisecting the distance between the upper aspect of the papillary aperture and the iris: 1 to 2 mm signals mild ptosis, 3 to 5mm moderate ptosis, and more than 5 mm severe ptosis. Levator function is measured by subtracting the levator aperture in down gaze from the aperture in up gaze; 10 to 15 mm indicates good levator function, 6 to 9 mm fair function, and less than 5 mm poor function. Measurements of up, primary, and down gaze should be done while immobilizing the brow to eliminate compensatory brow action. If ptosis is mild and levator function is good, a procedure such as a tarsal conjunctival müllerectomy may be indicated. If ptosis is severe and levator function is poor, something more complex, such as a frontalis sling procedure, may be necessary, although such procedures are typically less satisfying than procedures that do not rely on exogenous muscle action.

ANESTHESIA

Local, monitored anesthesia care (MAC), or general anesthesia can be used for this procedure.

POSITION AND MARKINGS

Preoperatively, the endogenous lid fold is delineated. If a new lid fold is to be created, the desired fold, often chosen to match the contralateral fold, is marked. For this procedure, the patient is placed in the supine position with the ability to be sat upright.

Incision and Exposure

Local anesthetic with epinephrine should be infiltrated using a 27- to 30-gauge needle along the upper lid and the planned incision. Topical anesthetic, such as tetracaine, should be instilled. Next, a protective lens may or may not be put in place, depending on the surgeon's preference. The incision that follows depends upon the procedure being performed and is discussed below.

DETAILS OF THE PROCEDURE

Tarsal Conjunctival Müllerectomy (Fasanella-Servat)

Tarsal conjunctival müllerectomy (Fasanella-Servat) is used for mild ptosis and is contraindicated in patients with dry eye syndrome or decreased tear production.

The upper lid is everted and the tarsal complex is clamped with 2 small, curved clamps, leaving 3 to 4 mm of tarsal plate. It is important to observe the sweeping contour of the upper lid and mimic this with the clamp placement. A monofilament suture is then passed from the skin to the conjunctiva and then woven lateral to medial below the clamps; at the end, the suture is brought back through the skin. Then, before or after the clamps are removed, the excess tissue above the suture line is resected. After the clamps have been removed, the lid is reverted, and the 2 ends of the suture are loosely tied together (Fig. 36-1).

Levator Tuck

The levator tuck is used for mild to early moderate ptosis with good to excellent levator function.

A cutaneous incision is made along the upper-lid crease, and dissection is carried down through orbicularis muscle to the levator aponeurosis. Dissection then proceeds cephalad along the levator aponeurosis, incising the orbital septum, so that the preaponeurotic fat pad is visualized (Fig. 36-2). Caudally, dissection proceeds along the aponeurosis to the tarsal plate. The levator aponeurosis may then be plicated cephalad to the tarsal plate with an absorbable suture such as a 5-0 Vicryl. Typically, the

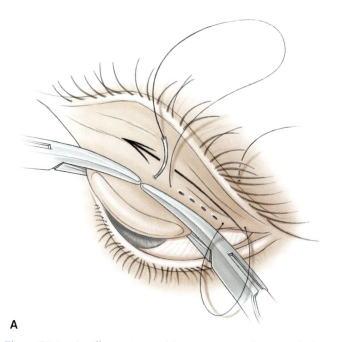

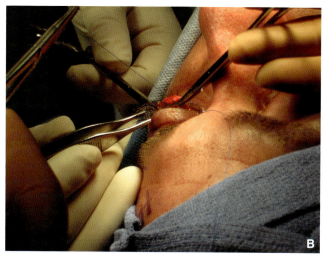

Figure 36-1   An illustration and intraoperative photograph demonstrating the clamping and suturing of the tarsal complex in a tarsal conjunctival müllerectomy.

medial aspect of the pupil is chosen as the apex of the eyelid curvature, and a plication suture should be placed here. Additionally, an interrupted suture may be placed both lateral and medial to this one, in keeping with the anatomic sweep of the upper eyelid. The resulting cuff may be resected so as to avoid cosmetically visible bulk,

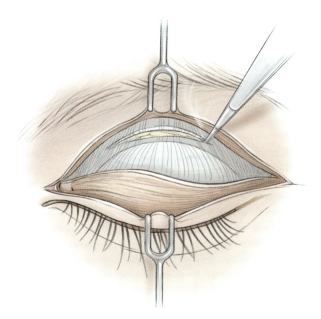

Figure 36-2   Cephalad dissection along the levator aponeurosis includes incision of the orbital septum. At this point fat pads become visible, and may be addressed if desired.

so long as the suture line is maintained. If resecting, it is important to firmly plicate the levator aponeurosis to avoid postoperative dehiscence.

Levator Advancement

Levator advancement is used for any degree of ptosis, including severe or congenital, in the presence of good to excellent levator function.

Dissection begins in the same way as a levator tuck procedure. The levator aponeurosis is then dissected off the tarsal plate caudal to cephalic. If possible, it is preferable to leave Müller's muscle behind with the tarsal plate. The medial and lateral horns of the levator muscle are then severed. Medial and lateral horn division, as well as complete cephalic dissection insure full mobility of the levator aponeurosis (Fig. 36-3). The aponeurosis is then advanced and reinserted into the tarsal plate, and fixed with a double-armed absorbable suture such as a 5-0 Vicryl (Fig. 36-4). The aponeurosis may be temporarily tied down to intraoperatively assess correction, and adjust the advancement as necessary. This is done by sitting the patient up, reducing ambient lighting to avoid squinting, and removing any protective lens. Once an ideal lid height and ptosis correction are achieved, the original suture, aligned with the nasal pupillary margin or the highest point of the lid corresponding to the contralateral side, can be permanently tied down. Single interrupted sutures may be placed both medially and laterally. Excess levator aponeurosis should then be resected. Attaching the upper and lower

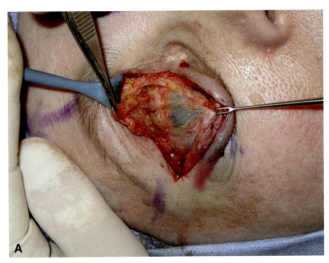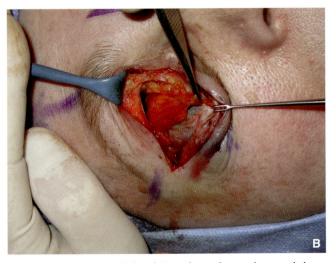

Figure 36-3   After medial and lateral horn division, the levator aponeurosis is optimally mobilized. It is then advanced toward the tarsal plate, and reinserted at the desired height.

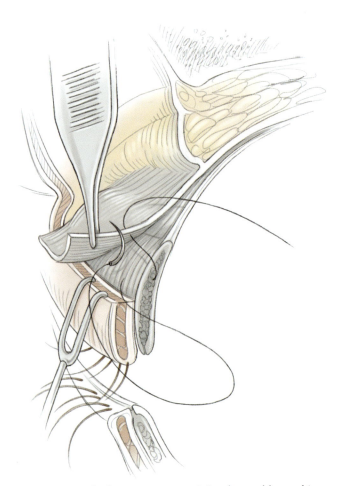

Figure 36-4   The levator aponeurosis is advanced beyond its previous insertion. The new place of insertion is then sutured directly to the tarsal plate.

skin margins to the levator aponeurosis at a chosen height can be done to accentuate a lid fold. Skin should then be closed intracutaneously as one would in an upper lid blepharoplasty.

In cases of levator dehiscence, one simply advances the levator without having to dissect it off the tarsal plate, and fixes it as described above.

Frontalis Sling

The frontalis sling is used for poor levator function.

Stab incisions are made medially, centrally, and laterally along the superior border of the eyebrow, and 3 mm superior to the lash line of the upper lid. A long, curved needle, such as a Wright needle, is then used to pass fascia from the medial and lateral brow incisions deep to the orbicularis muscle through the pretarsal area, and back to the brow (Fig. 36-5). Locking sutures are used to reinforce the sling ties, and it is generally helpful to slide the knots through the subcutaneous tunnels to eliminate potential extrusion. It is important to evert the upper lid to note whether there is any exposure or corneal penetration, before tying knots, as this could lead to corneal irritation and break down. Finally, closure should be performed in layers. A temporary tarsorrhaphy can then be used to protect the cornea immediately postoperatively. This is important in patients who have defective compensatory mechanisms for corneal coverage.

Closure

Closure differs for each procedure, and is discussed above (Figs. 36-6 to 36-9).

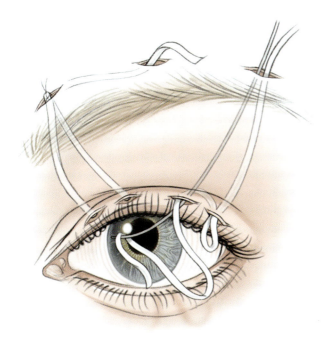

Figure 36-5 The upper incisions illustrated extend to the periosteum, while the lower incisions extend to the tarsal plate. A piece of fascia is then passed back and forth, with care given not to pierce the conjunctival surface of the lid. The illustrated technique requires that the facial strands be tied together and reinforced with an absorbable suture. The lid height should be at the limbus for patients with with good Bell's and lid protractor function, and lower for patients with poor protective mechanisms.

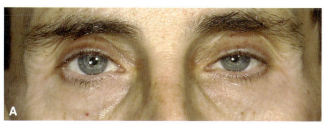
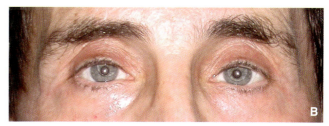

Figure 36-6 55 year old male with left eyelid ptosis before **A.** and after **B.** Tarsal Conjunctival Mullerectomy.

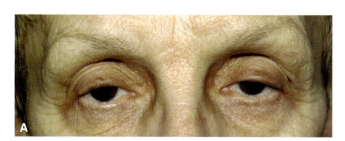
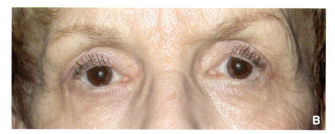

Figure 36-7 75 year old female with bilateral ptosis before **A.** and after **B.** Tarsal Conjunctival Mullerectomy.

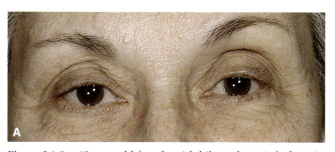
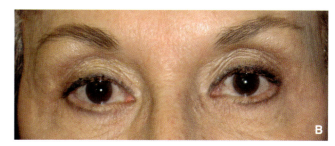

Figure 36-8 68 year old female with bilateral ptosis before **A.** and after **B.** Levator Advancement.

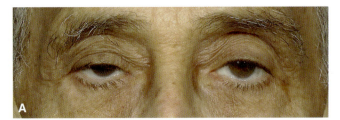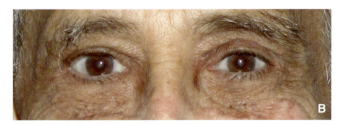

Figure 36-9   72 year old male with bilateral ptosis before **A.** and after **B.** Levator Advancement.

PITFALLS

One of the most important things to note when performing ptosis repairs are the physiologic changes the body makes in response to the local anesthetic and epinephrine infiltrated at the beginning of surgery. For example, the epinephrine stimulates contraction of Müller's muscle, so ultimately satisfactory ptosis repair may at the time of surgery appear slightly overcorrected. Additionally, local anesthetic distorts soft-tissue anatomy and impairs levator function. These agents also decrease frontalis function, making elevator action of a sling difficult to assess intraoperatively. In all cases, undercorrection is much more easily treated secondarily, via simple procedures such as a skin trim, than overcorrection.

PEARLS

An important biochemical aspect of levator function is concentration of circulating catecholamines, which changes throughout the day. Given this fact, ideally one should measure levator function on 2 separate occasions preoperatively.

In a tarsal conjunctival müllerectomy, sutures are typically left in place for 2 weeks. In the event that slight undercorrection has been achieved, sutures can be left in longer. The reverse is true for the case of overcorrection.

SUGGESTED READING

Spinelli HM. *Atlas of Aesthetic and Periocular Surgery.* Philadelphia, PA: Elsevier; 2004.

Chapter 37. Transconjunctival Lower Lid Blepharoplasty

Kimberly A. Swartz, BA; Robert C. Silich, MD, FACS;
Henry M. Spinelli, MD, FACS

INDICATIONS

The ideal candidate for this procedure is a younger patient who has no, or minimal, amount of skin redundancy but has prominent orbital fat pads. Another patient who is well suited for this procedure is the older individual who is unusually thin with minimal skin redundancy and does not have lower lid malposition. This technique allows nasojugal or lateral orbital rim depressions to be addressed through fat repositioning.

PREOPERATIVE PREPARATION

The transconjunctival approach is most successful in the younger patient, likely as a result of the greater skin elasticity when compared to an older patient. This elasticity allows conversion of the convex lid to a slightly concave lid to occur more easily. When the patient is older, it is best to plan to use this procedure as an adjunct to other procedures, such as laser procedures or a simple rhytidectomy with orbicularis suspension.

ANESTHESIA

Monitored anesthesia care (MAC) or general anesthesia can be used for this procedure.

POSITION AND MARKINGS

Generally there are no preoperative markings for the transconjunctival approach; however, standard medical photography is used intraoperatively. These photographs should include anterior, true lateral, and upward gaze views. The upward gaze views are particularly helpful in examining the periorbital fat pockets.

Incision and Exposure

Topical anesthetic (tetracaine) should be instilled into the conjunctival sac, and local anesthetic with epinephrine should be infiltrated using a 27- to 30-gauge needle by way of the transconjunctival route. This maneuver is accomplished by everting the lower lid with slight digital pressure on the inferior tarsus, or with an instrument such as a Desmarres retractor. A protective lens may or may not be put in place, depending on the surgeon's comfort. The conjunctiva and lower lid retractors are grasped near the fornix with a toothed forcep and engaged with a traction suture. The authors prefer a 5-0 fast absorbing catgut suture that can be later used for conjunctival closure. The lower lid is everted with an eyelid hook and a transconjunctival incision is made just below the tarsal plate with the conjunctiva and lower lid placed on cephalic traction. This incision should be made with a needle cautery (Fig. 37-1).

DETAILS OF THE PROCEDURE

Once the lower lid retractors are disengaged from the tarsal plate, the eyelid hook is replaced with a Desmarres retractor to engage the lower edge of the tarsal plate. Using insulated or plastic instruments reduces the risk of cautery burn injuries. Traction is placed cephalad and anteriorly, and dissection is carried out in front of the orbital septum in the preseptal, postobicularis plane down to the orbital rim. At this juncture an intact orbital septum, orbital rim, and suborbital tissues should be visible (Fig. 37-2). If adjuvant procedures or changes in other areas of the face are sought, dissection can be carried out inferiorly in a supraperiosteal or subperiosteal plane. To access the underlying fat compartments, the orbital septum may be incised in 3 distinct openings or by a wide transverse midseptal incision (Fig. 37-3). The latter is preferred to avoid tethering or strangulation of the fat pedicle. The inferior oblique muscle needs to be visualized and protected.

In fat resection, conservative resection of spontaneously herniated tissue is most appropriate. Special attention should be paid to the lateral fat pad, which is often underaddressed.

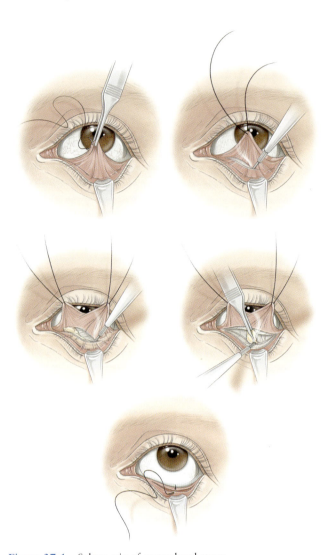

Figure 37-1   Schematic of procedural steps.

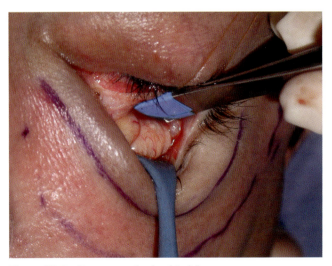

Figure 37-2   Exposure of suborbital fat.

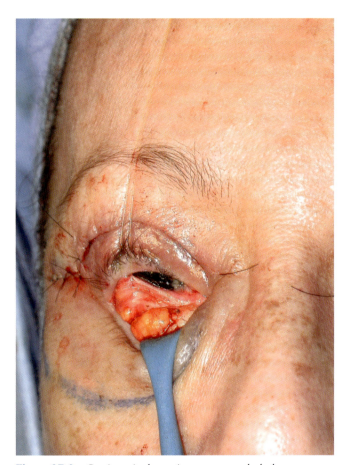

Figure 37-3   Conjunctival traction suture cephalad, Desmarres retractor exposure of fat compartments.

Closure

Hemostasis is usually spontaneous and complete. Closure requires only cutting the traction suture and allowing the conjunctival flap to spontaneously retract. The conjunctiva may then be apposed with a single interrupted suture using the aforementioned 5-0 catgut. The suture line should run lateral to the corneal surface. It is important to engage only the conjunctiva and not Tenon's capsule, which may lead to postoperative pyogenic granulomas. At this point the surgeon may proceed with adjuvant skin tightening procedures. The authors recommend using a topical antibiotic drop containing corticosteroid postoperatively when not contraindicated. This tends to lessen postoperative chemosis or conjunctival edema, and appears to shorten the recovery period.

PITFALLS

It is important to remember that because this procedure alone will not address severe skin laxity, it is best suited for the younger or very thin older patient (Fig. 37-4). Once the procedure has been undertaken, it is then important to address the lateral fat pad sufficiently and appropriately, as

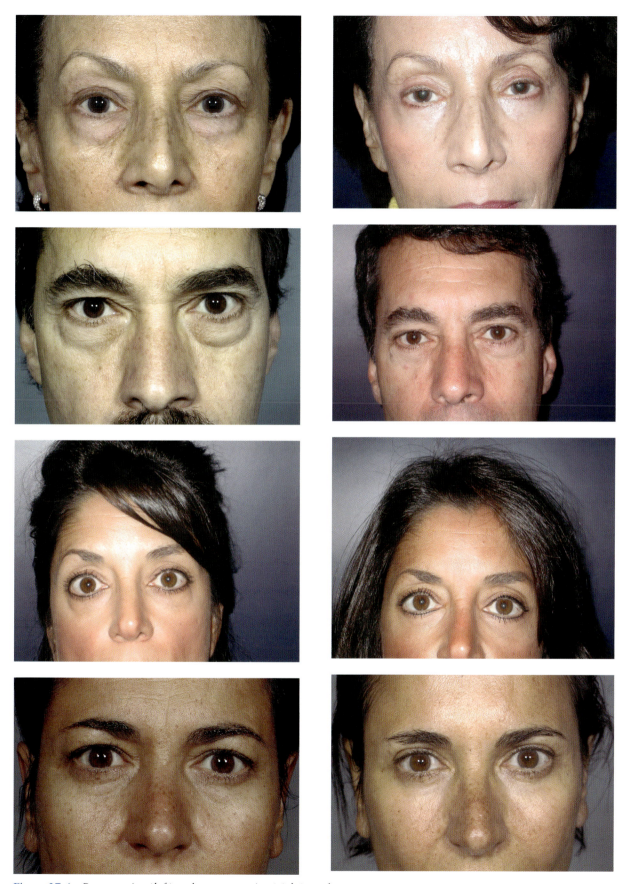

Figure 37-4 Preoperative (*left*) and post operative (*right*) results.

surgeons often fail to do so. When prescribing drops post-operatively, one must remember that topical steroids can raise intraocular pressure significantly. The best option is low concentrations (0.1%) of fluorinated preparations.

PEARLS

Rhytidectomy of the lower lid may be achieved without raising a cutaneous or myocutaneous flap. This can be done using a technique similar to that used at the beginning of the transcutaneous blepharoplasty with a wedge resection of the obicularis muscle near its raphe. In the transconjunctival approach, a cephalic traction suture on the conjunctiva allows for easy access to the postobicularis space. The lower fat pads can only be accessed after disinsertion of the lower lid retractors. Additionally, it is important to visualize the orbital septum to the orbital rim, and the inferior oblique muscle should be seen and preserved following incision of the septum. Using steroid-containing eyedrops can lessen postoperative chemosis.

SUGGESTED READING

Spinelli HM. *Atlas of Aesthetic and Periocular Surgery.* Philadelphia, PA: Elsevier; 2004.

Chapter 38. Subciliary Lower Lid Blepharoplasty

Christopher T. Chia, MD; Kimberly A. Swartz, BA;
Henry M. Spinelli, MD, FACS

INDICATIONS

The indications for the subciliary incision lower lid blepharoplasty (SLLB) include correction of dermatochalasis of the subciliary skin for aesthetic improvement of the periocular region, or in concert with fat resection or redistribution, canthal repositioning, or correction of other pathologic processes. This approach allows for resection of excess skin when indicated, as well as exposure of the underlying structures for other aesthetic and reconstructive techniques.

PREOPERATIVE PREPARATION

All patients undergo a complete history and physical examination with special consideration given to ophthalmologic conditions that may alter the surgical plan, such as prior surgery, dry eye, thyroid disease, blepharitis, and refractive corneal surgery. The lower lid position and vector, canthal support system, and integrity of the periocular adnexa need to be accurately determined in relation to the globe.

ANESTHESIA

Soft tissue injection of 1% lidocaine with epinephrine provides excellent analgesia and assists with hemostasis. This is often combined with conscious sedation or general anesthesia when performed alone or in conjunction with other procedures. Regional nerve blocks have been described as aiding postoperative analgesia.

POSITION AND MARKINGS

The patient is positioned with his or her head in a doughnut pillow supine in slight hyperextension with the head of the bed slightly raised. The lower eyelid incision is delineated by a line extending from the lateral canthus posteriorly in a natural skin fold 1 to 2 mm below the lash margin, anticipating leaving a cuff of pretarsal orbicularis.

DETAILS OF THE PROCEDURE

Following infiltration of the local anesthetic with vasoconstrictive agent, placement of corneal protectors and a standard prep and drape, the primary incision is made with a scalpel at the lateral extent of the surgical markings through the skin and orbicularis muscle. A Steven's scissor is inserted into the potential space just anterior to the orbital septum in the postorbicularis/preseptal plane. The scissor is opened gently from a lateral to medial direction to develop a space extending from the preseptal to pretarsal suborbicularis regions. One limb of a fine iris scissor is inserted into the incision with the other overlying the skin of the lower lid. The marginal aspect of the incision is made just below the lash line and extended to a point lateral to the medial punctum (Fig. 38-1). With skin hooks providing cephalic retraction and an assistant applying manual countertraction on the lower eyelid, a myocutaneous flap is elevated to the level of the orbital rim inferiorly. At this point, the orbital septum is easily visualized and incised to access the orbital fat pockets when resection, redistribution, or both are indicated (Figs. 38-2 and 38-3).

Once the fat pockets have been treated, the surgeon has the opportunity to correct any lower lid or midface issues, if appropriate. Redraping of the myocutaneous flap is done with a cephalic and lateral vector force running superiorly from the nasojugal groove through the lateral canthal area. Muscle is cut back at the edge of the flap to avoid bulging just below the lash line and a minimal amount of skin is removed (Fig. 38-4). At this point, an absorbable suspension suture to repair the orbicularis may be considered to reduce distraction forces on the lower lid closure. Skin closure is commonly done with running silk or nylon sutures to be removed in the early postoperative period (approximately 5 days) (Figs. 38-5 to 38-8).

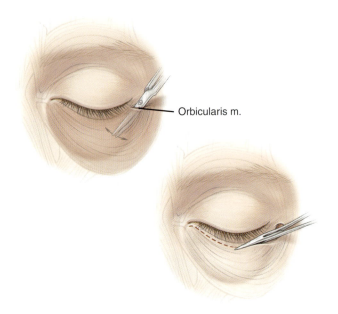

Orbicularis m.

Figure 38-1   The primary incision should be placed within a desired or potential fold. The preseptal postorbicularis plane may then be developed by gently pushing and spreading the small curved scissor. After the preseptal postorbicularis plane has been undermined, the scissors are inserted with one limb in the developed plane and the other on the skin surface beveled toward the eyeball. The secondary incision is made lateral to medial, ending just lateral to the lower-lid punctum. This is best done with inferior digital traction.

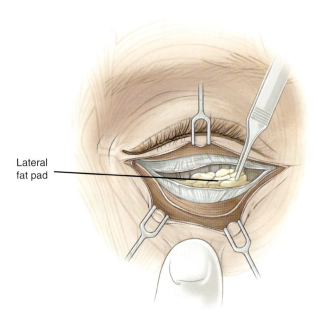

Lateral fat pad

Figure 38-2   The septum may be divided either with a wide transverse incision, or 3 separate (medial, central, and lateral) stab incisions.

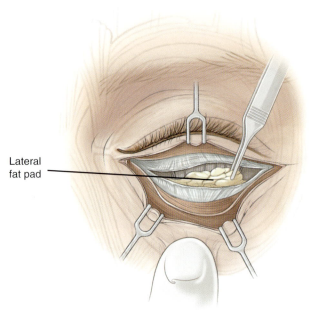

Lateral fat pad

Figure 38-3   The lateral fat pad is often underresected. Pressure on the upper lid causes the lateral orbital fat pad to bulge anteriorly, allowing for greater access and subsequent resection.

PITFALLS

- The orbicularis muscle (ie, orbicularis muscle at the lid margin) should be preserved when raising a skin muscle flap. Disruption of the muscular integrity may lead to unexpected alterations in the lower-lid/globe interface.

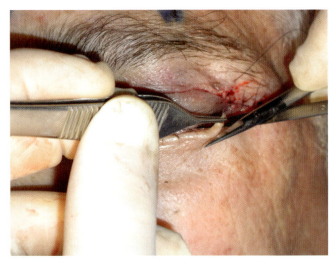

Figure 38-4   The myocutaneous lower lid flap is redraped with the muscle edge cut back to avoid bulging. A minimal amount of skin may be removed to provide tension-free apposition of the wound edges.

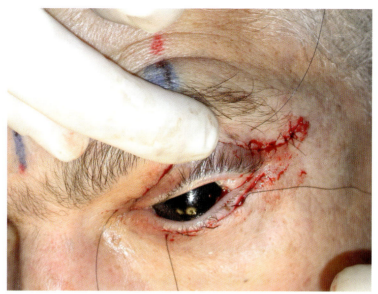

Figure 38-5 After hemostasis has been achieved, closure is completed with a running 6-0 silk for the transverse secondary incision, and an interrupted nylon for the lateral primary incision.

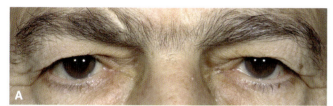
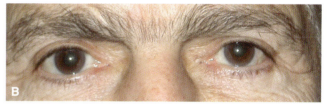

Figure 38-6 60 year-old man underwent upper blepharoplasty with upper lid approach browpexy and SLLB preoperatively **A.** and at one year postoperatively **B.**

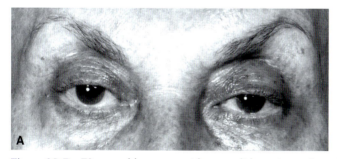
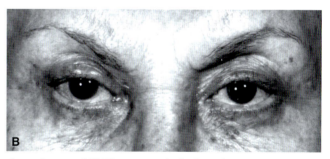

Figure 38-7 72 year-old woman with upper lid ptosis repair and blepharoplasty and SLLB preoperatively **A.** and at one year postoperatively **B.**

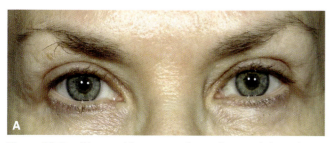
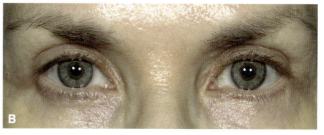

Figure 38-8 47 year-old woman who underwent bilateral SLLB preoperatively **A.** and at one year postoperatively **B.**

- Avoid overzealous resection of the medial and nasal orbital fat pads leading to a concave appearance and consider fat redistribution techniques in higher-risk patients. Conversely, the lateral orbital fat pad should be adequately addressed, as it is a frequently undertreated area, especially with the patient in the supine position.
- Orbicularis muscle suspension through the transcutaneous access route is the simplest but least effective method of increasing lower lid support.

PEARLS

- During myocutaneous flap elevation, superior lid traction applied by a small hook, preferably on the conjunctival side of the lower eyelid, with countertraction with a Desmarres retractor, provides excellent visualization.

- The key anatomic plane in any of the techniques for lower lid blepharoplasty is the preseptal postorbicularis space.
- Assessment of how much skin to resect from the flap edge is helped by having a cooperative patient look up and open his or her mouth to mimic naturally occurring increases in tension at the incision.
- Before closure, it is sometimes helpful to resect a few millimeters of orbicularis muscle at the superior aspect of the flap to avoid bulging just below the lash line postoperatively; this does not alter lid function.

SUGGESTED READING

Spinelli HM. Lower lid blepharoplasty. *Atlas of Aesthetic and Periocular Surgery*. Philadelphia, PA: Elsevier; 2004: 72-79.

Chapter 39. Canthal Fixation

Kimberly A. Swartz, BA; Martin I. Newman, MD, FACS;
Henry M. Spinelli, MD, FACS

INDICATIONS

There are many manifestations of a malpositioned eyelid, including ectropion, entropion, and retraction. The etiology of these conditions is often the attenuation of canthal tendons, evident in the descent of the lateral canthal tendon from the 10- to 15-degree incline, compared to the medial canthal tendon, seen in young patients, to a coplanar, or inferior position. The two most effective treatments for lax lateral canthal tendons are canthopexy, suitably for the young patient without extensive lid laxity, and canthoplasty, a more powerful treatment suitable for older patients who present with lid laxity, apparent on a snap back or pinch test.

PREOPERATIVE PREPARATION

In consultation, it is important to note any prior oculoplastic surgery. A history of cosmetic surgery can indicate cicatricial eyelid malposition, which may be accompanied by a deficiency in anterior lamella. In this case, a canthopexy or canthoplasty alone will not suffice, and a mid-cheek suspension, free skin graft, or transpositional graft may also be required for full correction.

ANESTHESIA

Monitored anesthesia care (MAC) or general anesthesia can be used for this procedure.

POSITION AND MARKINGS

Preoperatively, the desired position of the canthus is delineated in 3 planes: cephalic-caudal, anterior-posterior, and medial-lateral. Locations are all important, and when only one side is to be addressed, the contralateral side can serve as a guide.

Incision and Exposure

Local anesthetic with epinephrine should be infiltrated using a 27- to 30-gauge needle along the lower lid, and the planned incision. Next, a protective lens may or may not be put in place, depending on the surgeon's preference. The incision is then made using a no. 15 blade,

either along a lateral canthotomy incision or along an upper lid incision, which is often used in the case of concurrent procedures. At this point, division of the inferior crus of the lateral canthal tendon should be carried out to prepare it for lysis.

DETAILS OF THE PROCEDURE

Following severing of the inferior crus of the lateral canthal tendon, the lower lid then must be completely mobilized (Figs. 39-1 and 39-2). This is accomplished by lysing the lateral retinacular structures, including the lower lid retractors and the orbital septum. Once this has been done, a tarsal strip is created by circumferentially deepithelializing a lateral segment of the lower eyelid, which is backcut below the tarsal plate, ultimately isolating approximately 3 mm of distal tarsal plate. This tarsal strip should then be engaged with a double-armed, braided, nonabsorbable suture.

Meanwhile, the orbital rim periosteum is incised and then elevated from anterior to posterior within the orbital rim at Whitnall's tubercle, not dividing or raising any flaps. The tarsal strip is sutured to the internal orbital rim

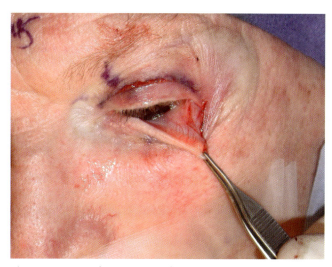

Figure 39-1 At this point, canthotomy and cantholysis are complete, as evidenced by the mobility of the lower lid.

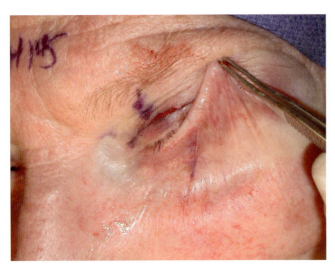

Figure 39-2   The full mobilization of the lower lid is evidenced by the ability to elevate it to the brow.

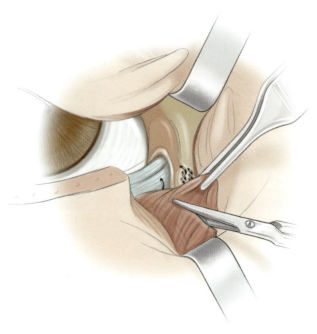

Figure 39-4   Excess muscle is resected and then the remaining muscle is fixed with absorbable sutures laterally and cephalad.

periosteum using the double-armed suture described above (Fig. 39-3). The new lower lid position should lie 1.5 to 2 mm above the lower limbus. Overelevation of the tendon will reduce the vertical visual axis, interfering with downward gaze.

If suturing the tarsal strip to the periosteum is not possible, other methods for fixation include bony fixation using devices such as the Mitek system (DePuy Mitek,

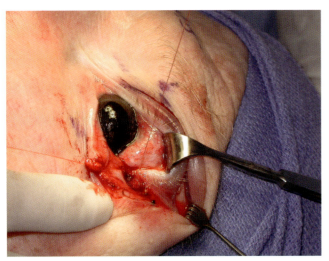

Figure 39-3   The denuded tarsal strip is engaged with a double-armed suture and fixed to the internal orbital rim periosteal flap.

Raynham, MA) or by creating a drill hole, passing both arms of the suture through the drill hole, and anchoring the tendons to the adjacent fascia. When sufficient bone is not present where appropriate fixation should occur, fixation via miniplates is an option. The lateral horn of the levator should be identified at this point because its accidental entrapment during suspension will result in upper lid retraction or lagophthalmos.

Once the tendon has been satisfactorily fixed, the lateral commissure should be refined. This includes trimming excess skin and/or obicularis muscle (Fig. 39-4), and aligning analogous structures of the upper and lower lid, such as lashes. It should be noted that skin conservation should be the goal, as secondary skin trim is always an option.

In younger patients, when it is not necessary to lyse the lateral canthal tendon, the tendon can simply be plicated, as seen in Figure 39-5, effectively shortening the length of the tendon. It is important to note that this procedure does not shorten the actual lid length at all; thus, it is not suitable in patients with lid laxity.

Both of these procedures, canthoplasty and canthopexy, can be performed on the inferior crus of the lateral canthal tendon, as described, or on the common canthal

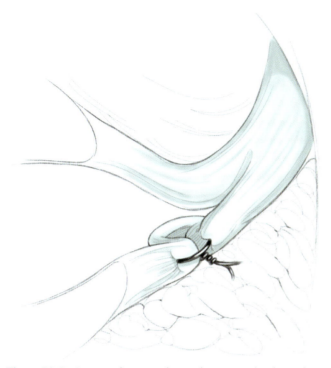

Figure 39-5 In a canthopexy, the tendon is simply plicated, and no resection is made. This operation is best suited for younger patients with minimum lid laxity.

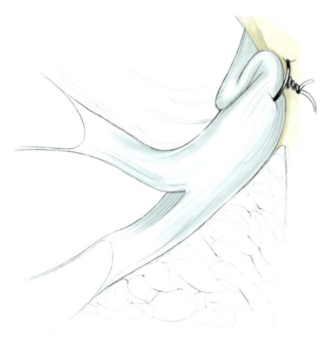

Figure 39-6 A common canthoplasty is a powerful tool for addressing the lower and upper lateral canthal tendons simultaneously.

tendon, shown in Figure 39-6. This latter procedure is most easily completed through an upper lid incision.

Closure

After the lateral canthal tendon has been fixed to either the periosteum or bone, as described above, the incisions should be close in accordance with standard closure of either a lateral canthotomy or upper lid incision. The preferred closure is 3 or 4 interrupted 6-0 nylon sutures.

PITFALLS

It is important to remember that moderate to severe lid laxity can only be corrected through lysis of the canthal tendon. Lower lid shortening procedures are not advocated because they ultimately decrease the intra-commissure distance, which is already decreased as a result of the attenuation of the canthal tendons. Furthermore, shortening produces additional inferomedial displacement of the lateral canthal complex. Identifying the pathophysiology of lower lid malposition is essential to creating a properly positioned lid, because different

etiologies require different considerations, that is, cicatricial origins and lamella deficiency (Fig. 39-7).

PEARLS

A fully mobilized lower lid can be identified by its ability to reach brow upon upward traction. Only once this has been done can optimal positioning of the lateral canthal tendon be achieved. These procedures can be used in conjunction with others, such as spacer grafts, palatal or synthetic, to correct more severe defects such as scleral show secondary to facial paralysis.

The place of fixation should be altered for patients with deep set or prominent eyes, to avoid changing the size of the lateral scleral triangle, which has the effect of producing "squinty" or narrow eyes. For patients with deep-set eyes (exophthalmometer measurements 15 mm or less), the point of fixation should be lowered. For patients with prominent eyes (exophthalmometer measurements 18 mm or greater), the point of fixation should be raised. Patients with prominent eyes may also require spacer grafts for optimal lower lid placement and support.

PREOPERATIVE AND POSTOPERATIVE PHOTOGRAPHS

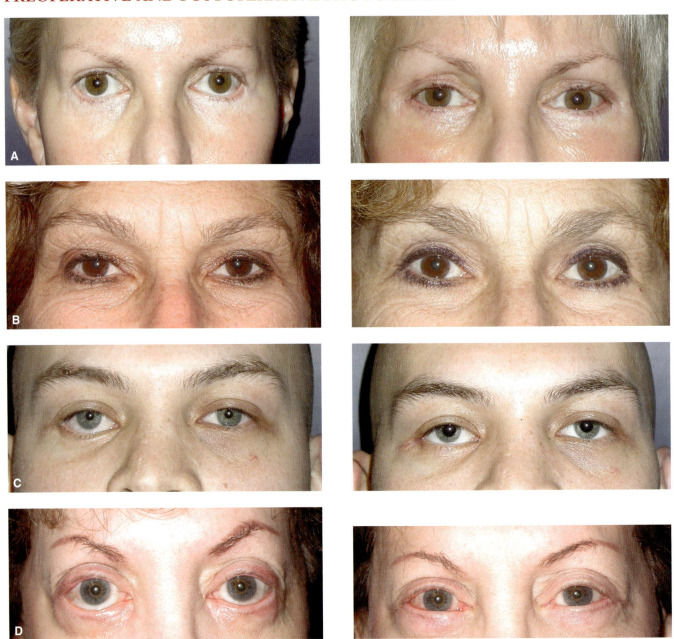

Figure 39-7   LEFT Preop and RIGHT Postop. **A.** 48 year old female 2 years status post upper and lower eyelid lid blepharoplasty elsewhere. Postop: Two years status post canthoplasty with bony fixation and palatal graft. **B.** 61 year old female with bilateral lower eyelid laxity. Postop: One year status post bilateral upper and lower eyelid blepharoplasty and lateral canthoplasty. **C.** 26 year old male status post right zygoma fracture treated elsewhere. Postop: One year status post right lateral cathoplasty. **D.** 86 year old female with orbital Grave's Disease and proptosis. Postop: Eighteen months status post palatal grafting and bilateral canthoplasty.

SUGGESTED READING

Bartsich S, Swartz KA, Spinelli HM. Lateral canthoplasty using the Mitek anchor system. *Aesthetic Plast Surg.* 2012; 36(1):3-7.

McCord CD, Boswell CB, Hester TR. Lateral canthal anchoring. *Plast Reconstr Surg.* 2003;112(1):222-237.

Spinelli HM. *Atlas of Aesthetic and Periocular Surgery.* Philadelphia, PA: Elsevier; 2004.

Spinelli HM, Tabatabai N, Nunn DR. Correction of involutional entropion with suborbicularis septal and lateral canthal tightening. *Plast Reconstr Surg.* 2006;117(5):1560-1567.

Chapter 40. Forehead Rejuvenation

Renato Saltz, MD, FACS; Omid Adibnazari, BS; Alyssa Lolofie, BS

INDICATIONS

Brow aesthetics cannot be generalized because of a changing of the ideal shape and position of the brow. Although the brow should be evaluated based on gender, ethnicity, orbital shape, and overall facial aging and proportions, the main factor to consider is the ratio of the visible eyelid to the palpebral fold. The best candidates for forehead rejuvenation are patients with eyebrow ptosis, asymmetry, temporal hooding and forehead wrinkles. Usually they also have short, flat foreheads and nonreceding hairlines (Fig. 40-1).

PREOPERATIVE PREPARATION

Assessment of the patient includes evaluation of both the medial and lateral brow position, the ratio from brow to upper eyelid, glabella and forehead lines, forehead shape and height, and the hairline. To assess the strength of the muscle action, movement, and depth of soft-tissue folds the patient should be asked to frown as well as to raise the eyebrows. The eyebrows should also be assessed for the thickness, shape, and position. In preoperative consultation the doctor should advise as to the number of incisions and type of fixations. Based upon the patient assessment, the operation can be planned. Patient inclusion is important in that brow lifts are individualized (Fig. 40-2).

The endoscopic technique is based upon the use of modern technology where the traditional eye-hand surgical coordination is done through a video-endoscopic system. Additional extensive training is necessary not only for the surgeon but all medical and nursing personnel involved in the surgical case. (Note from author: The novice should take his or her first assistant to cadaver workshops/courses to learn together.) The equipment, from endoscope to camera and monitors, are usually standard in centers where aesthetic surgeries are performed. It has become important to test each system, inspect each instrument and check for a backup system as a safeguard. The surgeon must have knowledge of the principles extending from training, mechanical equipment, and technical skills.

POSITION AND MARKINGS

In preparation for the procedure, the patient is marked from a standing position to utilize the natural positioning of the brows. Markings are made on both sides of the face outlining the temporal ridge, sentinel veins, and the

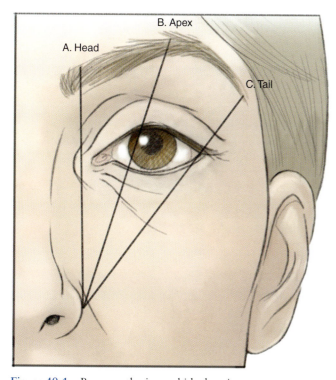

Figure 40-1 Brow aesthetics and ideal patients.

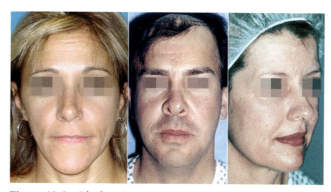

Figure 40-2 Ideal patient picture.

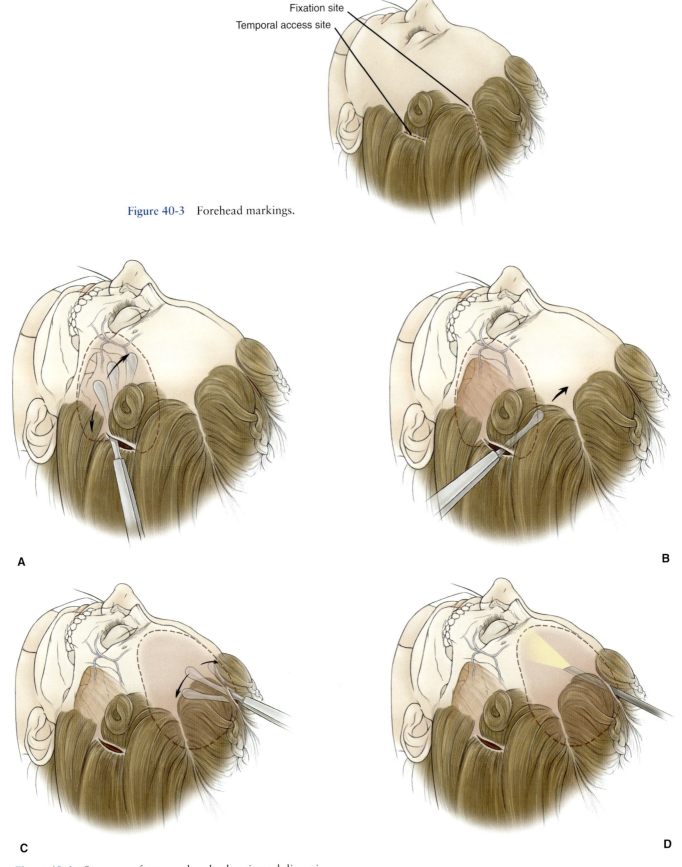

Figure 40-3 Forehead markings.

A

B

C

D

Figure 40-4 Sequence of temporal and subperiosteal dissections.

assumed position of supratrochlear and supraorbital nerve branches. If the sentinel vein cannot be found from an upright position, patients are asked to lie flat. Patients are then asked to clench their teeth, and with palpation, the temporalis muscle and temporal crest can be marked. Markings representing the incisions are made 1 to 2 cm beyond the temporal hairline, checking that the incisions will be over the temporalis muscle. The lateral incision markings should be parallel to the brow while the paramedian incision is radial along the midline of the face, forehead, and skull.

The 2 brow lift vectors are marked. They are determined by lifting the brow manually to the chosen aesthetic position. The lateral vector includes the tail of the brow while the medial vector includes the arch of the brow; both use the lateral canthus, mouth, and ala to determine placement. Before infiltration, the hair is cleansed and braided or stapled to either side of the chosen incision sites. This keeps the hair neatly away from the incision sites (Fig. 40-3).

ANESTHESIA

The most common approach for the patient is general anesthesia with an endotracheal tube that is attached with dental floss to the teeth. Infiltrate the site using a 20-gauge spinal needle in a tumescent fashion with a solution of 2% lidocaine, 20 mL of 0.25% Marcaine, and 1 mL of epinephrine in 140 mL of normal saline. The patient should then be prepped and draped in a standard sterile manner.

SURGICAL TECHNIQUE

Dissection

The procedure may begin after 20 minutes from infiltration to increase vascular constriction. An incision is made from the scalp to the temporal fascia; this allows visualization and dissection to remain on top of the deep temporal fascia. Dissection is carried down to the fusion ligament by preserving the sentinel veins if possible. Dissection is then turned medially by dividing the temporal crest with a periosteal elevator and continuing the dissection in a subperiosteal plane. At this point the dissection continues from the paramedian incisions communicating both pockets (deep temporal fascia with subperiosteal plane). A 4-mm 30-degree endoscope is once again calibrated with adequate focus, "white out," irrigation system down and inserted in the surgical field. The room lights are dimmed down to improve visualization on the screen (Fig. 40-4).

With the endoscope at the temporal incision, the sentinel veins are found and preserved when possible while the surrounding adhesions are removed. Following the caudal aspect of the temporal crest the "fusion ligament" (junction of deep temporal fascia and periosteum) is identified and divided with the endoscopic scissors. The supraorbital rim periosteum is divided from lateral to medial while identifying and preserving the

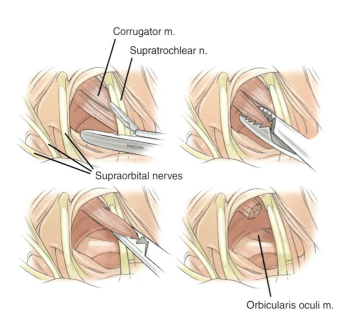

Figure 40-5 Corrugator resection.

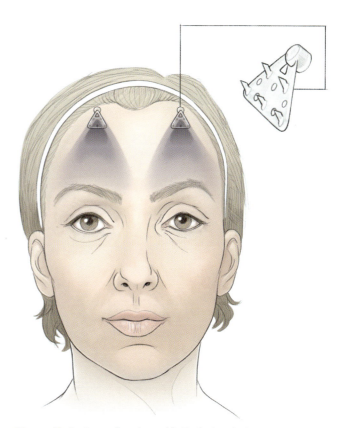

Figure 40-6 Brow fixation with Endotine device.

supraorbital neurovascular bundle. The periosteum is then divided from each lateral orbital rim, which serves to allow more lateral brow elevation and provide access to the glabellar musculature. An island of periosteum is preserved at the midline to avoid elevation of the most medial brow. The corrugator muscles are identified and excised/avulsed using endoscopic graspers. The assistant "pushes" the external skin to help with the corrugator resection and to allow the surgeon to visualize the dermis and avoid overresection, causing an external depression (Fig. 40-5). In case a depression is identified during the procedure, immediate fat grafting is recommended. The completion of the procedure can be tested by moving the brow up and down, which should be mobile at this point.

Fixation

The temporal fixations are accomplished using 3 interrupted sutures connecting the superficial temporal fascia and the deep temporal fascia using 3-0 Mersilene sutures. The excess skin is removed and the wound is closed with 4-0 plain gut. The paramedian fixation is accomplished with the Endotine device. The Endotine device is safely fixated to the outer table with a measured drill hole. The device is then securely inserted followed by digital pressure to hold the periosteum and galea in place. The patient is then assessed in a sitting position while still under general anesthesia. Measurements include pupil-to-brow and lateral canthus-to-tail of brow. The hair is washed and the patient is moved to the recovery room. No dressings are applied (Fig. 40-6).

Complications

Temporary paraesthesia and irregularities of the frontalis muscle will occur occasionally. However, it usually improves within 3 weeks. Cosmetic problems such as uneven movement of the brows, surface deformities, and elevation of the arch of the brows can sometimes arise. The "surprised look" can be avoided by keeping a bridge of periosteum undivided at the midline and by avoiding over elevation of the middle third of the brow. Alopecia can be eliminated through the abandonment of percutaneous screw fixations. Early detection of postoperative brow asymmetry (within 24 to 48 hours) can be improved by repositioning the paramedian fixation through reelevation and posterior displacement of galea/skin from the Endotine. Delayed temporary brow asymmetry can be improved with Botox. If the brow asymmetry persists and there is obvious recurrence of brow ptosis, reintervention is advised.

SUGGESTED READING

Nahai F, Saltz R, eds. *Endoscopic Plastic Surgery*. 2nd ed. St. Louis, MO: Quality Medical Publishing, Inc.; 2008.

Saltz R, Codner MA. Endoscopic brow lift. In: *Techniques in Aesthetic Plastic Surgery*. Philadelphia: Saunders Elsevier; 2009:133–142.

Chapter 41. Limited Incision, Nonendoscopic Foreheadplasty

David M. Knize, MD

INDICATIONS

This limited incision foreheadplasty procedure is appropriate for any patient at any age that has ptotic eyebrows and skin line formation of the forehead and glabellar areas produced by underlying muscle hypertonicity. It is particularly indicated for the patient who has frontal scalp baldness yet has adequate temporal scalp hair to conceal incision scars.

PREOPERATIVE PREPARATION

With the patient looking into a mirror, elevate each eyebrow to the planned postoperative level and confirm that the eyebrow position and shape are consistent with the patient's expectations. Evaluate the patient's general medical status for undergoing surgery.

ANESTHESIA

This procedure can be done under conscious sedation or general anesthesia, either of which should be administered by an anesthesia provider.

POSITION AND MARKINGS

With the patient positioned supine, prep the face and scalp and apply a head drape. Mark the palpable superior temporal line of the skull (STL) on the forehead skin as a future reference point for several deeper structures (Fig. 41-1). Visualize the 6-mm wide zone of soft-tissue adhesion to frontal bone medial to the STL that requires complete release. Mark the approximate course of the deep division of the supraorbital nerve on the forehead skin. This nerve runs over periosteum between 0.5 and 1.5 cm medial to and parallel with the STL to supply

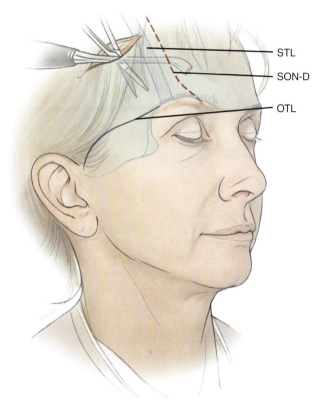

Figure 41-1 Soft-tissue release. The subperiosteal elevation extends across the frontal bone almost down to the level of the superior orbital rims. The temporal fossa dissection between the superficial and deep temporal fascial planes extends through the orbicularis-temporal ligament (OTL) down to the zygomatic arch level. The superior temporal line of the skull (STL) and the usual course of the deep division of the supraorbital nerve (SON-D) are labeled. Note the zone of soft-tissue adhesion to bone medial to the STL (*slant lines*) that must be completely released to adequately transpose a forehead flap.

181

sensation to the parietal scalp. Mark the suspension vector that will elevate the lateral eyebrow to the desired level, which is determined by elevating the lateral eyebrow using 1 finger. This vector line usually falls along the lateral side of the STL. At approximately 2 cm superior to the frontal hairline mark a 4-cm long line perpendicular the vector line, which will be the future temporal incision location on each side. The medial end of the incision should extend just over the STL; however, limit the extension to 0.5 cm medial to the STL to avoid transection of the deep division of the supraorbital nerve. No marking for medial eyebrow elevation is required, because elevation of the medial eyebrow is infrequently indicated. However, medial eyebrow elevation can be adequately obtained later, if necessary, by weakening the medial eyebrow depressor muscles. Finally, mark the area of excess eyelid skin in the usual manner for upper blepharoplasty, and then determine how much of this excess skin will be resuspended with the eyebrow elevation and mark that area for skin preservation.

DETAILS OF THE PROCEDURE

Infiltrate the forehead and temporal fossa areas with approximately 75 to 100 mL of 0.25% lidocaine with 1:400,000 epinephrine solution. The bilateral temporal scalp incisions are made as parallel to the axis of the hair shafts as possible to avoid injury to hair follicles. Initially, dissect between the superficial and deep temporal fascial planes (see Fig. 41-1) to the STL medially and to the orbicularis-temporal ligament inferiorly. This ligament is a 6- to 8-mm wide transverse band of adhesion between the superficial and deep temporal fascial planes that runs from the lateral margin of the superior orbital rim laterally toward the ear. Stop dissection at this ligament for now, because immediately inferior to it runs the superiormost ramus of the temporal branch of the facial nerve and further dissection through the ligament and on to the zygomatic arch requires different technique. This is a convenient time to remove a 2 × 2-cm area of deep temporal fascia just inferior to the scalp incisions to expose underlying temporalis muscle there. Next, free the 6-mm wide zone of soft-tissue adhesion along the medial side of the STL with a periosteal elevator and raise the periosteum over the frontal bone from both temporal scalp incisions. Initially, limit the inferior level of this elevation to 2 cm above the superior orbital rims to avoid injuring the deep division of the supraorbital nerve. Before dissecting further, locate this nerve and preserve it. This requires wearing a headlight and using a retractor in the scalp wound for exposure to make a vertical incision on the undersurface of the raised periosteum. This incision begins approx-

imately 4 cm above the superior orbital rim level along the approximate course of the deep division of the supraorbital nerve that was marked on the forehead skin earlier. Use gentle blunt dissection within the galeal fat superficial to the periosteum to find the nerve that usually runs with one smaller branch. Simply follow the nerve down to its bony exit point by progressively incising periosteum inferiorly to expose it. In 90% of patients, the bony exit point is the supraorbital notch where the deep branch divides from the supraorbital nerve trunk; however, this branch can exit bone up to 1.5 cm above the superior orbital rim anywhere over the lower frontal bone. When there is an atypical exit point, it will usually be just medial to the STL. With this nerve branch protected, continue elevating periosteum more inferiorly on the frontal bone and incise the periosteum horizontally at a level about 1 cm above and completely across the superior orbital rim on each side (Fig. 41-2). Then release the periosteal attachments along the lateral orbital rim.

Direct attention back to the temporal fossa area where earlier dissection stopped at the orbicularis-temporal ligament. Use careful blunt dissection to separate the fused superficial and deep temporal fascial planes that form this ligament, because the 6 to 8 rami that compose the temporal branch of the facial nerve run only 3 to 4 mm inferior to and parallel with this ligament. These rami pass within the superficial temporal fascia that forms the roof of the space created by this dissection as it extends down to the level of the zygomatic arch. Avoid any vertical spreading action of the dissection scissors, which could produce a traction injury to these rami. Finally, search with the index finger along the superior and lateral orbital rims for any bands of residual attachment to bone to ensure that the soft-tissue release is complete.

Adequate forehead flap release allows flap transposition with relatively little resistance. Transpose the flap cephalad until the lateral eyebrow is elevated to the desired level, which usually requires advancement of the leading edge of the flap between 2.0 and 2.5 cm above the scalp incision level. Through the incision, undermine scalp posterior to that level to expose underlying deep temporal fascia. At the level of forehead flap advancement, anchor the edge of the superficial temporal fascia lining the advanced flap to the deep temporal fascia (see Fig. 41-2) and leave a small suction drain tube under the forehead flap. At this point, the lateral eyebrow should be at the desired level of elevation. If it is not, repeat the flap anchoring process. The redundant scalp that now remains at the posterior side of the scalp incision can be trimmed, or it can simply be turned into a slight roll and the wound edges reapproximated with a running 4-0 nylon suture.

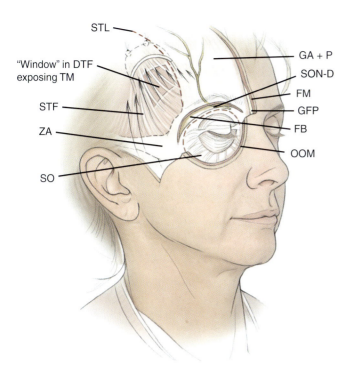

Figure 41-2 Suspension vectors. The superficial temporal fascia (STF) lining the advanced forehead flap is fixed with absorbable sutures to the deep temporal fascia (DTF) at a level that will suspend the lateral eyebrow as desired. The STF plane will form a scar bond with the temporalis muscle (TM) exposed through the resected area of DTF, which acts as an autologous anchor for lateral eyebrow segment position. The periosteum (P) lining that part of the advanced forehead flap medial to the superior temporal line of the skull (STL) will rebond to the underlying frontal bone and support the medial eyebrow segment to act as another autologous anchoring mechanism. The galea aponeurosis (GA) and P move cephalad with the transposed STF. Because the frontalis muscle (FM) takes origin from the GA, it moves cephalad with GA, which elevates the medial eyebrow through the attachments between the inferior margin of FM and the superior orbicularis oculi muscle (OOM), which is not shown here. Labeled are zygomatic arch (ZA), septum orbitale (SO), deep division of the supraorbital nerve (SON-D), and the galea fat pad (GFP).

Begin the upper blepharoplasty portion of the procedure by removing the area of upper eyelid skin marked for excision earlier. Incise the orbicularis oculi muscle horizontally across the eyelid approximately 2 mm superior to the inferior margin of the eyelid skin excision area. Do not excise muscle. Dissect cephalad between the orbicularis oculi muscle and the septum orbitale until the superior orbital rim is reached. Continue dissection over the superior orbital rim by transecting the galeal and periosteal attachments there. Retract the edges of

this opening and find the transverse head of the corrugator supercilii muscle. If this muscle is not immediately visible, find it adhered to the undersurface of the orbicularis oculi muscle. Cauterize the supraorbital vein to avoid unnecessary bleeding later. Transect the lateral end of the transverse head of the corrugator supercilii muscle, leaving a 1- to 2-mm stump. Resect the lateral one-half to two-thirds of this muscle (Fig. 41-3), leaving the

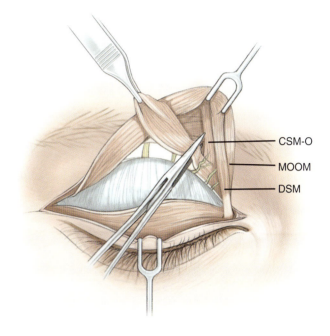

Figure 41-3 Transblepharoplasty glabellar muscle modification. The muscles that depress the medial eyebrow and that produce glabellar skin lines can be accessed through the upper blepharoplasty incision. Resection of the lateral half of the transverse head of the corrugator supercilii muscle is shown. The remainder of this muscle, along with the oblique head of the corrugator supercilii muscle (CSM-O) and the depressor supercilii muscle (DSM) will be carefully avulsed from around the supratrochlear nerve branches. A myotomy of the medial head of the orbicularis oculi muscle (MOOM) will also be done to further weaken this group of glabellar muscles that act to depress the medial eyebrow segment by antagonizing the frontalis muscle action that elevates the medial eyebrow. The procerus muscle (not shown) can be transected from the medial end of the blepharoplasty incision to further elevate the medial eyebrow by weakening this additional antagonist to frontalis action. The trunk of the supraorbital nerve is shown under the elevated lateral segment of the transverse head of the corrugator supercilii muscle. (Modified, with permission, from Knize DM. Limited incision foreheadplasty. In: Knize DM, ed. *Forehead and Temporal Fossa: Anatomy and Technique.* Philadelphia: Lippincott Williams & Wilkins; 2001:120.)

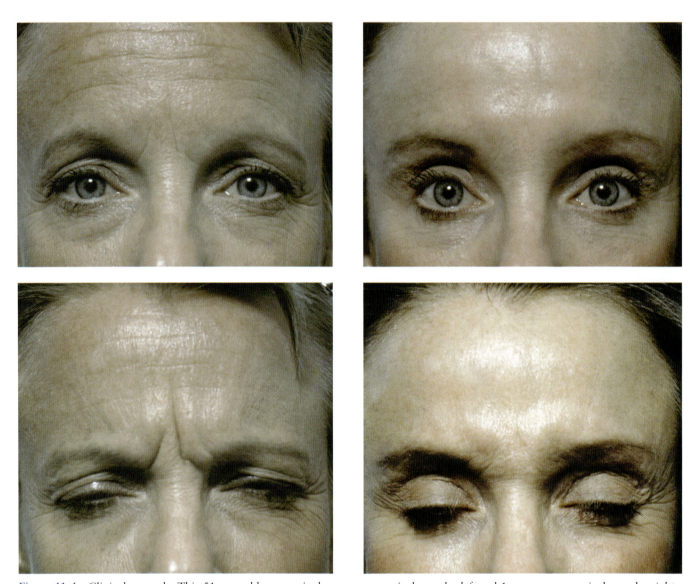

Figure 41-4 Clinical example. This 51-year-old woman is shown preoperatively on the *left* and 1 year postoperatively on the *right*. Her face is in the rest position above and frown position below. Note the smoothness of the forehead skin and her inability to form glabellar skin lines postoperatively. She had a concomitant lower blepharoplasty. (Reproduced, with permission, from Knize DM. Limited incision foreheadplasty. In: Knize DM, ed. *Forehead and Temporal Fossa: Anatomy and Technique*. Philadelphia: Lippincott Williams & Wilkins; 2001:127.)

branches of the supratrochlear nerve that run within the medial third portion. With a small hemostat, carefully avulse the muscle fibers of this medial portion from around the supratrochlear nerve branches. Similarly, avulse the rest of the muscle tissue on the superior-medial orbital rim. This avulsion process removes not only the medial portion of the transverse head of the corrugator supercilii but also that muscle's oblique head and the overlapping depressor supercilii muscle. Then remove a 1 × 1-cm section from the medial fibers of the orbicularis oculi muscle that is directly under the medial end of the

eyebrow. The effect of resecting these glabellar muscles ablates much of the medial eyebrow depressor action that produces vertical and oblique glabellar skin lines. Furthermore, these muscles antagonize frontalis muscle action, and the now unopposed frontalis muscle tone raises the medial eyebrows approximately 2 mm, which is usually all that is necessary. However, if the patient's medial eyebrows are particularly low or if deep transverse skin lines are present over the proximal nose, also transect the procerus muscle with a scissors from the medial end of the blepharoplasty wound. Weakening

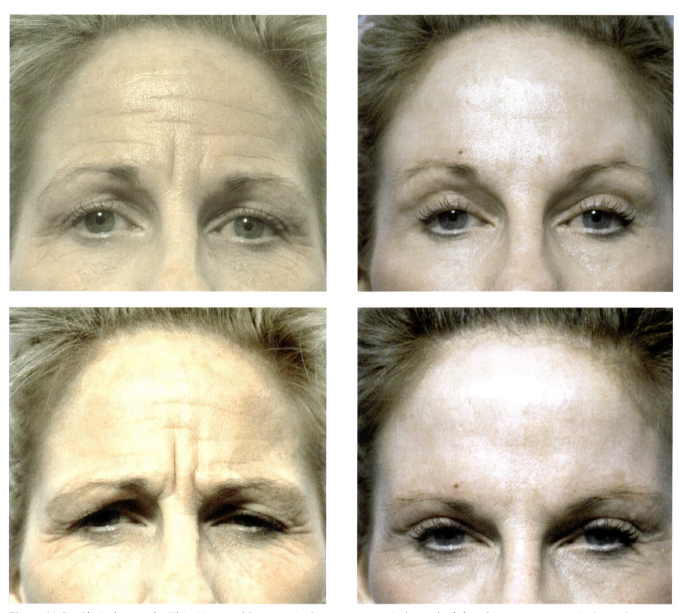

Figure 41-5 Clinical example. This 44-year-old woman is shown preoperatively on the *left* and 1 year postoperatively on the *right*. Her face is in the rest position above and frown position below. Note the smoothness of the forehead skin and her inability to form glabellar skin lines postoperatively. She had a concomitant lower blepharoplasty. (Reproduced, with permission, from Knize DM. Limited incision foreheadplasty. In: Knize DM, ed. *Forehead and Temporal Fossa: Anatomy and Technique*. Philadelphia: Lippincott Williams & Wilkins; 2001:128.)

procerus muscle antagonism of frontalis muscle action generally provides an additional 2 mm of medial eyebrow elevation from unopposed frontalis muscle tone. It is advisable to place a 1 × 1-cm fascial graft (made from the deep temporal fascia removed earlier) over the cut edges of the procerus muscle to prevent an overlying skin depression. It is unnecessary to place any graft material in the area of the other resected glabellar muscles because the surrounding glabellar fat pad in that area fills the void. Close the upper blepharoplasty wound to complete the procedure. (Figs. 41-4 and 41-5 show clinical results of this procedure.)

PITFALLS

Each patient can expect transient sensory loss over the forehead and parietal scalp for 3 to 6 weeks. Transient frontal palsy occurs in approximately 7% of cases, and the patient must be reassured that this function generally returns within 4 weeks.

PEARLS

- Importance of complete release of the forehead flap from bone cannot be overemphasized. Inadequate release will risk later loss of lateral eyebrow elevation.
- The ideal needle and suture for fixation of the advanced forehead flap is a G2 tapered needle on 2-0 polyglactic acid suture, although permanent suture material can be used if preferred.
- Leaving the redundant scalp on the advanced edge of the forehead flap and simply rolling this redundancy into a small tube before approximating the wound edges will result in minimal scars and minimal or no hair loss.

SUGGESTED READING

Knize, DM. Limited incision forehead lift for eyebrow elevation to enhance upper blepharoplasty. *Plast Reconstr Surg.* 1996;97:1334.

Knize DM. Limited incision foreheadplasty. In: Knize DM, ed. *Forehead and Temporal Fossa: Anatomy and Technique.* Philadelphia, PA: Lippincott Williams & Wilkins; 2001: 101-132.

Knize DM. Muscles that act on glabellar skin: a closer look. *Plast Reconstr Surg.* 2000;105:350.

Knize DM. Transpalpebral approach to the corrugator supercilii and procerus muscles. *Plast Reconstr Surg.* 1995;95:52.

Chapter 42. Chemodenervation

Douglas M. Sidle, MD, FACS

INDICATIONS

Injection of botulinum toxin type A is the most common cosmetic procedure performed in the United States. Although Botox (Allergan, Irvine, CA) Xeomin, San Mateo, CA and Dysport (Medicis, Scottsdale, AZ) have FDA approval for cosmetic use in the glabellar lines, it is common practice to use these drugs to inhibit muscle contraction all over the head and neck (Fig. 42-1). Off-label cosmetic indications for the use of botulinum toxin type A include horizontal forehead lines, "crow's feet," "bunny lines" on the nose, platysmal bands, and lines the perioral area. Certainly, the most common areas treated with Botox are the glabellar lines, "crow's feet," and horizontal forehead lines (Fig. 42-2).

PREOPERATIVE PREPARATION

Botox is supplied in a vial containing 100 U of a vacuum-dried neurotoxin complex. Manufacturer prescribing information recommends reconstitution with 2.5 mL of 0.9% nonpreserved saline, but many treating physicians use different dilutions, ranging from 2.5 to 4.0 mL per vial. Furthermore, preserved saline can be used. Once reconstituted, product efficacy has been shown to last up to 6 weeks if stored at 4°C (39.2°F). Other than standard precautions, no special handling precautions are necessary. Likewise, Dysport is supplied in a vial containing 300 U of neurotoxin complex. It is reconstituted in a similar fashion.

ANESTHESIA

Experienced injectors and patients who have had botulinum injections before may opt to have no anesthesia used during the procedure. However, a more pleasant experience can be offered with the use of a topical anesthetic, particularly in patients sensitive to needles. Topical

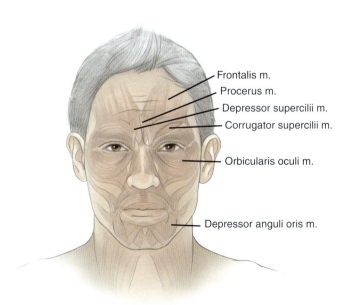

Figure 42-1 Muscles of facial expression that are commonly treated with injectable neurotoxins.

Frontalis m.
Procerus m.
Depressor supercilii m.
Corrugator supercilii m.
Orbicularis oculi m.
Depressor anguli oris m.

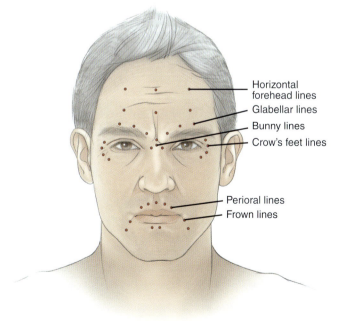

Figure 42-2 Basic injection strategy.

Horizontal forehead lines
Glabellar lines
Bunny lines
Crow's feet lines
Perioral lines
Frown lines

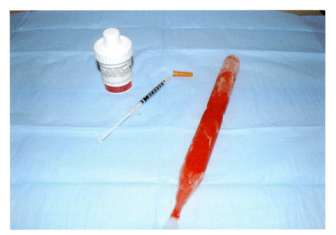

Figure 42-3 Topical anesthetic and ice can be used to improve patient comfort.

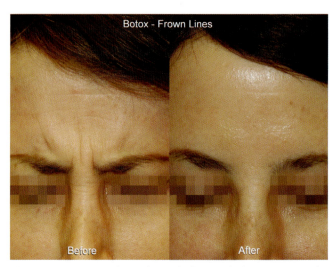

Figure 42-4 Frown lines shawn before and after injection of Botox cosmetic.

anesthetic techniques can be as simple as using EMLA (lidocaine 2.5% and prilocaine 2.5%; AstraZeneca, Wilmington, DE) applied for a minimum of 10 minutes prior to the procedure. In our practice we use BLT, a specially compounded cream of 20% benzocaine, 6% lidocaine, and 4% tetracaine. Likewise, ice applied to treatment areas prior to injection can result in reasonable hypesthesia, while reducing the risks of bleeding and ecchymosis. We use frozen popsicles that can be obtained from any grocer (Fig. 42-3).

POSITION AND MARKINGS

Because of the risk of a vasovagal syncope during any procedure, patients are treated in either a sitting or recumbent position. No markings are necessary.

DETAILS OF PROCEDURE

Once anesthesia has been obtained by a topical anesthetic, the areas to be treated are first cleansed using single-use alcohol prep pads. As stated earlier, botulinum toxin can be used at numerous locations in the face from "bunny lines" to the "pebbly" chin. For brevity, only the most commonly treated areas are discussed here. Table 42-1 is a brief overview of dosing guidelines for both Botox and Dysport as used in the most common

areas: the glabellar complex, the horizontal forehead lines, and the crow's feet area.

Glabellar Complex

The first step in treating this area is identifying the extent of action of both the corrugators and procerus muscles. Grasping the corrugators muscle between the nondominant index finger and thumb and elevating the muscle off of the underlying bone can reduce unwanted diffusion of neurotoxin. Five injection sites are used. The first is in the midline to treat the procerus. Then 2 additional sites are injected on each side above the brow (see Fig. 42-2). The skin and subcutaneous tissue is thick here, and the drug must be delivered deeply into the muscle. Avoid the periosteum. Figure 42-4 shows good reduction of the "frown lines."

Horizontal Forehead Lines

The frontalis muscle is a wide and thin muscle that is particularly sensitive to botulinum neurotoxin considering the area it covers. This is certainly an area that can be tailored to achieve a "frozen brow" or some element of lateral brow elevation. In general, injections are made at least 2 to 3 cm above the orbital rim to avoid brow and lid ptosis. The average number of injection points ranges from 4 to 6. Injections are delivered just beneath the dermis. Figure 42-5 shows good reduction of the "worry lines" of the brow.

Crow's Feet

The goal here is to weaken the muscles surrounding the lateral orbit without incurring asymmetry, paralysis, or dysfunction of the orbital complex. I recommend 3 injection sites on each side, but this can certainly be modified as the situation requires. The first is located

Table 42-1   General Dosing Guidelines

Site	Botox	Dysport
Glabellar complex	20 to 40 U	40 to 60 U
Horizontal forehead lines	10 to 30 U	20 to 40 U
Crow's feet	15 to 30 U	40 to 50 U

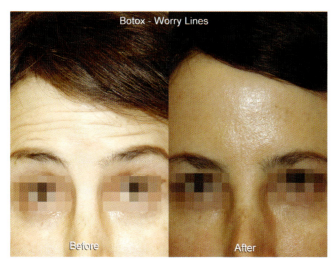

Figure 42-5 Injections delivered beneath the dermis to reduce the "worry lines" of the brow.

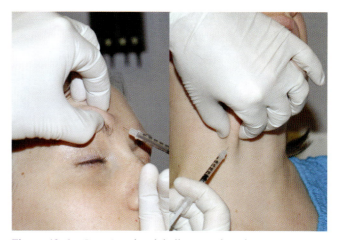

Figure 42-6 Grasping the glabellar muscle aids in prevention of ptosis. Grasping the platysma to deliver botulinum toxin. The same technique is used when treating the platysma bands in the neck.

approximately 1 cm lateral to the lateral canthus right over the orbital rim. Then 2 additional points, 1 cm above and 1 cm below, are injected. The skin in this area is very thin; thus, the drug is injected intradermally or just beneath the dermis.

PITFALLS

As with any medical procedure, a surgeon can eliminate dissatisfied patients simply through the process of proper patient selection. This starts with good communication between the surgeon and patient. A Glogau type 4 patient may ask for botulinum toxin as a quick fix for forehead lines, but may be better suited with a more aggressive treatment. There are, of course, exceptions, but botulinum neurotoxin type A is best used on younger patients.

As with any office-based injectable treatment, ecchymosis and pain at the site of injection are not uncommon. As described earlier, the use of topical anesthetics and pretreatment ice can help decrease the risk of these temporary setbacks.

Injection of neurotoxin into the glabellar complex to treat frown lines can result in ptosis of the eyelid caused by diffusion of the drug into the levator muscle. Anecdotally, some believe the newer Dysport has more diffusion potential, but clinical evidence shows similar diffusion and action halos between the 2 drugs. The risk of ptosis when using any drug may be mitigated by grasping the corrugator muscle and elevating it off the bone as shown in Figure 42-6.

Finally, unsatisfactory results often occur from under treatment rather than improper technique (see Table 42-1 for proper dosing guidelines).

PEARLS

A working knowledge and appreciation of overall facial aesthetics and facial harmony will aid the physician in both recommending and administering treatment using botulinum toxin. Although botulinum toxin can certainly be used on isolated muscles to reduce a specific wrinkle, it is best used as part of a comprehensive plan to restore facial harmony and symmetry. Combining an understanding of your patient's goals with good communication about the limitations of botulinum toxin will help eliminate many disappointed patients. Treatment with botulinum toxin is often best reserved for younger patients. Indeed, the drugs are only FDA approved for cosmetic use in patients younger than 65 years old. Glogau type 4 patients may not be the best candidates for this type of minimally invasive treatment.

At the time this chapter was written, there are 3 FDA-approved botulinum toxins approved for cosmetic use. Numerous other products, including a topical botulinum neurotoxin type A, are seeking approval. Not all formulations are identical and it is necessary to convert dose equivalents between the different drugs to achieve similar clinical results. A simple conversion between Botox and Dysport has been described by Karsai et al. They recommend a dose equivalent using a 2.5:1 ratio of Dysport to Botox.

In an effort to decrease the risk of ptosis when treating glabellar lines, we have found it helpful to grasp the corrugator muscle between the index finger and thumb of the noninjecting hand (Fig. 42-6). Elevating the muscle away from bone and ultimately away from the supraorbital foramen may decrease the risk of drug diffusion affecting the levator muscle.

SUGGESTED READING

Hexsel D, Dal'Forno T, Hexsel C, Do Prado DZ, Lima MM. A randomized pilot study comparing the action halos of two commercial preparations of botulinum toxin type A. *Dermatol Surg.* 2008;34(1);52-59.

Hexsel DM, de Almeida AT, Rutowitsch M, et al. Multicenter, double-blind study of the efficacy of injections with botuli-num toxin type A reconstituted up to six consecutive weeks before application. *Dermatol Surg.* 2003;29:523.

Karsai S, Raulin C. Current evidence on the unit equivalence of different botulinum neurotoxin A formulations and recommendations for clinical practice in dermatology. *Dermatol Surg.* 2009;35(1):1-8.

Chapter 43. Facial Fillers

Bernard T. Lee, MD, MBA; Jason S. Cooper, MD

INDICATIONS

Redistribution of subcutaneous facial fat results in volumetric deflation and signs of facial aging (ie, creases, folds, and wrinkles). Facial rejuvenation with soft-tissue fillers has been used to treat atrophy of the upper and lower lips, down-turning at the corner of the mouth, malar soft-tissue descent, and deepening of the nasolabial folds.

PREOPERATIVE PREPARATION

Patients should be provided with an informed consent form specifically related to soft-tissue fillers. The area to be treated is photographed and corroborated by the patient with a handheld mirror after makeup is removed. Both patient and surgeon should be well versed in the fillers intended to be injected. Before soft-tissue augmentation, it is recommended that patients refrain from medication that can inhibit platelet aggregation and potentiate ecchymosis for approximately 2 weeks prior to injection. Immediately prior to injection, the patient's vital signs should be checked, along with a recent history of medications taken and review of systems. The treatment area should be assessed with respect to its aesthetic deformity and the patient's goals for treatment. The surgeon should choose a filler based upon the anatomic area being treated; consideration should be given to type of filler, duration of effect, and intended depth of injection. For example, the lips are evaluated for fullness, tightness of upper lip relative to maxillary arch, projection, and degree of eversion. Youthful lips demonstrate a certain amount of vermilion bulk, whereas thin lips are exaggerated by bony retrusion and changing dentition. The marionette lines, mental groove, and the anterior jowl line must be assessed similarly to optimize lip and perioral aesthetics.

ANESTHESIA

Adequate cutaneous anesthesia can be obtained with various topical preparations. Local anesthesia and nerve blocks may be unnecessary in collagen products that they already contain lidocaine in the syringe. The majority of patients receive a combination of topical, local, and regional anesthetic prior to filler injection. Topical anesthetic creams include lidocaine, tetracaine, and benzocaine. Regional anesthesia includes infraorbital and mental nerve blocks with 1% lidocaine and 1:200,000 epinephrine. It is our experience that after injection of filler, ice-saline gauze can be applied topically to soothe the treated area and reduce pain.

POSITION AND MARKING

Dynamic wrinkles caused by muscle action (ie, glabellar, crow's feet, nasolabial, and forehead) are marked after asking the patient to activate those muscles. This action accentuates wrinkles and enables an outline of the intended treatment sites. Static wrinkles caused by sun damage, smoking, and gravity are marked with the patient sitting.

DETAILS OF PROCEDURE

Various facial filler techniques have been described and familiarity with the different techniques and soft-tissue filler products improves aesthetic results (Fig. 43-1).

When treating thin lips, a linear threading technique is preferred at the vermillion–cutaneous border and within the vermillion. The entire length of the needle is inserted into the middle of the crease, wrinkle, or mucosa to create a channel. The product is injected while the needle is slowly being advanced so that threads are deposited along the entire length. One can also inject the product in a retrograde fashion. We have found Juvederm (Allergan, Irvine, CA), a nonallergenic hyaluronic acid product derived from a nonanimal source, to work well for lip augmentation with results lasting up to 1 year posttreatment.

A technique similar to linear threading is called fanning. The needle is inserted in a fashion similar to linear threading; however, prior to removing the needle from the tissue, its direction is changed, enabling a new line of injection. Ideally, the fanning pattern of lines should be evenly spaced in a progressive direction. We find this technique to be well suited for use when augmenting the malar area. Radiesse (BioForm Medical, San Mateo, CA), a calcium hydroxylapatite (CaHA) suspension in a patented aqueous polysaccharide gel carrier, is our preferred filler for nonsurgically reelevating the malar eminence.

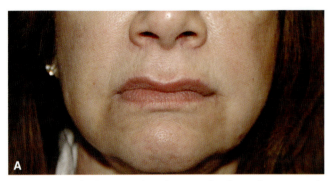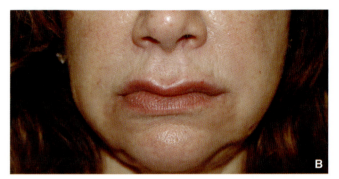

Figure 43-1   **A.** Preoperative photograph of a patient presenting for upper-lip rejuvenation. **B.** Enhancement of vermilion and philtral column with 1 mL of Juvederm.

Because CaHA is a normal constituent of bone, we inject it in a supraperiosteal plane and avoid superficial injection near the deep dermis.

When treating fine lines or wrinkles in the midface, we prefer to use multiple injections within the desired treatment area. Multiple injections in the same tissue plane enable the product to coalesce into a smooth continuous line. When small gaps exist after serial injections, postinjection molding and massage can be used to uniformly blend the material into an even layer. This technique is well suited for the glabella and philtral column. We frequently fill fine lines and perioral wrinkles with Restylane (Medicis Aesthetics, Scottsdale, AZ) or Juvederm. Restylane is a stabilized, partially cross-linked hyaluronic acid created via bacterial fermentation from *Streptococci* bacteria. Very small amounts of Restylane (0.5 mL) are needed to augment the upper lip.

Another technique to fill the perioral area is crosshatching. In this technique, the needle is inserted much like linear threading; however, premarked crosshatching lines are outlined to guide future injections. The pattern of lines is equally spaced in a progressive grid. We advocate this technique when a large area requires correction to optimize filler.

Lip rejuvenation involves volume enhancement and vermillion–cutaneous augmentation. Linear threading or serial puncture techniques are carried out via the oral commissure. The needle is inserted in a lateral to medial direction with careful attention paid to the preexisting width of the vermillion to avoid over-injection. Commissure elevation is achieved via a crosshatching technique around the oral commissure and marionette line. Because of the dynamic nature of the perioral area, concomitant injection of 2 to 4 U of Botox in the upper lip improves the longevity of lip rejuvenation. This blocks the action of the depressor anguli further aiding the lift effect from dermal injection. Postinjection smoothing is important to maintain a uniform contour and prevent subtle irregularities.

Nasolabial fold augmentation to soften a deep fold is an extremely useful adjunct to midface rejuvenation (Fig. 43-2). Serial puncture or linear threading to the middle and deeper portion of the dermis is essential when using a long-acting filler (ie, Radiesse). Injections should begin inferiorly and move superiorly, while layering product in a deep-to-superficial approach. Immediate massage to smooth uneven injections is critical to achieving a desirable result. Complete fold correction is not required and may actually appear unattractive. Instead a gradual

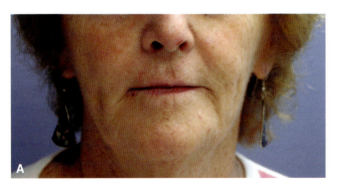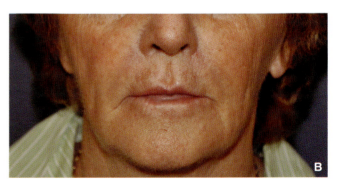

Figure 43-2   **A.** Preoperative photograph of a patient presenting for nasolabial, upper lip, and marionette line rejuvenation. **B.** Enhancement of nasolabial fold, upper lip, and marionette lines with 3 mL of Juvederm.

blunting of the deep nasolabial fold is our goal, starting at the upper third of the fold. When using hyaluronic acid, approximately 0.5 to 2.0 mL are used per patient in the nasolabial area. When deep creases within the nasolabial fold are addressed, serial puncture is used in the mid portion of the dermis. Finer lines around the midface can be augmented using a small particle hyaluronic acid filler at the dermal–epidermal junction (ie, Restylane). Forehead lines can be addressed via a linear threading technique. A downside to combining Botox A with a filler is that it more easily unmasks superficial injections.

The amount of filler needed in a specific area depends on the thickness of the skin, history of previous Botox injections in the area, and the depth and number of wrinkles. The malar eminence and tear trough are amenable to a number of injection techniques: serial puncture, cross-hatching, and linear threading. When treating the midface and periocular area, we start laterally and move medially. Product is injected in a supraperiosteal plane to avoid contour irregularities. Larger particle hyaluronic acid fillers (ie, Perlane [hyaluronic acid] [Medicis Aesthetics, Scotts-dale, AZ], fat, or CaHA) have been used successfully in this area to augment the cheek and blunt the tear trough.

Another excellent volumetric enhancer of the malar area is poly-L-lactic acid. Injectable poly-L-lactic acid is marketed as Sculptra (Sanofi-Aventis, Bridgewater, NJ). It is composed of crystalline, irregularly sized particles of poly-L-lactic acid. These particles are biocompatible, bio-degradeable, synthetic polymers from the α-hydroxy acid family. When using Sculptra, we inject into the subcutaneous plane of the malar area. Poly-L-lactic acid is meant to provide volumetric expansion through a foreign-body giant cell reaction that occurs several weeks to month after treatment. Collagen production resulting from product degradation leads to the desired volumetric expansion. Unlike other fillers products, multiple treatments are often needed to achieve the full extent of malar augmentation in our patients; however, the desired effect can last up to 2 years. Consequently, proper informed consent is particularly important when discussing both the short- and long-term trade-offs of this product with our patients. We often inject a treatment area at 6-week intervals for a total of 2 to 4 treatments, depending upon the amount of augmentation needed.

When injecting the tear trough area, it is important to avoid superficial injection as dermal injections tend to be easily visible and palpable. Gentle massage after injection enables the filler product to conform to the underlying skeletal and soft-tissue contours.

Postoperative instructions are given to patients prior to their filler procedures, providing appropriate patient expectations and ample time for questions regarding the preferred protocol. Ice-saline gauze is recommended for 15 minutes at a time during the first 24 to 48 hours to limit postinjection bruising and swelling. Patients are advised to sleep with their head elevated at approximately 35 degrees. Swelling from injections can persist up to 3 weeks.

PITFALLS

Potential adverse reactions include local bruising, purpura, erythema, tenderness, swelling, and itching. Major hypersensitivity and chronic granulomatous reactions have been reported after hyaluronic acid injection.

PEARLS

The thickness of the dermis has to be assessed prior to dermal filler injection. The depth of hyaluronic acid injection is a critical consideration in optimizing the aesthetic result. The small particle fillers are more easily injected into the superficial dermis and should be used in areas with thin dermis. Thicker facial areas, including the glabella, forehead lines, nasolabial folds, and atrophic scars, are best augmented at the middermal level with medium-size hyaluronic acid fillers. In the case of overfilling, hyaluronidase has been reported to dissolve hyaluronic acid products and can improve nodularity and granuloma-tous-like reactions.

SUGGESTED READING

Klein AW. Filler materials. In: Thorne CT, Beasley RW, Aston SJ, et al, eds. *Grabb and Smith's Plastic Surgery*. 6th ed. Baltimore, MD: Lippincott Williams & Wilkins; 2007:468-474.

Rohrich RJ, Ghavami A, Crosby MA. The role of hyaluronic acid fillers (Restylane) in facial cosmetic surgery: review and technical considerations. *Plast Reconstr Surg*. 2007;120 (6 Suppl):41S-54S.

Chapter 44. Chemical Peels

Olubimpe A. Ayeni, MD, MPH, FRCSC;
Samuel J. Lin, MD, FACS; Thomas A. Mustoe, MD

INDICATIONS

Chemical peels involve the application of a caustic solution to the skin to produce a controlled, partial thickness chemical burn and subsequent "resurfacing" with new epidermal and dermal connective tissue. Chemical peels induce exfoliation, which, in turn, stimulates inflammation, neocollagenesis, and collagen remodeling. The main indications for peels include rhytids, photodamage, actinic damage, acne scarring, and pigment changes. The process results in the appearance of fewer rhytids, improved skin texture, and more even pigmentation.

Chemical peels create a thinner, more compact stratum corneum, as well as a thicker epidermis and more uniform distribution of melanin. The increased volume of tissue tightens the superficial skin layers, leading to an improvement of skin appearance. Common skin problems such as ephelides, melasma, and epidermal hyperpigmentation can be treated with epidermal peels, but senile lentigines and lentigines simplex require deeper peels. Depth of wound mostly determines cosmetic result and is influenced by many factors, such as chemical concentration, duration of contact, number of layers applied, and agent.

CLASSIFICATION OF PEELS BY DEPTH

Superficial chemical peels penetrate the epidermis and can reach as far as the papillary dermis. These agents remove the stratum corneum without inducing necrosis. The deep-ithelialization stimulates epidermal growth and reduces fine lines, rhytids, and sun damage. The most commonly used superficial chemical peels are glycolic acid (40% to 70%), trichloroacetic acid (10% to 20%), Jessner's solution, salicylic acid, and tretinoin.

Medium-depth peels extend to the deep papillary dermis and often to the superficial reticular dermis. These peels are associated with greater collagen remodeling and longer durations of posttreatment erythema. In terms of the agents used, 35% trichloroacetic acid is often combined with solid CO_2, Jessner's solution, or 70% glycolic acid. A superficial peeling agent is applied, which acts to break the epidermal barrier and allow more complete penetration of the 35% trichloroacetic acid.

Deep chemical peels penetrate into the mid reticular dermis. These peels induce inflammation in the reticular dermis and stimulate production of ground substance and new collagen. The Baker-Gordon Phenol Peel (88% phenol, water, Septisol, and croton oil) is the most commonly used deep chemical peel. It resurfaces skin defects, but it requires special cardiac monitoring during application.

PRETREATMENT

Evaluation of skin type and complexion is very important to determine which chemical peels would be suitable for the patient and to avoid complications such as abnormal scarring and pigmentation abnormalities. The Fitzpatrick classification of skin types (I to VI) is useful for this purpose (Table 44-1). Patient selection is important to a successful outcome and the best results are seen in patients with fair skin (pigment changes less noticeable), nonoily skin (better peel), patients who have avoided sun exposure for 6 months, and females (ability to use cosmetic camouflage, thinner skin).

Table 44-1 Fitzpatrick Classification Scale

Skin Type	Skin Color	Characteristics
I	White; very fair; red or blond hair; blue eyes; freckles	Always burns, never tans
II	White; fair; red or blond hair; blue, hazel, or green eyes	Usually burns, tans with difficulty
III	Cream white; fair with any eye or hair color; very common	Sometimes mild burn, gradually tans
IV	Brown; typical Mediterranean caucasian skin	Rarely burns, tans with ease
V	Dark Brown; mid-eastern skin types	Very rarely burns, tans very easly
VI	Black	Never burns, tans very easily

Rubin MG. Photoaged and photodamaged skin. In: Rubin MG, ed. *Manual of Chemical Peels: Superficial and Medium Depth.* Philadelphia, PA: Lippincott Williams & Wilkins; 1995:3.

Before undergoing a chemical peel, a thorough history and physical examination should be performed. One to 2 weeks before the peel, retinoic acid (Retin-A) can be applied to decrease the height of the stratum corneum, increase the uniformity/penetration of peel, promote faster healing, and decrease postinflammatory hyperpigmentation by dispersing melanin through epidermis. Hydroquinone (4%) can also be used; it decreases the probability of postpeel hyperpigmentation. In any patient with a history of herpes simplex virus 2, acyclovir/Valtrex (valacyclovir) must be used 2 days before treatment until epithelialization occurs.

The patient should thoroughly cleanse the face with nonresidue soap the day before the peel and should not apply makeup or moisturizers. Immediately before starting the procedure, the skin is cleansed to remove any remaining traces of makeup or oils, using ether, acetone, or isopropyl alcohol. Cleansing the skin before a chemical peel is very important to prevent uneven penetration of the peeling agent.

PROCEDURE

The patient should sit in a comfortable position, at least at a 45-degree sitting angle, to observe natural gravitational effects on the face rather than being supine. The patient may wear a disposable hair cap, and should be instructed to keep the eyes closed during the procedure. A zinc oxide paste should be applied at the lip and eyelid commissures. Liquid products are better applied using a fan brush; gel products can be applied with cotton-tipped applicators or gloved fingers. Treatment should start on facial areas with thicker skin. The peeling agent is applied on the forehead first, from side to side, and then on the cheeks, the nose, and the chin. The periocular and perioral regions should be treated last. The face should be treated in cosmetic units with the goal of hiding demarcations between units; this means the peel should be extended beyond jaw line, vermillion border, and into hairline.

The depth of penetration of chemical peels can be determined by the following 3 changes:

1. Epidermal penetration is signaled by diffuse, homogeneous erythema.
2. A white frost indicates coagulative necrosis of the papillary dermis.
3. A gray-white frost indicates coagulative necrosis of the reticular dermis.

POSTOPERATIVE CARE

The healing process after a chemical peel must be as rapid as possible to avoid infections that may deepen the wounds, extending the peel from superficial to deep, with increased risks of scarring. Deep peels may be prophylactically treated with antimicrobials, but superficial and medium-deep peels are simply kept moist with the application of petrolatum-based products. After reepithelialization, and when skin appearance is back to normal, a regimen of α-hydroxyl acids, retinoic acid, bleaching creams, moisturizers, and sunscreens should be restarted. Sun exposure must be avoided for 6 weeks after the peel to minimize the risks of postinflammatory hyperpigmentation.

PITFALLS

Systemic isotretinoin use is a strict contraindication to peeling. This drug should be stopped at least 6 months before the procedure in patients with thick sebaceous skin and 1 year for patients with thin skin. Patients with a history of herpes simplex virus 2 infections should be pretreated prior to undergoing a chemical peel. For deeper peels, especially with the use of phenol, cardiac monitoring is essential because of the risk of cardiac arrhythmias.

PEARLS

Patient selection is crucial in obtaining the best post-peel results and avoiding complications. It is often necessary to combine chemical peeling with other skin rejuvenating and resurfacing techniques for best overall results.

SUGGESTED READING

Bernstein EF. Chemical peels. *Semin Cutan Med Surg*. 2002; 21(1):27-45.

Brenner MJ, Perro CA. Recontouring, resurfacing, and scar revision in skin cancer reconstruction. *Facial Plast Surg Clin North Am*. 2009;17(3):469-487, e463.

Fabbrocini G, De Padova MP, Tosti A. Chemical peels: what's new and what isn't new but still works well. *Facial Plast Surg*. 2009;25(5):329-336.

Fischer TC, Perosino E, Poli F, Viera MS, Dreno B. Chemical peels in aesthetic dermatology: an update 2009. *J Eur Acad Dermatol Venereol*. 2010;24(3):281-292.

Stone PA. The use of modified phenol for chemical face peeling. *Clin Plast Surg*. 1998;25(1):21-44.

Chapter 45. Hair Transplantation

Alfonso Barrera, MD, FACS

In the past 25 years, great advances have occurred in techniques of hair transplantation for the treatment of male pattern baldness, allowing for natural and aesthetic results. The most significant change has been the ability to transplant a large number of significantly smaller grafts (follicular unit grafts) in an artistic way that mimics nature.

This technique gradually evolved from the traditional hair plugs to the use of follicular unit grafts, which have become the gold standard today. The original hair plug or punch graft technique was described by Orentrech in 1959 for the treatment of male pattern baldness, and was the standard of care for many years. These 4-mm plugs contained 10 to 20 hairs and resulted on an artificial "corn row" appearance. We learned a lot from the use of hair plugs, specifically the "donor dominance concept," that is the fact that the longevity of hair growth is dependent on the genetic programming of the hair follicles (hair roots) of the *donor* area. The success of hair transplantation today rests on this concept: Transplanted hair will continue to grow on the transplanted site as long as it was going to do so on the donor area. Male pattern baldness occurs primarily on the top of the head and not on the occipital or temporal areas. The hair follicles on the top of the head are genetically sensitive to dehydrotestosterone (DHT), whereas the hair follicles on the occipital and temporal areas are not. This feature is maintained as they are transplanted to the bald area.

As the use of smaller and more numerous grafts were introduced, much better results were obtained. The first report of the use of single hair grafts on the scalp was that of Nordstrom in 1980. He described the benefit of such grafts camouflaging the scarring and unnatural appearance of hair plugs, finally allowing for natural-looking results. It was very time consuming working at the front hairline and it did not seem feasible at the time that the entire area of baldness could be treated with such small grafts. Uebel, in 1991, reported his technique using micrografts (1 to 2 hair grafts) and minigrafts (3 to 4 hair grafts) in large numbers (1000 to 1200 grafts) per session to graft large areas of hair loss such as the entire top of the head in cases of male pattern baldness (MPB).

In 1993, I became interested in hair transplantation based on the work of Nordstrom and Uebel, and this has become the most common procedure in my practice today. The key for a natural result has been doing a large number of very small grafts and using finer instrumentation to avoid detectable scarring both on the transplanted area, and on the donor site.

In 1984, Headington reported an interesting anatomical finding on hair follicle anatomy. He studied horizontal sections of scalp and found that hair follicles come in anatomic units of 1, 2, 3, or 4 hairs; they have their own blood supply, sebaceous glands, sweat glands, piloerectile muscle, and innervation and are surrounded by a sheath of collagen. This configuration is what we know as follicular units. They appear to be true physiologic units. As long as you do not use grafts larger than these the results are very natural looking. Of course, it is also important to transplant them artistically in terms of orientation and direction of hair growth.

There is a variable nomenclature regarding grafts, the most logical and common today is "follicular unit grafts," as mentioned above.

I have been working on improving the technique by further increasing the number of grafts transplanted in a single session, I frequently do well over 2000 and have done as many as 2900 in a single session for MPB patients, which works out to be approximately 6000 hairs in a single session.

I have found additional applications restoring natural looking hair in reconstructive cases such as iatrogenic alopecia (ie, as a result of facelift procedures), but also alopecia caused by burns, accidents, tumor resections, congenital deformities, etc.

PATIENT SELECTION

To date, we have no method to create new hair. All current techniques for hair restoration involve *redistributing* the patient's existing hair. Therefore, to be a candidate, the patient must have a favorable ratio between the donor-site surface area and density relative to the size of the area to be transplanted. Patients who have a higher donor density and a larger potential donor site area (occipital and temporal areas) and a smaller the surface area to be grafted have optimal ratios.

Unfortunately, MPB is a progressive condition. The rate of hair loss may slow down after the age of 40 years, but it never stops completely.

Therefore, the preoperative plan must ensure results that look natural both short- and long-term. Good communication with patients is essential to establishing realistic expectations.

Be conservative; design a mature hairline by leaving a reasonable degree of frontotemporal recession even in the young patient, as this will help the patient to look natural long term. Explain to the patient that it is not uncommon to have more than one session of grafts. I prefer to wait at least a year before a second session; density may be increased at that time by adding grafts between the ones done before.

Several centers worldwide are working on tissue engineering in an attempt to clone hair follicles or culture and multiply hair follicles in the laboratory setting. When successful, we will be able to treat patients with limited donor hair (the follicular-challenged patient), will only need to harvest a sample of hair follicles, and will eliminate the minimal donor-site morbidity and discomfort almost completely.

PREOPERATIVE PREPARATION

As in all other elective plastic surgical procedures the patient must be in good health and have no significant health problems. The patient needs to avoid aspirin, Plavix (clopidogrel), Coumadin (warfarin), and all types of anticoagulants for at least a week preoperatively. It is very important to have a normal clotting time.

Normally we only check a complete blood count (CBC). If there is a history of bleeding tendencies, then we check a coagulation profile, and specifically an Ivy bleeding time, which should be well below 6 minutes. If the bleeding time is longer than 6 minutes, do not operate.

The patient is told to have nothing by mouth (NPO) after midnight and comes to our clinic at 8 AM the next morning.

Typically we do 1000 to 2500 follicular unit grafts per session, depending on the degree of baldness and the availability of donor hair. The procedure usually takes us 4 to 5 hours, depending on the number of grafts.

ANESTHESIA

I use IV sedation and local infiltration. The patient is placed in the supine position and mildly sedated with midazolam (Versed) 2 to 10 mg and Sublimaze (fentanyl) 50 to 100 mcg, which are titrated for each patient. The patient's vital signs, electrocardiogram (EKG), and O_2 saturation are monitored throughout the procedure.

A ring block anterior to the proposed hairline is established with 0.5% bupivacaine (Marcaine) with 1:200,000 epinephrine (approximately 30 mL).

POSITION AND MARKINGS

Preoperative markings of the design and level of the proposed hairline and the occipital donor ellipse are done in our preoperative holding area. The donor ellipse is designed horizontally in the occipital area, 1 cm in width and as long as needed, often up to 25 to 32 cm, extending well into the temporal areas. Making the ellipse no more than 1 cm wide ensures closure without tension, and a safer and more predictable degree of minimal scarring.

There is no magic number as to the distance from the eyebrows to the ideal hairline, as there is a huge variety of head dimensions and craniofacial proportions. I draw it in advance to what seems appropriate and aesthetically pleasing, making sure to provide definite irregularity at the front, to better mimic nature.

DETAILS OF PROCEDURE

For cases of MPB, I typically do between 1000 and 2500 grafts per session, depending on the degree of hair loss. This labor-intensive procedure requires an organized and efficient surgical team.

My surgical team consists of 3 surgical assistants and myself. I remain in the operating room for the duration of the procedure and insert all grafts personally. It is clearly important to work efficiently when transplanting a large number of grafts in a single session to complete the job in a reasonable period of time (see video).

With the patient's head turned to the left, I harvest the right half of the donor ellipse with a no. 10 blade. Under 3.5 × loupe magnification, thin slices of 1.5- to 2.0-mm thickness are immediately dissected from the donor ellipse with Personna Prep blades over a sterile wooden board and handed to the assistants. I like a wooden board because it provides a nonslippery, firm surface.

The assistants, under magnification, prepare the final grafts from these slices, while the surgeon closes the right half of the donor strip. Careful dissection of the thin slices into 1 to 2 hair follicular unit micrografts and 3 to 4 hair follicular unit minigrafts is done with background lighting using a no. 10 blade and magnification. This is the most tedious part of the procedure and one of the most important steps, as the grafts obviously need to be handled gently and atraumatically. The darker and thicker the individual hair shafts, the easier it is to dissect the grafts. The ideal grafts have intact hair shafts all the way from the subcutaneous fatty tissue to the scalp surface and contain from 1 to 4 hairs. Again, they must be handled as atraumatically as possible. The grafts are handled with jeweler's forceps by the fatty tissue under the hair bulbs or by the tissue around them, not by the hair bulb or dermal hair papilla itself.

In cases of very-light-colored or white hair, we use microscopes (10×) for a safe dissection of the grafts; I prefer the Mantis microscope. The harvested scalp and all grafts are kept chilled in normal saline until transplanted.

The surgeon then turns the patient's head to the right to harvest the left half of the donor ellipse. The surgeon subsequently closes the left-side donor site and then finishes slicing the remaining segment of the donor ellipse into slides.

Several hundred grafts will have been dissected at this point. They are lined up in rows on a wet green or blue surgical towel and are now ready for insertion. The process of graft dissection and insertion continues until all the grafts are transplanted. It is imperative to keep the grafts wet, as desiccation damages the hair bulbs.

Three key points to remember in graft dissection are:

1. Maintain the follicular units as intact as feasible.

2. In patients with dark hair, 3.5 × loupe magnification is sufficient to dissect most grafts as follicular units.

3. In patients with light hair or gray hair, surgical microscopes and background lighting may be needed for more accurate dissection.

Graft Insertion

Infiltration of tumescent solution into the recipient area is important for several reasons; the most important step is to promote hemostasis and to produce temporary edema of the scalp, which facilitates graft insertion.

In a given case I generally use a total of 150 mL of 0.25% lidocaine with 1:200,000 epinephrine plus 40 mg of triamcinolone (Kenalog).

If good hemostasis is not obtained with this amount of solution, I increase the epinephrine strength to 1:100,000. Optimal hemostasis is often achieved if the tumescent solution is infiltrated in thirds. I first inject the anterior region once a large number of grafts have been inserted there; I proceed posteriorly doing the same for the middle third and, then, the posterior third. Having this sequence allows us to take advantage of the peak times of epinephrine effect.

As fibrinogen turns into fibrin, the grafts adhere better to the recipient slits and we repetitively return anteriorly to insert more grafts, packing them densely to minimizing the "popping out" of neighboring grafts. The epinephrine effect is often still adequate when returning to the anterior region to place additional grafts; otherwise, we may reinject local anesthesia.

I use 22.5-guage Sharpoint blades at 2 cm in front of the hairline to create a nice transition zone, intentionally making slight irregularities to mimic nature. The scars are undetectable every time with these blades; posterior to the hairline I prefer to use no. 11 Feather Personna blades.

I place the grafts initially approximately 5 mm from each other, beginning at the front hairline and proceeding posteriorly. As fibrinogen turns into fibrin (15 to 20 minutes later) the grafts become more secure in place.

Next, I go back anteriorly between the previously inserted grafts, placing them about 2.5 mm apart. If one tries to pack them densely too soon, they often "pop out," which is very frustrating and time-consuming as you need to reinsert them.

As fibrinogen turns into fibrin, I return to place more grafts between the first set of grafts, getting them closer and closer to each other until the distance is approximately 1 to 1.5 mm between grafts; at this point, this is "dense packing."

The surgeon must be working all along in various areas, periodically returning anteriorly and proceeding posteriorly, and so on and so forth until all the grafts are inserted.

Of course, if the main area of baldness is the crown and not the front hairline, I may then start the grafting on the crown and then work on the front; if the area also needs some grafts, going back and forth in the above-mentioned fashion achieves optimal grafting with minimal "popping out" of the grafts (Figs. 45-1 to 45-8).

PITFALLS

For the first 3 to 4 months after hair transplantation there is normally no visible improvement, in fact the patient's hair may even look thinner than prior to the procedure because of telogen effluvium.

Once the grafts shift into the anagen (growth) phase, after 3 to 4 months, fine villous hair appears and gradually thickens into terminal hair. A visually significant increase in hair density and growth does not occur until approximately 5 to 6 months postoperatively and often takes 10 to 12 months before the final result. In female patients, it may take a little longer.

PEARLS

- Spend sufficient time preoperatively with the patient to assure good communication.

- Answer all their questions and make certain they understand and have realistic expectations.

- Make sure the patient knows that there will be a definite improvement in one session but that it is not uncommon to require more than one session for an optimal result.

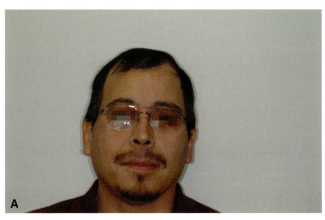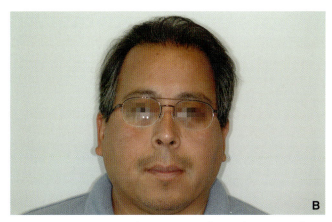

Figure 45-1 **A.** Patient no. 1 preoperative, front view. **B.** Same patient 2 years postoperative, front view. Had a single session of 2350 follicular unit grafts.

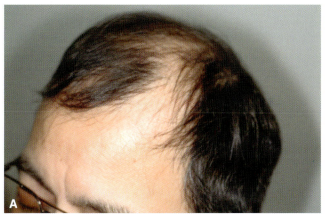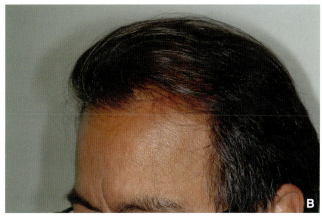

Figure 45-2 **A.** Patient no. 1 preoperative, left oblique view. **B.** Same patient 2 years postoperative, left oblique view. Had a single session of 2350 follicular unit grafts.

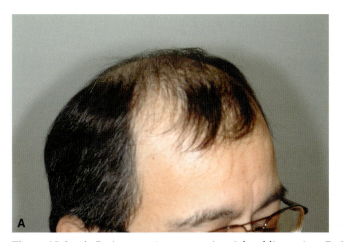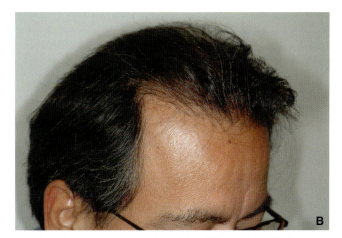

Figure 45-3 **A.** Patient no. 1 preoperative right oblique view. **B.** Same patient 2 years postoperative, right oblique view. Had a single session of 2350 follicular unit grafts.

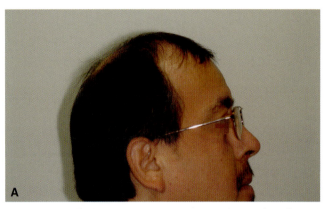
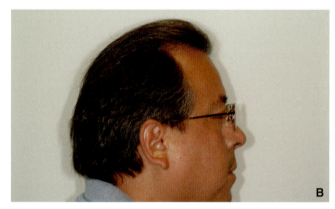

Figure 45-4   **A.** Patient no. 1 preoperative view, right side. **B.** Same patient 2 years postoperative, view right side. Had a single session of 2350 follicular unit grafts.

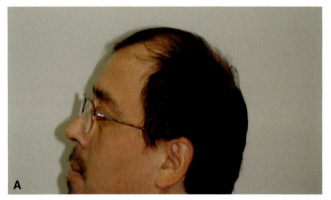
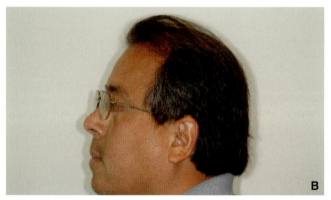

Figure 45-5   **A.** Patient no. 1 preoperative left side view. **B.** Same patient 2 years postoperative, view, left side. Had a single session of 2350 follicular unit grafts.

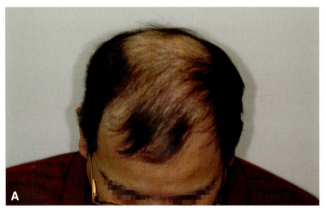
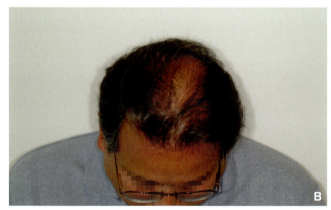

Figure 45-6   **A.** Patient no. 1 preoperative top view. **B.** Same patient 2 years postoperative, top view. Had a single session of 2350 follicular unit grafts.

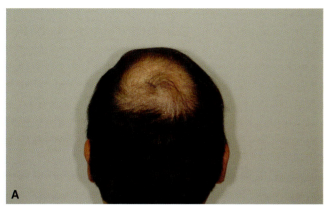
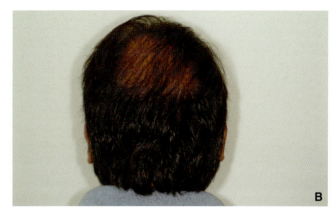

Figure 45-7   **A.** Patient no. 1. preoperative view of the back of the head **B.** Same patient 2 years postoperative, view of the back of the head. Had a single session of 2350 follicular unit grafts.

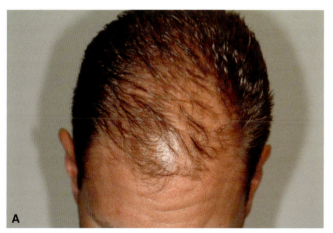
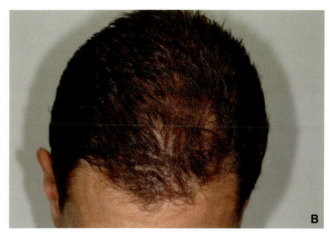

Figure 45-8   **A.** Patient no. 2 preoperative view of the frontal scalp. **B.** Same patient 1 year postoperative, view of the frontal scalp. Had a single session of 1800 follicular unit grafts.

SUGGESTED READING

Barrera A. *Hair Transplantation—The Art of Micrografting and Minigrafting.* St. Louis, MO: Quality Medical; 2002.

Barrer, A: Micrograft and minigraft megasession hair transplantation results after a single session. *Plast Reconstr Surg.* 1997;100(6):1524.

Barrera A. Micrograft and minigraft megasession hair transplantation: review of 100 consecutive cases. *Aesthet Surg J.* 1997;17(3):165.

Barrera A. Refinements in hair transplantation: micro and minigraft megasession. *Perspect Plast Surg.* 1998;11(1):53.

Headington JT. Transverse microscopic anatomy of the human scalp. *Arch Dermatol.* 1984;120:449.

Nordstrom REA. Micrografts for improvement of the frontal hairline after hair transplantation. *Aesthetic Plast Surg.* 1981;5:97.

Orentreich N. Autografts in alopecias and other selected dermatological conditions. *Ann NY Acad Sci.* 1959;83:463.

Uebel CO. Micrografts and minigrafts: a new approach to baldness surgery. *Ann Plast Surg.* 1991;27:476.

Chapter 46. Fat Grafting

Kenneth B. Hughes, MD

INDICATIONS

Structural fat grafting is used to enhance contour in virtually any area amenable to grafting, and the indications are continually expanding. The first and most common indication for structural fat grafting is breast reconstruction defect. With the increased popularity of fillers for facial augmentation, fat grafting for facial augmentation has been a result of the plentiful nature of filler material available and decreased cost, particularly for larger volume needs or as an adjunctive measure in facelifts.

Less common indications include buttock augmentation, breast augmentation, and hand rejuvenation. Fat grafting has also received attention for volume restoration in acquired or congenital conditions such as HIV lipodystrophy, Parry-Romberg syndrome, and craniofacial microsomia.

ANESTHESIA

As with many liposuction procedures, the choice for anesthesia is largely dictated by amount of tissue to be harvested, the number of harvest sites, the number of areas to be augmented, and the volume to be instilled. Some minor revisions can be performed under local anesthesia alone. Tumescent anesthesia may allow the donor site surface area to be increased. However, there is a theoretical concern of disruption of fatty tissue and concomitant decreased survival with these methods.

In addition, the manner of liposuction and technique utilized should be considered. Removal through smaller volume Luer-Lok syringes is theoretically less traumatic to the fat and less painful to the patient as compared to fat harvest through traditional suction cannulae with much greater suction pressures.

DETAILS OF PROCEDURE

Typical donor sites for fat grafting include the abdomen and thighs. They are convenient access points in the supine position, as breast reconstruction defects and facial augmentation are the most common indications. This also permits a 2-team approach in which one can harvest, while the other can inject. However, almost any site with readily accessible fat will serve as an adequate donor site.

Incisions for access should be placed in relaxed skin tension lines, skin creases, previous scars, striae, or hirsute areas, although creating the most optimal contour in donor areas, particularly in large-volume aspiration, should be the guiding principle. Avoidance of contour deformities should trump the concern over the addition of small incisions.

A common approach to fat harvesting utilizes blunt-tipped Coleman cannulae applied to Luer-Lok syringes. Some surgeons prefer 10 mL syringes (Coleman), whereas others opt for larger syringes because of faster harvest times. Once the fat is harvested, the specimen is centrifuged and separated to create the fat sample to be injected for augmentation. A typical protocol observed by Coleman is to use 10 mL syringes centrifuged at 3000 RPM for 3 minutes. After separation by centrifugation, the top layer contains oil, the middle layer contains viable fat, and the bottom layer contains other more dense liquid materials, primarily the local infiltrate. Decanting after gravity sedimentation is another variant for creation of an appropriate specimen for injection.

Once the harvested fast is prepared, injection can be performed with 1 mL syringes for face and hand injections because of the need for precision; 3 mL syringes may be more appropriate for breast reconstruction defects or buttock augmentation. However, the volume to be injected into an area should be the guide. An HIV lipodystrophy patient who may require 40 mL of fat augmentation to one side of his or her face may be more efficiently augmented with 3 mL syringes initially, followed by 1 mL syringes for final refinements. More important, large volumetric amounts injected in a single pass should be discouraged as this leads to greater fat necrosis, greater potential for infection, and poorer graft survival. The gauge of the cannulae to be introduced for fat grafting in the face should be in the 18 gauge range, although eyelids may require smaller bore cannulae.

The principles of placement as articulated by Coleman center around the concept that harvested fat must be positioned so that the greatest surface area of contact between it and host tissue is created. This technique is performed so as to encourage as much diffusion, oxygen exchange, and nutrient exchange as can be obtained.

Blunt-tip cannulae are usually used and fat is injected upon withdrawal. Coleman recommends 0.1 mL maximum volume per pass to minimize potential for irregularities and maximize surface contact with host tissue.

Fat is much harder to shape with digital manipulation than many of the filler agents. As such, precise placement is recommended.

These procedures can produce a considerable recovery period of 2 to 4 weeks, which may be longer than most patients expect. The persistent swelling associated with these injections is greater than that associated with Botox or conventional filler treatments to which many patients are accustomed. As such, patients should be educated about convalescence time.

PITFALLS

- Most common complications include surface irregularities as a result of errors in technique, migration, and patient healing characteristics.
- Fat necrosis, infection, and abscess formation are more prevalent in single, large-volume fat injections.
- Microcalcifications after fat grafting for breast augmentation may lead to greater numbers of biopsies and unnecessary surgical procedures because of difficulties in mammographic interpretation.

PEARLS

- Fat embolus may be avoided by epinephrine injection into the area to be augmented, as well as the use of the use of blunt cannulae.

- Sharper cannulae may be more appropriate for freeing adhesions and augmenting scarred or fibrous beds, but these cannulae still carry greater inherent risk to surrounding structures.
- Most important in structural fat grafting is Coleman's principle that fat must be positioned so as to ensure the greatest surface area of contact between it and host tissue. Small volumes injected upon cannula withdrawal through multiple passes minimize the potential for irregularities and complications and maximize graft survival.

SUGGESTED READING

Coleman SR. Avoidance of arterial occlusion from injection of soft tissue fillers. *Aesthet Surg J*. 2002;22:555-557.

Coleman SR. Structural fat grafting. In: Thorne CH, Bartlett SP, Beasley RW, Aston SJ, Gurtner GC, Spear SL, eds. *Grabb and Smith's Plastic Surgery*. 6th ed. Philadelphia, PA: Wolters Kluwer Health/Lippincott Williams & Wilkins; 2007:480-485.

Coleman SR. *Structural Fat Grafting*. St. Louis, MO: Quality Medical; 2004.

Coleman SR. Structural fat grafts: the ideal filler? *Clin Plast Surg*. 2001;28(1):111-119.

Tanna N, Wan DC, Kawamoto HK, Bradley JP. Craniofacial microsomia soft-tissue reconstruction comparison: inframammary extended circumflex scapular flap versus serial fat grafting. *Plast Reconstr Surg*. 2011;127(2):802-811.

Wang C-F, Zhou Z, Yan Y-J, Zhao D-M, Chen F, Qiao Q. Clinical analyses of clustered microcalcifications after autologous fat injection for breast augmentation. *Plast Reconstr Surg*. 2011;127(4):1669-1673.

Safety Checklists for Providers and Patients

Richard Urman, MD, MBA, Fred E. Shapiro, DO

Appendix

The Institute for Safety in Office-Based Surgery (ISOBS) has developed a template for a safety checklist to be used in an office where procedures are being performed, based on the work of the World Health Organization (WHO). This template can be customized to meet the needs of the specific subspecialty and office setting and these checklists can be designed for use by both healthcare providers and patients.

Improving patient safety in the office-based setting should be of paramount concern. In recent years, the economic pressures of medicine have incited a paradigm shift in health care delivery, such that surgical procedures are moving from the hospital to the office-based setting. Often called the "wild west of health care," office-based procedures continue to increase at a rapid pace, with an estimated more than 10 million procedures performed in 2010. A recent study from the WHO found that a comprehensive checklist used in an interdisciplinary, team-based setting resulted in a reduction in surgical complications as well as cost savings. Development of such a checklist and education of practitioners, patients, and office personnel is the mission of the Institute for Safety in Office-Based Surgery. An independent, non-profit organization, ISOBS, has developed a safety checklist for use in the office-based setting.

SAFETY CHECKLIST FOR HEALTHCARE PROVIDERS

The checklist, shown in Figure 1, calls on engagement from all healthcare providers physicians, physician assistants, medical assistants, and nurses to ensure safe care. This template is fully customizable to fit the needs in a variety of office-based settings, including plastic surgery. In addition, ISOBS is developing web-based educational modules for practitioners and personnel on using the checklist.

THE PATIENT'S CHECKLIST FOR OFFICE-BASED PROCEDURES

The latest innovation in improving patient safety is the ISOBS Patient Checklist (ISOBS 'P.C.') shown in Figure 2. It is designed to empower the patient with the knowledge needed to make educated decisions about the provider and the office facility. This checklist enables the patient to ask the "right" questions about their provider's qualifications, facility credentialing, recovery, and emergency planning.

For further information, see www.ISOBS.org

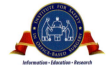

Introduction
Preoperative encounter;
with practitioner and patient

Patient

Patient medically optimized for the procedure?
☐ *Yes*
☐ *No, and plan for optimization made.*

Does patient have DVT risk factors?
☐ *Yes, and prophylaxis plans arranged.*
☐ *No*

Procedure

Procedure complexity and sedation/analgesia reviewed?
☐ *Yes*

NPO instructions given?
☐ *Yes*

Escort and post-procedure plans reviewed?
☐ *Yes*

Setting
Before patient in procedure room;
with practitioner and personnel

Emergency equipment check complete (e.g. airway, AED, code cart, MH kit)?
☐ *Yes*

EMS availability confirmed?
☐ *Yes*

Oxygen source and suction checked?
☐ *Yes*

Anticipated duration ≤ 6 hours?
☐ *Yes*
☐ *No, but personnel, monitoring and equipment available*

Operation
Before sedation/analgesia;
with practitioner and personnel*

Patient identity, procedure, and consent confirmed?   ☐ *Yes*

Is the site marked and side identified?
☐ *Yes* ☐ *N/A*

DVT prophylaxis provided?
☐ *Yes* ☐ *N/A*

Antibiotic prophylaxis administered within 60 minutes prior to procedure?   ☐ *Yes* ☐ *N/A*

Essential imaging displayed?
☐ *Yes* ☐ *N/A*

Practitioner confirms verbally:
☐ **Local anesthetic toxicity precautions**

☐ **Patient monitoring (per institutional protocol).**

☐ **Anticipated critical events addressed with team.**

☐ **Each member of the team has been addressed by name and is ready to proceed.**

Before discharge
On arrival to recovery area;
with practitioner & personnel

Assessment for pain?
☐ *Yes*

Assessment for nausea/ vomiting?
☐ *Yes*

Recovery personnel available?
☐ *Yes*

Prior to discharge:
(with personnel and patient)

Discharge criteria achieved?
☐ *Yes*

Patient education and instructions provided?
☐ *Yes*

Plan for post discharge follow-up?
☐ *Yes*

Escort confirmed?
☐ *Yes*

Satisfaction
Completed post-procedure;
with practitioner and patient

Unanticipated events documented?
☐ *Yes*

Patient satisfaction assessed?
☐ *Yes*

Provider satisfaction assessed?
☐ *Yes*

Figure 1   Safety Checklist for Office-Based Surgery.
Adapted from the WHO Surgical Safety Checklist. © 2010 Institute for Safety in Office-Based Surgery (ISOBS), Inc – All Rights Reserved – www.isobs.org

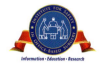

Inquire	**What are my doctor's credentials?**	Does the doctor have privileges to perform the same procedure at a hospital? □ Yes □ No
		In what specialty is the doctor board-certified? □ _____
		How many times recently has the doctor performed this type of procedure? □ _____
		What is the doctor's reputation? □ _____
		Who will be giving sedation/anesthesia, if needed, and who will be monitoring me during the procedure? □ _____
Stable	**Are my medical conditions stable?**	Are my medical conditions under control? □ Yes □ No
Office	**Is the office accredited and licensed?**	Is the office accredited and certificate posted? □ Yes □ No
		Who inspects and certifies the office for safety and infection control? □ _____
Best	**Is this office the best place for my procedure?**	For my procedure, Is the office or the hospital the best setting? □ Yes □ No
Suited	**Can this office handle an emergency?**	Is the office staff properly trained and equipment available in case of an emergency? □ Yes □ No
		If I need additional medical care, where will I be transferred? □ _____
Plan	**After the procedure, what is the plan for my recovery?**	Who will monitor my recovery and who will supervise my discharge home? □ _____
Communication	**After the procedure, who should I call if I have questions?**	Who will contact me after the procedure for follow-up? □ _____
		If I have questions, whom do I call? □ _____

Figure 2   Patient's Checklist for Office-Based Procedures.

Adapted from the WHO Surgical Safety Checklist. © 2011 Institute for Safety in Office-Based Surgery (ISOBS), Inc – All Rights Reserved – www.isobs.org

Index

Note: Page numbers followed by *f* and *t* indicate figures and tables respectively.